The Complete Book of Ayurvedic Home Remedies

ALSO BY THE AUTHOR

Ayurveda Cooking for Self-Healing (with Usha Lad)

The Yoga of Herbs (with David Frawley)

Ayurveda: The Science of Self-Healing

Secrets of the Pulse

The Complete Book of Ayurvedic Home Remedies

Vasant D. Lad, B.A.M.S., M.A.Sc.

Illustrations by Vasant D. Lad

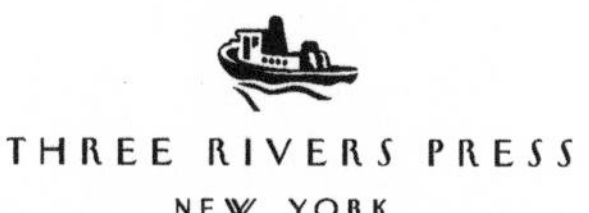

THREE RIVERS PRESS
NEW YORK

Although the information contained in this book is based on Ayurvedic principles practiced for thousands of years, it should not be taken or construed as standard medical diagnosis or treatment. For any medical condition, always consult with a qualified physician.

Published by Three Rivers Press, New York, New York.
Member of the Crown Publishing Group.

Random House, Inc. New York, Toronto, London, Sydney, Auckland
www.randomhouse.com

Originally published in hardcover by Harmony Books in 1998.
First paperback edition printed in 1999.

Printed in the United States of America

Design by Susan Hood

Library of Congress Cataloging-in-Publication Data
Lad, Vasant, 1943–
The complete book of Ayurvedic home remedies / by Vasant D. Lad.—1st ed.
Includes bibliographical references and index.
1. Medicine—Ayurvedic. I. Title.
R605.L263 1998 615.5'3—dc21 97-27802

ISBN 0-609-80286-0

10 9 8

This book is dedicated with all my heart to my most loving wife,
Usha, and my children, Aparna and Pranav.

Contents

Part III: SECRETS OF AYURVEDIC SELF-HEALING: AN ENCYCLOPEDIA OF ILLNESSES AND REMEDIES

Acknowledgments

The author would like to acknowledge those whose dedication and insight brought the knowledge of Ayurveda to the world, especially his teachers who lovingly showed the way and shared their knowledge and experience. He would also like to express his gratitude to the following people, without whose contributions this book would not exist. To his loving wife, Usha, and his children, Pranav and Aparna, for their love, patience, and support during the writing of this book. To Wynn Werner and the Ayurvedic Institute staff for their help with the original outline, the various drafts, and for raising important points during this process. To Jack Forem for proposing the idea for the book, and for help writing, organizing, and editing the material in a clear and enjoyable style. At Harmony Books, appreciation to Leslie Meredith and Peter Guzzardi for believing in the project, and to Joanna Burgess for her exacting attention in bringing the book to production.

Introduction

The Need for Healing

Ayurveda is the art of daily living in harmony with the laws of nature. It is an ancient natural wisdom of health and healing, a science of life. The aims and objectives of this science are to maintain the health of a healthy person and to heal the disease of an unhealthy person. Both prevention (maintenance of good health) and healing are carried out by entirely natural means.

According to Ayurveda, health is a perfect state of balance among the body's three fundamental energies, or *doshas (vata, pitta, kapha)* and an equally vital balance among body, mind, and the soul or consciousness.

Ayurveda is a profound science of living that encompasses the whole of life and relates the life of the individual to the life of the universe. It is a holistic system of healing in the truest sense. Body, mind, and consciousness are in constant interaction and relationship with other people and the environment. In working to create health, Ayurveda takes into consideration these different levels of life and their interconnectedness.

As a science of self-healing, Ayurveda encompasses diet and nutrition, lifestyle, exercise, rest and relaxation, meditation, breathing exercises, and medicinal herbs, along with cleansing and rejuvenation programs for healing body, mind, and spirit. Numerous adjunct therapies such as sound, color, and aromatherapy may also be employed. The purpose of this book is to acquaint you with these natural methods, so you can make the lifestyle choices and learn the self-healing modalities that are right for you in order to create, maintain, or restore health and balance.

Ayurveda is a Sanskrit word that means "the science of life and longevity." According to this science, every individual is both a creation of cosmic energies and a unique phenomenon, a unique personality. Ayurveda teaches that we all have a constitution, which is our individual psychobiological makeup. From the moment of conception, this individual constitution is created by the universal energies of Space, Air, Fire, Water, and Earth.

These five elements combine into the three fundamental energies, or *doshas*. Ether and air constitute vata, which is the energy of movement; fire and water constitute pitta, the principle of digestion or metabolism, the transformation of matter into energy; and water and earth make up kapha, the energy of structure and lubrication. When the male sperm and the female egg join at the time of fertilization, the vata–pitta–kapha factors from the parents' bodies that are most active and predominant at the moment, due to the season, the time, the emotional state, and the quality of their relationship, form a new individual with a particular constellation of qualities.

In modern terms we speak of this blueprint of the individual as our inherited genetic code; from ancient times Ayurveda has called it our *prakruti* or individual constitution, a constant factor that does not change throughout life. It is our own unique pattern of energy, our combination of physical, mental, and emotional characteristics and predispositions.

Though the underlying structure of our *prakruti* remains a fixed reality, our home base or essential individuality, it is constantly bombarded by numerous forces. Changes in age and in our external environment, alternating heat and cold as the seasons pass, our endlessly shifting thoughts, feelings, and emotions, and the quality and quantity of the food we eat continuously affect us. Unhealthy diet, excess stress, insufficient rest or exercise, and repressed emotions all disturb our *doshic* balance. Depending on the type of changes and the individual's underlying constitution, various ailments may develop:

- Some individuals experience an increase or aggravation of kapha, leading to conditions such as colds, congestion, sneezing, and allergic manifestations, as well as attachment, greed, and possessiveness.
- A pitta individual may become highly critical, angry, or perfectionistic, or may develop physical symptoms such as acid indigestion, heartburn, diarrhea, dysentery, hives, rash, or acne.
- Vata imbalances may manifest as constipation, abdominal distention, sciatica, arthritis, or insomnia, along with psychological symptoms such as fear, anxiety, and insecurity.

All these illnesses and conditions, in addition to the countless others that lead to human suffering, are due to alterations in the body's inner ecology. These upset the individual's balance, creating subtle biochemical changes that ultimately lead to disease. This is why the Ayurvedic system of medicine speaks of the need for healing for every individual in every walk of life.

As the internal and external conditions of our lives change, if we are going to remain healthy we need to constantly adjust in order to maintain equilibrium. Some of this adjusting takes place automatically due to the beautiful wisdom and intelligence with which our bodies have been designed. But much demands conscious choice.

To maintain health and balance, we have

to juggle with the three doshas, taking action to increase or decrease vata, pitta, or kapha as conditions demand. This requires moment-to-moment awareness, moment-to-moment consciousness, moment-to-moment healing.

Thus healing—healthy, balanced, conscious living in the fullness of the present moment—is really a way of life. Ayurveda is not a passive form of therapy but rather asks each individual to take responsibility for his or her own daily living. Through our diet, our relationships, our job, our numerous responsibilities, and our daily life as a whole, we can take simple actions for prevention, self-healing, wholeness, and growth toward fulfillment.

According to Ayurveda, our life has a purpose. Simply stated, that purpose is to know or realize the Creator (Cosmic Consciousness) and to understand our relationship with That, which will entirely influence our daily living. This great purpose is to be achieved by balancing four fundamental aspects of life: *dharma,* which is duty or right action; *artha,* material success or wealth; *kama,* positive desire; and *moksha,* spiritual liberation. These are called the four *purusharthas,* the four great aims or achievements in the life of any individual.

The foundation of all these facets of life is health. To maintain *dharma* and carry out our duties and responsibilities to ourselves and others, we must be healthy. Likewise, in order to create affluence and achieve success in action, good health is indispensable. To have creative, positive desire, we need a healthy mind and consciousness, a healthy body, and healthy perception. (Desire—*kama*—is sometimes translated as sex and refers to progeny and family life, but it is really the positive energy or force of desire that generates and propels any creative work.) And *moksha* or spiritual liberation is nothing but perfect harmony of body, mind, and consciousness or soul. Thus the whole possibility of achievement and fulfillment in life rests on good health.

In the quarter century that I have been practicing medicine, I have worked in surgery, gynecology, obstetrics, and pediatrics, as well as in general medicine, treating thousands of individuals in all stages and walks of life. I have repeatedly observed that lifestyle choices, such as diet, exercise, and daily routine, can be a potent source of healing as well as a cause of disease. Many health problems seem intertwined with the stresses of daily life, family and relationship problems, and worries about job and money. Others are directly connected to eating the wrong kinds of food or getting too much or too little exercise.

I have also grown more and more aware that illness provides us with an invitation for self-transformation, an opportunity to change our way of thinking, feeling, eating, and in general caring for ourselves and our lives. It never ceases to amaze and delight me how quickly and powerfully life can be set on the right track and balance restored simply through a proper diet, herbal medicines, meditation, an appropriate exercise program, and other purely natural means.

The remedies in this book come from my own practical clinical experience, based on principles and practices developed over centuries. The tradition of Ayurveda extends back over more than five thousand years of continuous daily practice, from ancient times to the present day. It is not a recently developed system of "alternative healing" but an enduring science of life that has never lost its integrity and essential nature. You can imagine how much wisdom it contains and how much practical knowledge it has accumulated over a span of five millennia!

About three thousand years ago (around 900 B.C.), the long oral tradition of Ayurveda took new form when three great scholars—Charaka, Sushruta, and Vagbhata—wrote down the principles of this ancient wisdom. Their textbooks are still used by students, practitioners, and teachers in Ayurvedic medical schools and colleges throughout India.

In a profound sense, Ayurveda is the mother of all healing systems. From its eight principal branches (pediatrics, gynecology and obstetrics, ophthalmology, geriatrics, otolaryngology, toxicology, general medicine, and surgery) have come the main branches of medicine as it is practiced today, as well as many modern healing modalities, including massage, diet and nutritional counseling, herbal remedies, plastic surgery, psychiatry, polarity therapy, kinesiology, shiatsu, acupressure and acupuncture, color and gem therapy, and meditation. All these have roots in Ayurvedic philosophy and practice.

The great sage-physician Charaka, one of the founders of Ayurvedic medicine, said, "A physician, though well versed in the knowledge and treatment of disease, who does not enter into the heart of the patient with the virtue of light and love, will not be able to heal the patient." To the best of my ability, I have followed this advice all my life, and I would urge you to follow it in using this knowledge to help others and to heal yourself.

Love is the essence of our life. I have written this book with love, and I offer it to you, dear reader, with the hope that the suggestions offered here will become a vital part of your self-healing and continued well-being.

Part I

The Science of Life

Chapter 1

Ayurveda: Body, Mind, and Soul

Like other great ancient civilizations, India never separated science from philosophy and religion. Rather, it viewed all knowledge as part of a whole designed to promote human happiness, health, and growth.

Philosophy is the love of truth. *Science* is the discovery of truth through experiment. *Religion* is the experience of truth and application of it in daily living.

Ayurveda, the science of life, is both systematized knowledge and practical wisdom, an art of healthy living that encompasses all phases of life, body, mind, and spirit. Like all sciences, it includes both a practical and a theoretical aspect. In order to make best use of the practical recommendations that come later in this book, it will help if you understand the essentials of Ayurvedic theory. This first chapter may seem a bit abstract, but please be patient and read it carefully, as it forms the basis of all that is to follow.

The Universe and How We Are Connected

According to Ayurveda, the source of all existence is universal Cosmic Consciousness, which manifests as male and female energy. *Purusha,* often associated with the male energy, is choiceless, passive, pure awareness. *Prakruti,* the female energy, is active, choiceful consciousness. Both *Purusha* and *Prakruti* are eternal, timeless, and immeasurable. These two energies are present in all living organisms, including every man and woman, as well as inanimate objects.

Purusha is formless and beyond attributes. Unmanifested pure existence, beyond cause and effect, beyond space and time, *Purusha* takes no active part in creation but remains a silent witness.

Prakruti, which has form, color, and attributes, is the divine creative will that dances the dance of creation. *Prakruti* is the One that becomes many. *Purusha* is the lover, *Prakruti* the beloved. Creation of this universe happens through their love. All of nature is the child born from the womb of *Prakruti*, the Divine Mother.

In the manifestation of nature from *Prakruti*, the first expression is *Mahad* (or *Mahat*), intelligence or cosmic order. (In human beings, it is referred to as *Buddhi*, intellect.) Next is *Ahamkar* or ego, the sense of self-identity, the center in our consciousness from which we think, act, and react. *Ahamkar* expresses itself in three universal qualities:

Sattva is stability, purity, wakefulness, essence, clarity, and light.

Rajas is dynamic movement and causes sensations, feelings, and emotions.

Tamas is the tendency toward inertia, darkness, ignorance, and heaviness. *Tamas* is responsible for deep sleep and periods of confusion. It also leads to the creation of matter.

From the essence of *Sattva* are born the mind, the five sense faculties and their organs (ears to hear, skin to perceive touch, eyes to see, tongue to taste, nose to smell), and the five motor organs or organs of action: the mouth (for speech), the hands, feet, reproductive organs, and organs of excretion.

Rajas is the active force behind the movement of both the sensory and motor organs.

Tamas gives rise to the five elements, which form the basis of material creation: space (ether), air, fire, water, and earth.

Man, a creation of Cosmic Consciousness, is considered to be a microcosm of the macrocosm that is the universe. Whatever is present in the cosmos, the same is present in human beings. Man is a miniature of nature.

The Five Elements: Building Blocks of Nature

The concept of the five elements is one of the most fundamental in Ayurvedic science. These five elements (space, air, fire, water, and earth) exist in all matter, both organic and inorganic. As man is a microcosm of nature, the five elements also exist within each individual. Our psychological tendencies, as well as our five senses and the various aspects of our body's functioning, are all directly related to the five elements.

According to Ayurveda, the five elements manifest sequentially, beginning with space, from the pure, unified, unmanifested Cosmic Consciousness that is the source of all.

SPACE

Sometimes referred to as "ether," space is empty, light, subtle, all-pervading, omnipresent, and all-enclosing. It is universal, nonmoving, and formless. Space is nuclear energy. It appears when the pure unmanifest consciousness begins to vibrate and is associated with sound and the sense of hearing. We need space in order to live, move, grow, and communicate. Spaces in the body include the mouth, nose, gastrointestinal tract, respiratory tract, abdomen, and thorax. Psychologically, space gives freedom, peace, and expansion of consciousness and is responsi-

THE SANKHYA PHILOSOPHY OF CREATION

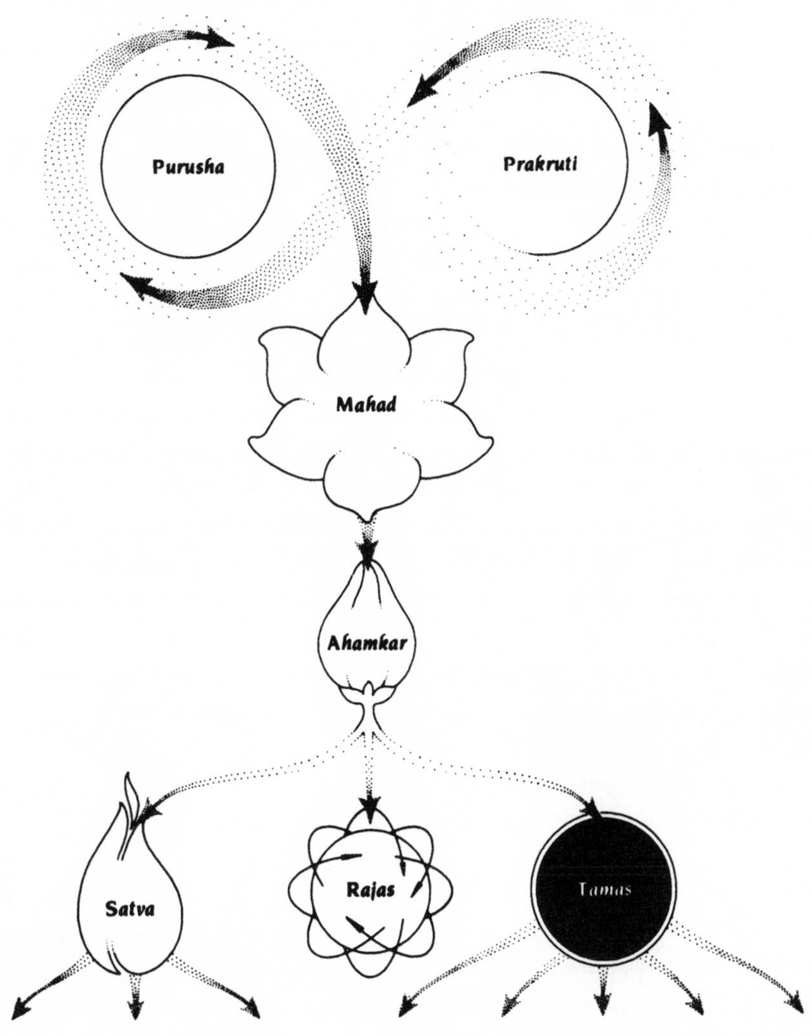

Five Sense Faculties	Five Motor Organs	Mind	Sound	Touch	Sight	Taste	Smell
organs of cognition	*organs of action*	*an organ of both action and cognition*	is the *guna* of Space	is the *guna* of Air	is the *guna* of Fire	is the *guna* of Water	is the *guna* of Earth
ears	mouth						
skin	hands						
eyes	feet						
tongue	reproductive organs						
nose	excretory organs						

ORGANIC

INORGANIC

ble for love and compassion as well as feelings of separation, isolation, emptiness, ungroundedness, insecurity, anxiety, and fear.

AIR

Air is dry, light, clear, and mobile. The second manifestation of consciousness, air moves in space. Air is electrical energy—the electron moves because of the air element. It is formless, but it can be perceived by touch, to which it is related. The principle of movement, air expresses itself in the movements of the muscles, the pulsations of the heart, the expansion and contraction of the lungs. Sensory and neural impulses move to and from the brain under the influence of the air principle, which is also responsible for breathing, ingestion, the movement of the intestines, and elimination. The flow of thought, desire, and will are governed by the air principle, which gives us happiness, freshness, joy, and excitation. It is, along with space, also responsible for fear, anxiety, insecurity, and nervousness.

FIRE

Fire is hot, dry, sharp, penetrating, and luminous. When air begins to move, it produces friction, which generates heat or fire. Fire is radiant energy. On the atomic level, the atom radiates heat and light in the form of a quantum wave. Fire is active and changeable. In our solar system, the sun is the source of fire and light. In the body, our biological "fire" in the solar plexus regulates body temperature and metabolism: digestion, absorption, and assimilation. Fire is associated with light and with vision. Fire is intelligence. It is necessary for transformation, attention, comprehension, appreciation, recognition, and understanding. Fire is also responsible for anger, hatred, envy, criticism, ambition, and competitiveness.

WATER

The next manifestation of consciousness, water is fluid, heavy, soft, viscous, cold, dense, and cohesive. It brings molecules together. Water is chemical energy (it is the universal chemical solvent). Water is associated with the sense of taste; without moisture the tongue cannot taste anything. Water exists in the body as plasma, cytoplasm, serum, saliva, nasal secretion, cerebrospinal fluid, urine, and sweat. It is necessary for nutrition and to maintain life; without it, our cells could not survive. Water is contentment, love, and compassion. It creates thirst, edema, and obesity.

EARTH

Earth is heavy, hard, rough, firm, dense, slow-moving, and bulky—the most solid of the five elements. It is neither hot nor cold. Earth is mechanical or physical energy. According to Ayurveda, it is nothing but crystallized or solidified consciousness. It gives strength, structure, and stamina to the body. All the body's solid structures (bones, cartilage, nails, teeth, hair, skin) are derived from the earth element. Earth is associated with the sense of smell. It promotes forgiveness, support, groundedness, and growth. It also creates attachment, greed, and depression, and its absence produces feelings of ungroundedness.

In our body, the electrical energy of the neuron becomes the physical energy of the movement of muscles, mediated through the neurotransmitter, which is chemical. Indeed, all the five elements are present on every level of our physiology, starting with a single cell. Within the cell, the cell membrane is earth, cellular vacuoles are space, cytoplasm is water, nucleic acid and other chemical components of the cell are fire, and movement of the cell is due to the air principle. Every single cell also has mind, intelligence, and consciousness, through which it manifests selectivity and choice. From all the possible nutrients in its environment, every cell chooses its own food—that choice is intelligence at work.

Both in our outer environment and within us, the proportion and balance of these elements is forever shifting, changing with the seasons, the weather, the time of day, the stage of one's life. For health, and often for sheer survival, we have to continuously accommodate ourselves to these changes, through what we eat, what we wear, where we live, and so on. This is a balancing act, playing elements against each other. We use solid earth to build homes, to protect ourselves against changes in air, heat (fire), and water. We use fire to prepare food (made of water and earth).

The Three Doshas: Vata, Pitta, and Kapha

These five great elements combine into three basic energies or functional principles, which are present, in varying degrees, in everything and everybody. Space (ether) and air constitute vata. Fire and water combine to make up pitta. Water and earth constitute kapha.

In our bodies, these three doshas or humors govern our psychobiological functioning. Vata–pitta–kapha are present in every cell, tissue, and organ. When in balance, they create health. When out of balance, they are the cause of disease.

These three doshas are responsible for the huge variety of individual differences and preferences, and they influence all we are and all we do, from our choices of food to our modes of relating to others. They govern the biological and psychological processes of our body, mind, and consciousness. They regulate the creation, maintenance, and destruction of bodily tissue, and the elimination of waste products. They also govern our emotions. When in balance, they generate noble qualities such as understanding, compassion, and love. When their balance is disturbed by stress, improper diet, environmental conditions or other factors, they can give rise to negative emotions such as anger, fear, and greed.

In Ayurveda, vata is the bodily air principle. It is the energy of movement. Pitta is the principle of fire, the energy of digestion and metabolism. And kapha is the principle of water, the energy of lubrication and structure.

All people have all of these three doshas, but one of them is usually primary, one secondary, and the third least prominent. Thus, each person has a particular pattern of energy, an individual combination of physical, mental, and emotional characteristics that make up his or her constitution (*prakruti*). Just as everyone has an individual fingerprint that can be identified by a trained practitioner, so everyone has an energy print—a balance or proportion of vata, pitta, and kapha—that is uniquely his or her own.

Health depends on maintaining this proportion in balance. Balance is the natural order of things; imbalance provokes and reflects disorder. Within our bodies there is a constant interplay between order and disorder, which determines our state of health.

Health is order; disease is disorder. The internal environment of the body is ceaselessly reacting to the external environment. Disorder occurs when these two are out of harmony with each other. But since order is inherent within disorder, the wise person learns to be aware of the presence of disorder and sets about to reestablish order.

In chapter 2 we will see how the three fundamental doshas combine to create the seven constitutional types of Ayurveda, and you will learn your own body type, the key to making lifestyle choices for self-healing and maximum well-being. For the moment, let us look a little more deeply into the characteristics of these three basic energies of life.

VATA

Vata is the energy of movement. Although it is the air *principle,* it is not considered the same as actual air in the external environment, but rather as the subtle energy that governs biological movement.

Vata is intimately related to our vital life essence, known as *prana. Prana* is the pure essence of vata. It is the life-force, the play of intelligence. That flow of intelligence is necessary for communication between two cells, and it maintains the life function of both. On a cosmic level, *prana* is said to be the attraction between *Purusha* and *Prakruti.*

As the principle of mobility, vata regulates all activity in the body, both mental and physiological. It is responsible for breathing, the blinking of our eyes, the beating of our hearts, and all movement in the cytoplasm and cell membranes. All the impulses in the vast networks of our nervous system are governed by vata.

When vata is in balance, it promotes creativity and flexibility and evokes feelings of freshness, lightness, happiness, and joy. Out of balance, vata produces fear, nervousness, anxiety, even tremors and spasms.

Vata is dry, light, cold, subtle, clear, mobile, and dispersing. We shall soon see how these qualities are expressed in a person with a vata constitution.

PITTA

Pitta is translated as fire, but this is not meant literally. Rather, it is the *principle* of fire, the energy of heating or metabolism. Pitta governs all the biochemical changes that take place within our bodies, regulating digestion, absorption, assimilation, and body temperature. From the standpoint of modern biology, pitta comprises the enzymes and amino acids that play a major role in metabolism.

Pitta regulates body temperature through the chemical transformation of food. It promotes appetite and vitality.

Not only food is metabolized by us. Every impression coming in from the outside is also processed or "digested" and made a part of us. Thus pitta (when in balance) promotes intelligence and understanding and is crucial in learning. Out-of-balance pitta may arouse fiery emotions such as frustration, anger, hatred, criticism, and jealousy.

Pitta is hot, sharp, light, oily, liquid, pungent, sour, and spreading. These qualities occur in various ways in people of pitta constitution.

KAPHA

Kapha combines water and earth. It is the energy that forms the body's structure, the glue that holds the cells together. Kapha also supplies the liquid needed for the life of our cells and bodily systems. It lubricates our joints, moisturizes the skin, helps to heal wounds, and maintains immunity. Kapha provides strength, vigor, and stability.

Psychologically, excess kapha is responsible for the emotions of attachment, greed, lust, and envy. When kapha is in balance it expresses itself in tendencies toward love, calmness, and forgiveness.

The qualities of kapha include heavy, slow, cool, oily, damp, smooth, soft, static, viscous, and sweet. Kapha individuals display these qualities in various ways.

Together, these three doshas govern all the body's metabolic activities. Kapha promotes anabolism, the process of building up the body, the growth and creation of new cells as well as cell repair. Pitta regulates metabolism, which is digestion and absorption. Vata triggers catabolism, the necessary deterioration process in which larger molecules are broken down into smaller ones.

Vata, the principle of movement, moves both pitta and kapha, which are immobile. Thus when vata is out of balance, it influences and disturbs the other doshas. The majority of illnesses have aggravated vata at their source.

The whole of life's journey is divided into three major milestones. From birth to age 16 is the kapha age. From 16 to 50 is the age of pitta, and from 50 to 100 the age of vata.

In childhood, kapha and the process of anabolism are predominant, as this is the time of greatest physical growth and the structuring of the body. Kapha disorders, such as lung congestion, cough, colds, and mucus secretions, are common at this time. In adulthood, a time of activity and vitality, pitta is most apparent. Vata and the catabolic processes of deterioration take over in old age, bringing vata disorders such as tremors, emaciation, breathlessness, arthritis, and loss of memory.

The Twenty Qualities: An Important Key to Healing

Now we come to another important aspect of Ayurvedic theory, which will help you to make intelligent choices for self-healing. Ayurveda delineates twenty fundamental qualities, which appear in ten pairs:

The Twenty Basic Attributes or Qualities

Heavy—Light	Cold—Hot
Oily—Dry	Slow—Sharp
Stable—Mobile	Soft—Hard
Slimy—Rough	Dense—Liquid
Gross—Subtle	Cloudy—Clear

These qualities are found both in the world around us and in our bodies. Today's weather may feel light or heavy, and it may be liquid or dry, mobile (windy) or stable, hot or cold, cloudy or clear. Food we eat can partake of any of these qualities. Ice cream, for example, is heavy, oily, cold, soft, and liquid. Our skin may be oily or dry, rough or smooth. Our moods, too, can be heavy or light, cloudy or clear; our thinking may be slow or sharp, our mind quiet and stable or mobile and hyperactive, clear or cloudy.

We are constantly affected by changes in these qualities. Cold, windy, clear, dry weather aggravates vata dosha and may lead to colds and any number of vata ailments such as insomnia, constipation, or arthritis. Hot, humid weather aggravates pitta and may lead to outbreaks of irritation and anger as well as physical complaints like acne, eczema, or skin rashes. Cloudy, gray, humid or rainy weather can aggravate kapha, leading to colds and coughs, depression, lethargy, overeating and oversleeping, and weight gain.

Each of these paired qualities represents the extreme on a continuum. The two qualities in each pair influence or affect one another according to two fundamental principles of Ayurveda:

1. Like increases like.
2. Opposites decrease each other.

These principles are a key to healing with Ayurveda. When an imbalance has manifested, *successful treatment requires increasing opposite qualities*. For example, if there is too much heat (excess pitta), a cool drink, a swim, or some herbs with cooling properties will greatly help pacify pitta and reduce the heat. A person suffering from too much heat will not be helped by playing tennis in the sun, eating spicy foods, or taking a sauna. Similarly, if you are cold and shivering from exposure to cold windy weather, have a bowl of warm soup, wrap up in a blanket, or take a hot bath. These simple remedies immediately make sense when we hear them because they are so natural.

Ayurvedic physicians have carefully observed nature and located these qualities within all things, both organic and inorganic. Ayurvedic treatment consists to a great extent of identifying a person's disorder in terms of these qualities, and setting right any imbalances.

How is this done? Speaking in very general terms, excessive dryness in the body—constipation, dry skin, emaciation, and so on—is frequently associated with aggravated vata; excessive heat—burning urine, irritated eyes, fever, inflammation, anger, or a critical attitude—with aggravated pitta; and undue heaviness—lethargy, overweight, congestion, and excess mucus—with unbalanced kapha. Whatever the symptoms may be, for self-treatment you need to understand them and then adjust your lifestyle—diet, exercise, and so on—to restore a state of balance and health.

The hundreds of remedies in Part III of this book will help you to do this, but essentially it is your own moment-to-moment awareness and self-observation, your sensitivity to your own constitution and your own unique requirements for health, and perhaps most importantly, your willingness to act on your knowledge, that will make all the difference between poor health and a vital, happy, healthy, long life.

Chapter 2

Discover Your Mental and Physiological Type

This chapter will take you further on your journey toward radiant health as we begin to apply the principles from chapter 1 to discover and understand your own unique constitution.

According to Ayurveda, there are seven main body types:

- Vata
- Pitta
- Kapha } Mono types
- Vata–Pitta
- Pitta–Kapha
- Kapha–Vata } Dual types
- Vata–Pitta–Kapha } Triple type

All three doshas are present in each individual at all times, but their proportion varies from person to person. Thus, ten vata individuals, or ten kapha–pitta individuals, will have ten different temperaments, ten unique sets of qualities and characteristics. Maintaining our individual qualitative and quantitative proportion of the doshas is our challenge if we are to remain healthy. When we maintain this proportion our health is good, but when the balance is upset, disease may result.

Prakruti and Vikruti

At the time of conception, each person's combination and proportion of vata, pitta, and kapha is determined according to the genetics, diet, lifestyle, and current emotions of the parents. As mentioned in the Introduction, the doshas predominant in the parents combine to form the constitution of the new life they are creating.

If, for example, the father is pitta predominant and the mother vata predominant, and the pitta factor is stronger than the vata, and the union is taking place on a hot summer night after eating a spicy meal, then the baby that is born will have a constitution that is pitta predominant. Or if both parents are kapha, and they have a kaphagenic diet and are making love in kapha season, then their child will have a predominance of kapha dosha.

A few fortunate individuals are born with a constitution in which all three doshas are equally present, which gives them the likelihood of exceptionally good health and a long life span, but most of us have one or two doshas predominant.

NOTE: When Ayurveda says health comes from balancing your doshas, this does not mean you should try to have equal amounts of vata, pitta, and kapha. Rather, it means *maintaining the balance with which you were conceived.*

The unique and specific combination of the three doshas at conception is called your *prakruti,* which means "nature." It is your psychobiological temperament. *Prakruti* does not change during a person's lifetime. Your *prakruti* may, for example, be predominantly pitta, with vata secondary and a little kapha. (This can be written as $V_2P_3K_1$.) For you, maintaining balance means keeping this proportion. If your vata or kapha should increase, moving toward an equal proportion of the doshas, it would not be healthy for you.

As conditions change—due to weather, dietary choices, fatigue, stress, emotional state, exercise or lack of it—the balance of the doshas in our mind-body system also changes. This altered state of the doshas, reflecting the current state of our health, is called our *vikruti.* If your health is excellent, your current doshic status will be the same as your *prakruti.* But more likely there will be a discrepancy, and it is this difference between the two that gives a direction for healing. Your aim will be to reestablish the balance indicated by your *prakruti.*

I know you are eager to find out what your constitution is, so let's move on to that. Afterward, we will look more deeply into the characteristics of each doshic type.

How to Determine Your Constitutional Type

The chart on pages 18 to 19 is a self-assessment that will enable you to determine your unique constitution according to Ayurveda.

Please remember that this can provide only a rough guideline. The subtleties of each person's mental, emotional, and physical makeup are manifold and can be accurately assessed only by a physician thoroughly trained and experienced in Ayurvedic diagnosis. So please do not draw any absolute conclusions about yourself based on the self-assessment or the descriptions of the doshas; rather, use this information to help you grow in self-understanding, and as a guide to plan your diet, exercise regimen, and other aspects of your lifestyle for maximum health.

It is best to fill out the self-evaluation twice. (You might want to photocopy it, to have it available for others or for future use.) First, base your choices on what is most consistently true about your life as a whole, over many years. This indicates your *prakruti*. Then fill it out a second time, considering how you have been feeling recently, in the last month or two. This is your *vikruti* or present condition.

It often helps to have a spouse or good friend verify your answers, as they may have good insights and some objectivity to offer as you make your responses.

After filling out the chart, add up the number of marks under vata, pitta, and kapha to discover your own balance of the doshas in your *prakruti* and *vikruti*. Most people will have one dosha predominant, a few will have two doshas approximately equal, and even fewer will have all three doshas in equal proportion.

After adding up the numbers, make them into a ratio, with 3 as the highest number. For example, suppose you come out with V = 10, P = 6, K = 3. This would translate into $V_3P_2K_1$.

Once you have determined your predominant doshas, studying the following characteristics of vata, pitta, and kapha will help you gain a deeper and more comprehensive understanding.

Characteristics of the Vata Individual

Vata individuals have light, flexible bodies. Their frame is on the small side, with light muscles and little fat, so that they tend to be slim or even underweight. They often appear to be "too tall" or "too short," or they may appear physically underdeveloped, with flat chests and less strength and stamina than the other types. Their veins and muscles are often quite prominent.

Vatas generally have dry skin tending toward roughness. Their circulation is poor, with the result that their hands and feet are often cold. Because vata dosha is cold, dry, light, and mobile and people with a vata constitution tend to lack insulating material (the fatty tissue under the skin), they are uncomfortable in cold weather, especially if it is dry and windy, and they much prefer spring and summer.

These individuals have a variable appetite and thirst and variable digestive strength. They are often attracted to astringent food such as salads and vegetables, but their bodies actually need sweet, sour, and salty tastes. (We will discuss the effect of tastes in chapter 8.) Raw vegetables increase, rather than balance, vata. Vata individuals often experience digestive difficulties and problems with absorption of nutrients. They tend to produce scanty urine, and their feces are hard, dry, and small in size and quantity. Constipation is one of their most common ailments.

Vatas are the most likely of the body types to fast or to eat very little, but this actually increases vata and tends toward imbalance.

Other physical characteristics typical of vata types include small, recessed eyes, which are often quite lusterless; dry, thin hair, often curly or kinky; dry, rough skin and nails; cracking, popping joints; and teeth that may be irregular, broken, or protruding.

Vatas walk quickly and are always in a rush. Due to the mobile quality of vata, they

GUIDELINES FOR DETERMINING YOUR CONSTITUTION

OBSERVATIONS	V	P	K	VATA	PITTA	KAPHA
Body size	☐	☐	☐	Slim	Medium	Large
Body weight	☐	☐	☐	Low	Medium	Overweight
Skin	☐	☐	☐	Thin, Dry, Cold, Rough, Dark	Smooth, Oily, Warm, Rosy	Thick, Oily, Cool, White, Pale
Hair	☐	☐	☐	Dry Brown, Black, Knotted, Brittle, Thin	Straight, Oily, Blond, Gray, Red, Bald	Thick, Curly, Oily, Wavy, Luxuriant, All colors
Teeth	☐	☐	☐	Protruding, Big, Roomy, Thin gums	Medium, Soft, Tender gums	Healthy, White, Strong gums
Nose	☐	☐	☐	Uneven shape, Deviated septum	Long pointed, Red nose-tip	Short Rounded, Button nose
Eyes	☐	☐	☐	Small, Sunken, Dry, Active, Black, Brown, Nervous	Sharp, Bright, Gray, Green, Yellow/red, Sensitive to light	Big, Beautiful, Blue, Calm, Loving
Nails	☐	☐	☐	Dry, Rough, Brittle, Break easily	Sharp, Flexible, Pink, Lustrous	Thick, Oily, Smooth, Polished,
Lips	☐	☐	☐	Dry, Cracked, Black/brown tinged	Red, Inflamed, Yellowish	Smooth, Oily, Pale, Whitish
Chin	☐	☐	☐	Thin, Angular	Tapering	Rounded, Double
Cheeks	☐	☐	☐	Wrinkled, Sunken	Smooth Flat	Rounded, Plump
Neck	☐	☐	☐	Thin, Tall	Medium	Big, Folded
Chest	☐	☐	☐	Flat, Sunken	Moderate	Expanded, Round
Belly	☐	☐	☐	Thin, Flat, Sunken	Moderate	Big, Potbellied
Belly button	☐	☐	☐	Small, Irregular, Herniated	Oval, Superficial	Big, Deep, Round, Stretched
Hips	☐	☐	☐	Slender, Thin	Moderate	Heavy, Big
Joints	☐	☐	☐	Cold, Cracking	Moderate	Large, Lubricated
Appetite	☐	☐	☐	Irregular, Scanty	Strong, Unbearable	Slow but steady

OBSERVATIONS	V	P	K	VATA	PITTA	KAPHA
Digestion	☑	☐	☐	Irregular, forms gas	Quick, Causes burning	Prolonged, Forms mucus
Taste, healthy preference	☑	☐	☐	Sweet, Sour, Salty	Sweet, Bitter, Astringent	Bitter, Pungent, Astringent
Thirst	☑	☐	☐	Changeable	Surplus	Sparse
Elimination	☑	☐	☐	Constipation	Loose	Thick, Oily, Sluggish
Physical activity	☐	☑	☐	Hyperactive	Moderate	Sedentary
Mental activity	☐	☑	☐	Always Active	Moderate	Dull, Slow
Emotions	☑	☐	☐	Anxiety, Fear, Uncertainty, Flexible	Anger, Hate, Jealousy, Determined	Calm, Greedy, Attachment
Faith	☐	☐	☑	Variable, Changeable	Intense, Extremist	Consistent, Deep, Mellow
Intellect	☐	☑	☐	Quick but faulty response	Accurate response	Slow, Exact
Recollection	☑	☐	☐	Recent good, remote poor	Distinct	Slow and sustained
Dreams	☑	☐	☐	Quick, Active, Many, Fearful	Fiery, War, Violence	Lakes, Snow, Romantic
Sleep	☐	☑	☐	Scanty, Broken up, Sleeplessness	Little but sound	Deep, Prolonged
Speech	☐	☑	☐	Rapid, Unclear	Sharp, Penetrating	Slow, monotonous
Financial	☑	☐	☐	Poor, spends on trifles	Spends money on luxuries	Rich, Good money preserver
TOTAL	10	16	6			

do not like sitting idle but prefer constant activity. They also like to do a lot of traveling. Not doing anything is a punishment for them. They are attracted to jogging, jumping, and vigorous physical activity, but because they tend to have less stamina, they can easily get strained or overtired.

Vatas are drawn toward a lot of sexual activity. But excess sex is one of the causes of aggravated vata. Vatas generally have a difficult time prolonging sex, and vata men may experience premature ejaculation.

Vata individuals sleep less than the other body types and have a tendency toward interrupted sleep or insomnia, especially when vata is aggravated. Nevertheless they generally wake up feeling alert and fresh and ready to go.

Psychologically, vatas are blessed with quick minds, mental flexibility, and creativity. They have excellent imaginations and excel at coming up with new ideas. When in balance, they are joyful and happy. Vatas tend to talk quickly and to talk a lot. They are easily excited, alert, and quick to act—but may not think things through before acting, so they may give a wrong answer or make a wrong decision with great confidence!

Vatas are quite loving people, but may love someone out of fear and loneliness. In fact, fear is one of the symptoms of unbalanced vata. These individuals may experience fear of loneliness, darkness, heights, and closed spaces. Anxiety, insecurity, and nervousness are also common among them. They are worriers.

One of the main psychological qualities of vata individuals is readiness to change or, to put it the other way, difficulty with stability and commitment. They often change furniture, housing, jobs, or towns, and get easily bored. They don't like to stay in any place more than a year! Their faith is also quite variable. Vatas may be low on willpower and often feel unstable or ungrounded.

Clarity is one of the attributes of vata, and vata individuals generally are clear-minded and even clairvoyant. Along with their lively minds and fertile imaginations, they are usually highly alert and grasp new ideas quickly. However, they are also quick to forget. They think and speak quickly, but are restless and easily fatigued. They generally have less tolerance, confidence, and boldness.

Vata types tend to make money quickly, but they spend it quickly, too, often impulsively or on trifles. A vata may go to the flea market and come home with a lot of junk! They are not good savers. Nor are they good planners, and as a consequence they may suffer economic hardship.

The word *vata* is derived from a root that means "to move," and this gives an important clue to the character of vata individuals. As the principle of mobility, vata provides the motive power for all our mental and bodily processes. It regulates all activity in the body, from the number of thoughts we have to how quickly and efficiently food moves through our digestive tract.

The behavior that vatas are drawn to—travel, erratic hours, continual stimulation, frequent change—can easily upset their balance and lead to vata disorders such as constipation, gaseous distention, weakness, arthritis, pneumonia, excessively dry skin, dry lips, dry hair, dry, cracked nipples, and cracked heels. Nerve disorders, twitches

The Attributes of Vata Individuals

Following are the main attributes of vata dosha and how they are expressed in the physical, mental, and behavioral characteristics of a vata individual.

ATTRIBUTES	MANIFESTATIONS IN THE BODY
Dry	Dry skin, hair, lips, tongue; dry colon, tending toward constipation; hoarse voice
Light	Light muscles, bones, thin body frame, light scanty sleep; underweight
Cold	Cold hands, feet, poor circulation; hates cold and loves hot; stiffness of muscles
Rough	Rough, cracked skin, nails, hair, teeth, hands and feet; cracking joints
Subtle	Subtle fear, anxiety, insecurity; fine goose pimples; minute muscle twitching, fine tremors; delicate body
Mobile	Fast walking, talking, doing many things at a time; restless eyes, eyebrows, hands, feet; unstable joints; many dreams; loves traveling but does not stay at one place; swinging moods and shaky faith
Clear	Clairvoyant; understands and forgets immediately; clear, open mind, experiences void and loneliness
Astringent	Dry choking sensation in the throat; gets hiccoughs, burping; loves oily, mushy soups; craving for sweet, sour, and salty tastes

and tics, mental confusion, palpitations, and breathlessness, as well as muscle tightness, low backache, and sciatica, are also due to aggravated vata. Excess vata makes the mind restless and hyperactive. Loud noises, drugs, sugar, caffeine, and alcohol also derange vata dosha, as does exposure to cold weather and cold foods.

Excess vata is a major factor in PMS (premenstrual syndrome). When, as her period approaches, a woman experiences bloating, low back ache, pain in the lower abdomen, cramps, pain in the calf muscles, and insomnia, and emotionally she feels anxiety, fear, and insecurity, this is due to aggravation of vata dosha.

Like the wind, vata types have a hard time settling down and staying grounded. When their vata becomes aggravated, it is difficult to calm them down. Sticking to a routine is difficult for them, but it is vital if they are to remain healthy.

The dry, cold, windy seasons of autumn and winter tend to increase and aggravate vata dosha, so at these times vata individuals need to be particularly careful to stay in balance. They need to dress warmly and eat warm, heavier foods. Warm, moist, slightly oily foods are beneficial, as are most warming spices. Steam baths, humidifiers, and moisture in general are helpful.

General Guidelines for Balancing Vata

Keep warm
Keep calm
Avoid raw foods
Avoid cold foods
Avoid extreme cold temperatures
Eat warm foods and spices
Keep a regular routine

Characteristics of the Pitta Individual

The pitta body type is one of medium height and build, though some individuals are slender with a delicate frame. They seldom gain or lose much weight. Their muscle development is moderate, and they are generally stronger physically than vata types. Pitta eyes are bright and may be gray, green, or copper-brown, and their eyeballs are of medium prominence. These individuals tend to have ruddy or coppery skin and may have reddish hair, which tends to be silky. They often experience early graying or hair loss, so that a pitta man frequently has a receding hairline or a big, beautiful bald head!

Moles and freckles are common on pitta skin, which tends to be oily, warm, and less wrinkled than vata skin. Pittas have sharp, slightly yellowish teeth and frequently have bleeding gums.

The normal body temperature of people with a pitta constitution is a little higher, and their hands and feet are usually warm and may be sweaty. Pittas may feel quite warm when both vatas and kaphas are cold. They perspire quite a lot, even when it's 50 degrees, while a vata person will not perspire even at a much higher temperature. Their body perspiration often has a strong, sulfury smell; their feet also perspire and may have a strong smell.

This heat is the main characteristic of pitta types, which is not surprising as the word pitta is derived from the Sanskrit word *tapa,* which means to heat. (The word can also be translated as "austerity," and pitta individuals can be quite austere.) They have a low tolerance for hot weather, sunshine, or hard physical work. Although they are a fiery type, their sex drive may not be very strong. Pittas may use sex to release anger.

Pittas have a strong appetite, strong metabolism, and strong digestion. They consume large quantities of food and drink, and they also produce large quantities of urine and feces, which tend to be yellowish and soft. When out of balance, they crave hot spicy dishes, which are not good for them. They should eat food with the sweet, bitter, and astringent tastes. When hungry, a pitta person needs to eat soon, otherwise he or she will become irritable and hypoglycemic.

Pitta sleep is of medium duration, but it is uninterrupted and sound. These individuals like to read before they go to sleep and often fall asleep with a book on their chest.

Girls with a pitta constitution begin menstruating and reach puberty early. They can start menstruation as early as the age of ten.

Pitta physical ailments tend to be related to heat and the fire principle. They are prone to fevers, inflammatory diseases, acid indigestion, excessive hunger, jaundice, profuse perspiration, hives and rashes, burning sensations, ulceration, burning eyes, colitis, and sore throats. All "itises" are inflammatory disorders and are due to excess pitta. These individuals are susceptible to sunburn and do not like bright light.

Pitta-type PMS symptoms include tenderness in the breasts, hot flashes, hives, urethritis, and sometimes a burning sensation when passing urine.

Pitta individuals are alert and intelligent and have good powers of comprehension and concentration. Their intellects are penetrating and keen, and their memories are sharp. They have good, logical, investigating minds. They love to go deeply into problems and find solutions. Their minds are always at work, and they like to solve problems and puzzles of all kinds. They also tend to be good speakers. They are lovers of knowledge and have a great capacity for organization and leadership.

Pittas are night people. They become alert around midnight and love to read late at night.

Orderliness is important to them. A pitta person's home or room is always clean and neat. Clothes are kept in a designated place, shoes are in orderly rows, and books are arranged according to height or another definite system.

Pittas love noble professions. They are doctors, engineers, lawyers, judges—very bright, brainy people. They have good administrative abilities and like to be in a leadership role. They are good planners and are ambitious and disciplined. Aggressive by nature, they easily take charge of situations. They may become political figures. They have a lot of charisma. People are attracted to them.

Pittas are often wise, brilliant people, but they can also have a controlling, dominating personality. They have a tendency toward comparison, competition, and aggressiveness, and they are meticulous and perfectionistic. Everything has to be done on time, and correctly! Pitta individuals never yield an inch from their principles, which sometimes leads to fanaticism. They tend to be critical, especially when pitta dosha is aggravated; if there is no one to criticize, pitta people will criticize and judge themselves.

A pitta's life span is only moderately long. These individuals burn their life energy through too much mental activity, perfectionism, aggressiveness, and the constant search for success. They have a deep-seated fear of failure. They don't like the words *no* or *fail* and therefore may be highly stressful. They are the typical workaholics.

Pittas generally seek material prosperity and tend to be moderately well off, though they spend rather than save their money. They like to live in luxurious homes and drive fancy cars; they love perfumes, gems, jewelry, and other costly items; and they enjoy exhibiting their wealth and possessions.

A number of factors can increase pitta to the point of aggravation. One is simply eating too much spicy food, including black pepper, cayenne pepper, curry peppers, and

The Attributes of Pitta Individuals

Following are the main attributes of pitta dosha and how they are expressed in the physical, mental, and behavioral characteristics of a pitta individual.

ATTRIBUTES	MANIFESTATIONS IN THE BODY
Hot	Good digestive fire; strong appetite; body temperature tends to be higher than normal; hates heat; gray hair with receding hairline or baldness; soft brown hair.
Sharp	Sharp teeth, distinct eyes, pointed nose, tapering chin, heart-shaped face; good absorption and digestion; sharp memory and understanding; irritable
Light	Light/medium body frame; does not tolerate bright light; fair shiny skin, bright eyes
Oily	Soft oily skin, hair, feces; does not like deep-fried food (which may cause headache)
Liquid	Loose liquid stools; soft delicate muscles; excess urine, sweat and thirst
Spreading	Pitta spreads as rash, acne, inflammation all over the body or on affected areas; pitta subjects want to spread their name and fame all over the country
Sour	Sour acid stomach, acidic pH; sensitive teeth; excess salivation
Bitter	Bitter taste in the mouth, nausea, vomiting; repulsion toward bitter taste; cynical
Pungent	Heartburn, burning sensations in general; strong feelings of anger and hate
Fleshy smell	Fetid smell under armpits, mouth, soles of feet; socks smell
Red	Red flushed skin, eyes, cheeks and nose; red color aggravates pitta
Yellow	Yellow eyes, skin, urine and feces; may lead to jaundice, overproduction of bile; yellow color increases pitta

jalapeño peppers. Pitta can also be increased by sour and citrus fruits, such as grapefruits and sour oranges. Eating rancid yogurt, smoking cigarettes, and drinking sour wine can also be harmful. Working near fire or lying in the sun are causes of increased pitta.

Eating fatty fried food, or oily food such as peanut butter, can create nausea or headaches for a pitta.

Summer is the most difficult time for pitta individuals. In hot humid weather pitta dosha can easily become aggravated. Heat builds up in the system, and pitta individuals become more susceptible to the heat-related ailments mentioned above. They may become quite irritable and are easily agitated and angered. Tempers flare. Their sharp minds become hypercritical and judgmental. Jealousy and envy may blaze up. They need to cool down!

General Guidelines for Balancing Pitta

Avoid excessive heat
Avoid excessive oil
Avoid excessive steam
Limit salt intake
Eat cooling, nonspicy foods
Drink cool (but not iced) drinks
Exercise during the cooler part of the day

Characteristics of the Kapha Individual

Kapha people are blessed with a strong, healthy, well-developed body. Their chests are broad and expanded, and they have strong muscles and large, heavy bones. With their larger frames and constitutions dominated by the water and earth elements, kaphas tend to gain weight and have difficulty taking it off. To complicate matters, kaphas generally have a slow digestion and metabolism. As a result, they tend to carry excess weight and to be on the chubby side. A kapha person may even do a water fast and gain weight!

In addition to their large frames, kapha individuals have strong vital capacity and stamina and tend to be healthy. Their skin is soft, smooth, lustrous and thick, and it tends to be oily. Their eyes are large, dark, and attractive, with long, thick lashes and brows. The whites of their eyes are very white. They have large, strong, white teeth. Their hair tends to be thick, dark, soft, wavy, and plentiful. They have hair everywhere!

Individuals with a kapha body type have a steady appetite and thirst, though digestion is slow. They can comfortably skip a meal or work without food, while it is difficult for a pitta person to concentrate without eating.

Because of their slow metabolic rate, kaphas who maintain health and balance generally enjoy a long span of life, longer than the other two doshic types, who tend to "burn out" more quickly. However, if kapha dosha is allowed to become aggravated, the person is likely to become obese, which is one of the main causes of diabetes, hypertension, and heart attack. Such a person cannot live a very long life.

Kaphas have quite a sweet tooth and love candy, cookies, and chocolate. They are generally attracted to sweet, salty, and oily foods, but these contribute to water retention and weight gain; their bodies need lighter fare and do better with the bitter, astringent, and pungent tastes.

Because of the cloudy and heavy qualities of kapha, these individuals often feel heavy and foggy in the morning and may find it hard to get going without a cup of coffee or tea. Morning is not their time. They prefer midday, yet might feel like taking a nap after lunch; they often feel lethargic after a full meal. Unfortunately, daytime sleep increases kapha and is not good for them.

Kaphas evacuate slowly and their stools tend to be soft and pale in color. Their perspiration is moderate, more than vatas but less than pitta types. Their sleep is deep and prolonged.

Despite their strong bodies and great stamina, kaphas shun exercise. Vigorous exercise is good for them, but they prefer to sit, eat, and do nothing! Rather than jog, they prefer to walk—slowly! Kaphas do tend to like swimming, but it is not particularly good for them, as their bodies will absorb some water. When they do exercise, they become hungry afterward and will want to eat. After a workout at the gym they will go to a restaurant for a snack.

Kapha dosha is slow and steady in every way. These individuals move slowly and talk slowly (their speech pattern may become monotonous). They eat slowly and are slow to decide and slow to act. They move slowly and gracefully.

Kapha individuals are blessed with a sweet, loving disposition. By nature they are peaceful, patient, tolerant, caring, compassionate, and forgiving. They love to hug people. Kaphas are stable, solid, and faithful. Their spiritual or religious faith is deep and abiding, and their minds calm and steady.

One of the dominant qualities of kapha is softness, which manifests as soft skin, soft hair, soft gentle speech, a soft nature, and a soft, gentle, loving look. A pitta person's look is sharp and penetrating. A vata's look is spacy! But a kapha person looks calm, quiet, grounded, stable. He or she is *here,* right now!

Kaphas can be slow to comprehend, but once they know something, that knowledge is permanently retained. They have excellent long-term memories.

Although a kapha individual is forgiving, if you insult them or hurt their feelings, they will forgive you, but they will never forget! A kapha person will tell you, "On the twenty-fourth of January, 1972, at three-thirty in the afternoon, when we were having tea, you said such and such to me—but I have forgiven you!"

Their tendencies toward groundedness and stability help them to earn and hold on to money, and they are good at saving. Their extravagances are minor, mostly in the area of spending a little on cheese, candy, and cakes.

A kapha person has a steady sex drive, and he or she can enjoy sex for hours at a time, without dissipation of energy, without orgasm or ejaculation of semen. It may take them some time to become interested, but once they are stimulated, they tend to stay that way.

Kapha dosha is aggravated by kapha-producing food, such as watermelon, sweet fruits, candy, cookies, yogurt, and other dairy products. Cold and frozen food and chilled water, sleeping in the daytime, and sitting and doing nothing all increase kapha. Sedentary work, especially when combined

The Attributes of Kapha Individuals

Following are the main attributes of kapha dosha and how they are expressed in the physical, mental, and behavioral characteristics of a kapha individual.

ATTRIBUTES	MANIFESTATIONS IN THE BODY
Heavy	Heavy bones, muscles, large body frame; tends to be overweight; grounded; deep heavy voice
Slow	Slow walk, talk; slow digestion, metabolism; sluggish gestures
Cool	Cold clammy skin; steady appetite and thirst with slow metabolism and digestion; repeated cold, congestion and cough; desire for sweets
Oily	Oily skin, hair and feces; lubricated, unctuous joints and other organs
Damp	Congestion in the chest, sinuses, throat and head
Smooth	Smooth skin; gentle calm nature; smoothness of organs
Dense	Dense pad of fat; thick skin, hair, nail and feces; plump rounded organs
Soft	Soft pleasing look; love, care, compassion and kindness
Static	Loves sitting, sleeping and doing nothing
Viscous	Viscous, sticky, cohesive quality causes compactness, firmness of joints and organs; loves to hug; is deeply attached in love and relationships
Cloudy	In early morning mind is cloudy and foggy; often needs coffee as a stimulant to start the day
Sweet	The anabolic action of sweet taste stimulates sperm formation, increasing quantity of semen; strong desire for sex and procreation; abnormal function may cause craving for sweets
Salty	Helps digestion and growth, gives energy; maintains osmotic condition; abnormal function may create craving for salt, water retention

with steady munching at the desk, produces too much kapha in the body. Excess kapha slows digestion and metabolism and lowers the digestive fire, and the person may become chubby or even obese.

The difficult time of year for kapha individuals is winter and early spring, when the weather is heavy, wet, cloudy, and cold. Then kapha accumulates in the system and leads to physical, emotional, and mental imbalances of the kapha variety. Physical problems will tend to be related to the water principle, such as colds, flu, sinus congestion and other diseases involving mucus, such as bronchial congestion. Sluggishness, excess weight, diabetes, water retention, and sinus headaches are also common.

Emotionally, when kapha becomes unbalanced, these individuals may suffer from greed, attachment, envy, possessiveness, lust, and laziness, leading to kapha-type depression.

Interestingly, kapha can become aggravated as the moon gets full because, as biologists have discovered, there is a tendency toward water retention in the body at that time.

Kapha women may suffer from PMS symptoms such as excessive emotionality, water retention, white vaginal discharge, and overurination. They may feel attachment, greed, and lethargy at that time and will probably have a tendency toward excess sleep.

General Guidelines for Balancing Kapha

Get plenty of exercise
Avoid heavy foods
Keep active
Vary your routine
Avoid dairy foods
Avoid iced food and drinks
Avoid fatty or oily foods
Eat light, dry food

How to Use This Knowledge

Knowing your Ayurvedic constitution (*prakruti*) has many benefits for your life and health:

• Self-understanding, which is the foundation of life, is greatly increased. Ayurveda says that every person is a unique and divine book. To read that book is a great art. The knowledge of *prakruti* can help you to read your own book, which is your life. By understanding your constitution, you can better understand your psychological tendencies, your strengths, and your weaknesses, as well as your physiological strong and weak areas.

• You may see that your habits and tendencies, such as erratic lifestyle and schedule (*vata*), irascibility (*pitta*), or laziness (*kapha*), or physical problems such as overweight (*kapha*), ulcers (*pitta*), or constipation (*vata*), are directly related to your constitution. The tendency toward such imbalances is inherent in the way your mind-body system is designed.

• When you can anticipate the kinds of illnesses and imbalances you are likely to have, you can take precautions to prevent them from arising. You can adjust your lifestyle—daily routine, diet, amount or type of exercise, and so on—to keep your doshas in balance and your health at its best.

• You can also use the knowledge of constitutional types to understand others with whom you are related, whether in your personal life or at work. To succeed in relationships, which is such a confused and problematic area today, it is helpful to know the constitution of your husband or wife, boyfriend or girlfriend. Understanding one another brings clarity; clarity brings compassion, and compassion is love. Such a relationship brings happiness, joy, and longevity.

Using this knowledge of *prakruti,* if your spouse is upset and angry you can say to him or her, "Honey, it's not you, it's your pitta!" That will open a new dimension of understanding of emotional reactions in the relationship.

Use the knowledge of your *prakruti* as a baseline, to see where you should be. Then look at your *vikruti,* your current imbalances, as a clue to help you restore balance, using the food charts, yoga postures, herbs, recommended exercises, and the like, presented throughout this book.

For instance, if your *vikruti* shows more pitta than your *prakruti,* you will want to follow the guidelines for pacifying pitta. If you have a disorder that is caused by excess vata, pitta, or kapha, follow the guidelines for pacifying that dosha. For sinus congestion, for example, follow a kapha-reducing diet until the condition subsides.

If your *prakruti* and *vikruti* seem about the same, then choose the diet and lifestyle guidelines for your strongest dosha.

Finally, remember that "balance" does not mean equal amounts of vata, pitta, and kapha; rather, it means maintaining *your proportion* of the three doshas, according to your constitution. It is not a static state, but a dynamic equilibrium that needs constant renewal.

Chapter 3

Why We Get Sick

What is health? What is disease? Are sickness and health just a matter of luck, or of which bacteria you happen to encounter in your daily life? What can we do to maintain a positive state of health and avoid getting sick?

These are questions that the five-thousand-year-old tradition of Ayurvedic medicine has considered in depth. The answers, drawn from deep insight and generations of practical experience, can help us prevent illness from developing and heal it if it arises.

Let's begin by examining the Ayurvedic understanding of health. Then we will look at ten potential causes of illness and how you can counteract them. Once you are aware of the factors that can either maintain health or disturb your body's equilibrium and set the disease process in motion, you can organize your life for health and balance. Finally, we will consider the Ayurvedic understanding of how illness develops, from its earliest, invisible stages until it is fully grown.

The Definition of Health

According to Ayurveda, health is not simply the absence of disease. It is rather a state of balance among body, mind, and consciousness.

> Health consists of a balanced state of the three humors (doshas), the seven tissues *(dhatus)*, the three wastes *(malas)*, and the gastric fire (agni), together with the clarity and balance of the senses, mind, and spirit.

Although you will not need to master all these terms and considerations in order to effectively use the remedies in Part III, an acquaintance with them will give you a bigger picture of the depth and practicality of this science.

You are already familiar with the three doshas, the biological humors or principles that govern all activity in the body:

vata, the energy or principle of movement; pitta, the energy of digestion and metabolism; and kapha, the principle of lubrication and structure. Balance of the three doshas maintains health; imbalance leads to disease.

The *dhatus* are the basic bodily tissues. They are responsible for the entire structure of the body and the functioning of the different organs and systems. Crucial to the development and nourishment of the body, the *dhatus* unfold successively as follows, starting with the nourishment derived from the product of digestion:

1. *Rasa* (plasma or cytoplasm) contains nutrients from digested food and subsequently nourishes all tissues, organs, and systems.
2. *Rakta* (blood) governs oxygenation in all tissues and vital organs and thus maintains life-function.
3. *Mamsa* (muscle) covers the delicate vital organs, performs the movements of the joints, and maintains the physical strength of the body.
4. *Meda* (fat) maintains the lubrication of the tissues and serves as insulating material to protect the body's heat.
5. *Asthi* (bone and cartilage) gives support to the body's structure.
6. *Majja* (bone marrow and nerves) fills up the bony spaces, carries motor and sensory impulses, and facilitates communication among the body's cells and organs.
7. *Shukra* and *artava* (male and female reproductive tissues) contain the pure essence of all bodily tissues and can create a new life.

Each *dhatu* is dependent on the previous one. If the raw materials of digestion are inadequate, or if there is a problem in any stage, each successive *dhatu* will not receive the nourishment it needs and the respective tissues or organ systems will suffer. So for good health, all seven *dhatus* must develop and function properly.

The three waste products (*malas*) are feces, urine, and sweat. The body must be able to produce these in appropriate amounts, and to eliminate them through their respective channels.

Agni is the biological fire or heat energy that governs metabolism. It can be equated with the digestive enzymes and metabolic processes involved in breaking down, digesting, absorbing, and assimilating our food. Agni maintains the nutrition of the tissues and the strength of the immune system. It destroys microorganisms, foreign bacteria, and toxins in the stomach and intestines. It is an extremely vital factor in maintaining good health.

Agni sustains life and vitality. An individual endowed with adequate agni lives long and has excellent health. But when agni becomes impaired because of an imbalance in the doshas, metabolism is adversely affected. The body's resistance and immunity are impaired, and the person begins to feel unwell. When this vital fire is extinguished, death soon follows.

In addition to these bodily factors, the senses, mind, and spirit also play a vital role in maintaining good health, as we will discuss in the next section. When all these factors are balanced, it produces a state called *swastha*, which means "totally happy within oneself."

Agni

There is a saying in Ayurveda that a person is as old as his or her agni. According to the *Charaka Samhita*, one of the great classics of Ayurvedic medicine:

"The span of life, health, immunity, energy, metabolism, complexion, strength, enthusiasm, luster, and the vital breath are all dependent on agni (bodily fire). One lives a long healthy life if it is functioning properly, becomes sick if it is deranged, or dies if this fire is extinguished. Proper nourishment of the body, *dhatus, ojas,* etc., depends upon the proper functioning of agni in digestion.

"The five types of agni, corresponding to ether, air, fire, water, and earth, digest the respective components of the food.... In this way, balanced agni cooks the appropriately chosen and timely consumed food, and leads to promotion of health....

"Agni is necessary for the normal process of digestion, and the subtle energy of *agni* transforms the lifeless molecules of food, water, and air into the consciousness of the cell."

This state of happiness and balance can be created and sustained by maintaining a healthy lifestyle in accordance with nature and the requirements of your own constitution. Proper nutrition, proper exercise, healthy relationships, positive emotions, and a regulated daily routine all contribute to a healthy life. On the other hand, wrong diet, inadequate exercise, troubled relationships, negative or repressed emotions, and an erratic schedule are at the root of disease. These causative factors upset the balance of the doshas, weaken agni and the *dhatus,* and lead to poor health.

Ten Factors in Health and Illness

Illness does not suddenly appear. There is a direct causal link between the factors that influence us and the effects they produce. *The cause is the concealed effect, and the effect is the revealed cause.* The cause is like a seed, in which the as-yet-unmanifested tree is concealed. The tree is the expressed value of the seed. Health is the effect of a healthy lifestyle and healthy habits; disease is the "tree" sprouted from unhealthy habits.

According to the *Charaka Samhita,*

> Both the patient and the patient's environment need to be examined in order to arrive at an understanding of the disease and the causes of disease. It is important to know where the patient was born and raised, and the time of onset of the imbalance. It is also important to know the climate, customs, common local diseases, diet, habits, likes and dislikes, strength, mental condition, etc.

This enumeration opens the door to the wide variety of factors constantly influencing our health. Let us consider some of them.

LIKE INCREASES LIKE

The first important principle in considering the potential causes of disease is "Like increases like." A dosha is increased by experiences and influences (such as food, weather, and seasons) with qualities similar to it. Dry foods, dry fruit, running, jogging, jumping, always being in a rush, and working too hard are all factors that aggravate vata in the system. Pittagenic factors, such as hot spicy food, citrus fruit, fermented food, and hot humid weather, provoke excess pitta. Cold, cloudy, damp weather, eating dairy products, wheat, and meat, and sitting and doing nothing increase kapha.

The antidote to "like increases like" is "opposite qualities decrease or balance." This is the key to healing.

> NOTE: In general, one's *prakruti* indicates one's disease proneness. Individuals of pitta constitution, for example, tend to have pitta diseases. But this is not inevitable. A person of vata constitution who eats a lot of hot spicy food, drinks alcohol, lies in the sun, smokes cigarettes, and represses anger will definitely get a pitta disease. If he or she eats candy, cookies, ice cream, and other dairy products and is exposed to cold weather, there will be a susceptibility to congestive kapha disorders.

FOOD AND DIET

We have already touched on the effects of food on the doshas, and chapter 8 will discuss this important topic in depth, so we won't go into it at length here. The principle is simply that eating the right kinds of food for your *prakruti* maintains vitality and balance, while eating the wrong kinds creates imbalance in the doshas, the first step in the genesis of disease.

Eating spicy food or sour or citrus fruit and drinking alcohol all increase heat and acidity in the body, something a pitta person cannot afford. For a vata individual, dried fruits, beans (including garbanzo, pinto, and aduki) are hard to digest and will provoke vata. Raw salads, which are cold and astringent, will likewise increase vata. For a kapha individual, dairy products, cold drinks, and fatty fried foods definitely add to kapha. So a vata person eating a vatagenic diet, a pitta person eating a pitta-provoking diet, and a kapha person eating kapha-aggravating food are definitely creating imbalance and sowing the seeds for ill health.

Wrong food combinations (see table page 101), stale food, food with chemical additives, and wrong eating habits, such as eating too much late at night or eating in a rush, also contribute to imbalance and lead to poor digestion and poor health. Diet is thus one of the main potential causes of ill health—but by understanding these principles and eating according to the guidelines for our constitutional type, it is also one of the major ways we can take control of our lives and maintain healthy balance.

SEASONS

Ayurveda classifies the seasons according to their predominant dosha. The windy, cool, dry weather of autumn is largely vata, followed by the dark, heavy, damp, cloudy kapha qualities of winter. Early spring is still primarily kapha, but as late spring arrives, the increased warmth, light, and brightness express pitta qualities, which blossom in their full intensity in the summer.

Each of these seasons brings its own challenges to health. The predominant dosha of the season will tend to build up at that time and can cause aggravation especially in someone of the same *prakruti*. If we act intelligently, we can avoid this accumulation and aggravation.

For example, because autumn and early winter tend to increase vata, individuals with a vata-predominant constitution need to eat warm foods, dress warmly, avoid cold food and drinks, and stay out of nasty weather. Otherwise they will fall prey to vata illnesses and discomforts, such as constipation, insomnia, and lower back pain. If pitta individuals want to remain free of anger, as well as hives, rash, and diarrhea, they need to keep cool in the summer, avoiding spicy foods, overexertion, and overexposure to the hot sun. Kaphas need care in the heart of winter and early spring if they are going to avoid colds, coughs, allergies, and sinus congestion in the damp, cool, heavy weather.

We will look further at the seasons, their effects, and how we can best live in harmony with their rhythms and changes in chapter 5, where we discuss the ideal Ayurvedic lifestyle, including daily and seasonal routines.

EXERCISE

Exercise is another factor that can profoundly influence your health for better or worse. Regular exercise improves circulation and increases strength, stamina, and immunity. It helps one to relax and to sleep peacefully. It benefits the heart and lungs, is vital for effective digestion and elimination, and helps the body purify itself of toxins through sweating and deep breathing. Exercise increases the rate of combustion of calories, so it is good for maintaining body weight and for weight loss. It also makes the mind alert and sharp and develops keen perception.

On the other hand, insufficient exercise, overexertion, or exercise that is inappropriate for one's constitution can lead to ill health.

Lack of exercise eventually brings a loss of flexibility and strength and puts one at greater risk for many diseases, such as diabetes, hypertension, osteoporosis, and heart disease.

Some amount of sweating helps to eliminate toxins, reduces fat, and makes you feel good. But overexertion may cause dehydration, breathlessness, chest pain, or muscle aches, ultimately leading to arthritis, sciatica, or a heart condition.

Yoga stretching and some aerobic exercise are valuable for all body types, but the amount and intensity of your exercise should be based upon your constitution. Kaphas can do the most strenuous exercise, pittas can handle a moderate amount, and vatas require the gentlest exercise. Even though fast-moving vatas are attracted to active sports, quieter exercises such as walking and yoga stretching are better for them. They should leave jogging, fast bicycling, aerobic dancing, and fast walking to pitta and kapha types. Kaphas are the most reluctant exercisers, preferring to do little or nothing, but it is important for them, or they will tend to put on weight and feel emotionally heavy and dull.

So here again, self-knowledge—knowledge of your constitution—plus a few pieces of vital information give you the opportunity and the challenge to maintain good health or fall into imbalance and illness.

You will find additional information about exercise in Part II, where we discuss the Ayurvedic daily routine.

AGE

As briefly mentioned in chapter 1, Ayurveda divides the human life span into three stages. At each stage, certain diseases and types of disease are more common. Childhood is the age of kapha. Children's bodies are growing and building up their structure, so kapha dosha is more predominant. Their bodies are soft and gentle (qualities of kapha), they require more sleep than adults, and they are susceptible to kapha illnesses such as colds and congestion.

Adulthood exhibits more characteristics of pitta. Adults are more competitive, aggressive, and ambitious than children; they work hard, they require less sleep, and they fall prey to pitta-type disorders such as gastritis, colitis, and peptic ulcers.

Old age is the age of vata. Elderly people sleep quite a bit less, and their sleep is broken. They tend to get constipation, cracking and popping of joints, degenerative diseases such as rheumatoid arthritis and Alzheimer's disease, and suffer from forgetfulness, all characteristic of vata dosha.

This shows that our age and stage of life are factors that have to be considered in the choices we make to keep our doshas in balance and remain healthy. Elderly people, for example, should not engage in strenuous exercise, and if possible they should minimize travel, among many factors that increase vata. They should favor a vata-balancing diet, with more warm, moist foods, more oil, and less salad and dried fruit.

MENTAL AND EMOTIONAL FACTORS

Our life is a whole, consisting of body, mind, and pure consciousness. Both health and disease have psychological as well as physical origins. Illness may begin in the mind and emotions and then affect the body; mental imbalance creates physical imbalance. Equally, physical disorders and imbalances can generate mental disorders. Because of this, mind and body are never considered separately in Ayurveda.

Every perception, thought, feeling, and emotion, whether positive or negative, is a biochemical event that influences the doshas and affects the cells, tissues, and organs of the body. Fear, anger, grief, hatred, envy, possessiveness, and other negative emotions disturb our doshic balance; likewise, when the doshas are already out of balance, they may give rise to these same negative emotions.

- Increased vata is associated with anxiety, insecurity, fear, nervousness, restlessness, confusion, grief, and sadness.

• *Increased pitta* is associated with anger, envy, hate, ambition, competitiveness, criticism, judgmental attitude, sharp speech, perfectionism, and the need to be in control.

• *Increased kapha* is associated with greed, attachment, possessiveness, boredom, laziness, and lethargy.

Emotions have an affinity with certain organs: grief and sadness with the lungs, anger with the liver, and hatred with the gall bladder. The kidneys may become the seat of fear, and the heart (as well as the lungs) the abode of grief and sadness. Nervousness is associated with the colon, while the stomach is the home of agitation and temptation, and the spleen may be related to attachment.

As we have discussed, emotions have a physical as well as a psychological aspect. Emotions are reactions to situations. If we do not understand and maintain clear awareness of the total movement of an emotion, from its arising to its dissolution, it will tend to adversely affect a particular organ, causing stress and weakness and creating what is known as a "defective space" *(khavaigunya)*, where a future disease may manifest. (See page 38, "How Disease Develops.")

STRESS

Modern medicine often views stress as the result of a particular lifestyle, or of overwork, emotional trauma, and so on. Ayurveda considers stress less as a result or condition than as a causal factor in disease. A regular daily routine, nourishing diet, positive emotions, and loving relationships result in strength and health. But keeping late hours, eating food that is aggravating to one's constitution, traveling a lot, using the mind or stimulating the senses too much, repressing negative emotions such as anger or fear, and maintaining problematic relationships all put stress on the body and mind. In addition, toxins in food, water, air pollution, excessive noise, and many other environmental factors are also stressful.

Stress is a major factor in many diseases. It may trigger allergies, asthma, and herpes, and it may even lead to heart conditions.

Stress disturbs the doshas and can create disequilibrium of vata, pitta, or kapha, depending on the individual's constitution. Vata individuals may develop vata conditions such as anxiety or fearfulness. Pitta individuals may react to stress in the form of anger, or they may suffer from hypertension, peptic ulcer, ulcerative colitis, and other pitta disorders. Kapha individuals under stress tend to eat and eat and eat.

In Part III you will find many suggestions to minimize the impact of stress on your life, and to relieve symptoms caused by stress if they develop.

OVERUSE, UNDERUSE, AND WRONG USE OF THE SENSES

Our senses give us great pleasure as well as vital information. Through ordinary experience our senses of taste, touch, smell, sight, and hearing can nourish us, and we can also find healing through sense therapies such as aromatherapy, color therapy, mantras and other healing sounds, massage, and the tastes in herbs and foods.

But because all our perceptions, as well as

our thoughts and feelings, are biochemical events as well as experiences in consciousness, improper use of the senses can create imbalance or damage in the body and result in illness.

Overuse of the senses strains and stresses our nervous system. To use a simple example, repeated exposure to bright light hurts the retina and strains the optic nerve, which triggers pitta, and sooner or later a person's eyesight will be affected or neuritis-like symptoms will arise. If we listen to loud music or hear loud sounds, the eardrum and the rest of our hearing apparatus are hurt and weakened; if it occurs often, the person can become deaf. Loud sounds also affect systemic vata dosha, giving rise to vata symptoms such as arthritis or degenerative changes in the bones. Lying in the sun strains the sense of touch, aggravates pitta, and may lead to skin cancer.

Misuse of the senses means using them in a wrong way, such as trying to read very small letters, or looking through a microscope or telescope (which creates a strain on the eyes), or reading while lying down (which changes the angle of focus and builds up stress on the muscles of the eyeball), which will eventually result in pitta or vata disorders. Eating a large quantity of wrong food, such as hot, spicy, stimulating food containing cayenne pepper, is a misuse of the taste organ. Listening to loud sounds over the telephone, and long phone conversations, both aggravate vata. Exposing the senses to wrong inputs, such as watching violent movies on television, is also a misuse of the senses.

Underuse of the senses means not perceiving with total attention, ignoring what we perceive, or not making full use of our wonderful sensory equipment. This can lead, for example, to accidents. SAD (seasonal affective disorder) is a form of depression that affects people who don't get enough sunlight during the winter—a kind of underuse of the sense of sight. "Cabin fever," the discomfort and restlessness born of staying indoors for a long time, is at least partly the result of sensory deprivation. Prolonged fasting—underuse of the sense of taste—aggravates vata.

"KNOWING BETTER"

Very often we get sick because we disregard our own knowledge or wisdom. Understanding our *prakruti*, our psychobiological constitution, is self-knowledge; understanding how certain foods, for instance, can disturb the balance of our mind-body system and lead to illness, while other food is balancing and strengthening for us, is knowledge we can use to remain healthy. And yet often we follow the impulses of the moment and choose foods that will cause us problems.

If a person who knows that her constitution is largely pitta decides to eat hot spicy food for lunch and then spends the rest of the summer afternoon working in the garden, she is disregarding her intelligence and understanding and asking for trouble.

As individuals, we are all part of the Cosmic Consciousness, the universal intelligence that so beautifully organizes all of nature. That intelligence is within us, and by following the time-tested principles of Ayurveda and paying attention to our own intuition and inner wisdom about what is right for us, we can regulate our lives in harmony with it.

RELATIONSHIPS

Our life is relationship. We are related to the earth, the moon, the sun, the air we breathe, the water we drink, the food we eat. You are related to your friends, your parents and children, your spouse, and your co-workers, as well as to your own body, your thoughts and feelings, your job, and your bank account. In our daily life, relationships are most important.

Often we use our personal relationships as a sort of power game, to control others. Then relationships become a battlefield rather than a field of love. When a negative emotion comes up in a relationship, such as resentment of a past hurt or insult, anger, fear, anxiety, or criticism, pay attention to the feeling. Don't judge the other person or yourself. When your spouse says something and you feel hurt or angry, look inside to see what your thoughts and feelings are saying to you. Be honest. Out of honesty, clarity comes.

When clarity is lacking, feelings are repressed, or communication is absent at times of crisis in our relationships, stress builds up, and this is one of the causes of illness. Stress disrupts our inner biochemistry, the doshas are thrown out of balance, and the seeds of disease are sown.

Husband and wife, brother and sister, parent and child—all our relationships must be absolutely clear. Clarity in relationships develops compassion, and compassion is love. Therefore love is clarity. And as we all know, love is the key to successful relationships.

If you look back over the ten factors presented in this section, you will see that you have a great deal of choice and control over whether they will create a potentially disease-producing imbalance in the doshas. This is true even of such apparently uncontrollable factors as the seasons and the weather: if it is cold, you can dress warmly; if it is hot, you can take it easy and stay out of the sun.

How Disease Develops

According to Ayurveda, illness is the end result of a long process that can be detected and addressed at any stage. This process has been thoroughly studied and its phases delineated in great detail.

The disease process begins with disturbances in the balance of the doshas. Temporary imbalances are common and quite normal; problems arise if the aggravated condition is not corrected. In the normal course of events, vata, pitta, and kapha go through cycles of change in three stages: accumulation, provocation or aggravation, and pacification. Pitta, for example, begins to build up and accumulate in the late spring. It is provoked or aggravated in the hot summer months, and it naturally becomes pacified when the weather cools down in the autumn.

If the increased dosha isn't pacified naturally through a change in seasons, it undergoes further changes and disease may result. If a person with a predominantly vata constitution experiences some degree of increased vata in the fall due to the cool, dry, windy weather, but it returns to normal soon after,

How to Transform Negative Feelings

Negative feelings can cause hurt both to ourselves and to others. If we express anger or criticism, for example, we inflict pain on someone else. On the other hand, repressing such feelings creates problems for ourselves, as the stressful biochemistry affects the internal organs and systems down to the cellular level.

If both expressing and holding back negative feelings can be harmful, what shall we do when these emotions boil up in us? Ayurveda offers a way to learn from such situations and resolve them in a positive manner.

At the moment the feeling comes up, look into it. Let's suppose it is a feeling of anger. Take a long, deep breath, let yourself feel the anger, and exhale it out. Give the feeling total freedom to express itself *within you,* so that you look at it honestly and feel it. Breathe into it, surrender to it, and be with it. Breathe into it, and breathe out. Soon it will dissolve by itself.

You have to be aware not only of the external thing—what your spouse or friend is saying—but at the same time you have to bring awareness to your inner self. When awareness goes both ways, outer and inner, understanding is total. This approach doesn't put a scar on the mind.

Look at the feeling—any feeling or emotion—without labeling it or naming it. Then the observer and the observed become one. Observe with total awareness, with no division between subject and object, no separation between yourself and the feeling. Give freedom to the feeling; let it flower; let it fade away.

disease will not develop. The person can aid the process of restoring balance, for example, by eating moist, warming foods and dressing warmly in the windy weather.

If the condition of aggravated vata continues, vata will move into the general circulation and into the deep connective tissue, where it will generate pathological changes. Disease will develop. Imbalance is disorder, and disorder is disease.

Disease is like a child. It has its own creation within the womb of the body, according to a process known as *samprapti* or pathogenesis, literally "the birth of pain." In brief, this is how it happens:

1. ACCUMULATION

Due to various causes, such as diet, weather, seasons, emotions, and others we have discussed, the doshas begin to accumulate in their respective sites: vata in the colon, pitta in the intestines, and kapha in the stomach. This is the easiest stage at which to treat any incipient health problem. A trained Ayurvedic physician can feel the imbalance in your pulse even at this stage, and you may be able to detect it yourself.

Vata accumulation may be experienced as constipation, abdominal distension, or gases in the colon. Pitta buildup may be felt as heat around the belly button area and can be observed as a slightly yellowish discoloration in the whites of the eyes, or dark yellow-colored urine. The person will be very hungry and will crave candy and sugar. Accumulated kapha leads to feelings of heaviness, lethargy, and loss of appetite.

At this stage the individual is still quite healthy, and when a dosha starts to build up, the body's intelligence creates an aversion to the causal factor and a craving for opposite qualities, which can restore balance. For example, if you've eaten ice cream three days in a row and kapha is building up, the thought of more ice cream will not be appealing; rather, your body will crave cayenne pepper or other spicy food to burn up the kapha and counteract it. One should listen to this wisdom and not continue increasing the cause.

2. AGGRAVATION

The accumulated dosha continues to build up in its own site. The stomach gets brimmed up with kapha, the intestines fill with pitta, or the colon overflows with vata. These accumulated doshas then try to move from their sites. Kapha tries to go up into the lungs, pitta tries to move into the stomach and gallbladder, and vata tries to move into the flanks.

You can feel this stage, too. For example, if you eat too much kapha food on Saturday night, you might feel full when you wake up on Sunday and think to yourself, "Maybe I should fast or eat very lightly today." But then someone invites you out for Sunday brunch, and you eat heavily again. The next day you might get a cough or a feeling of congestion in the lungs as the kapha starts to move upward. Excess pitta in the second stage may cause heartburn or acid indigestion, even nausea. Vata rising up may cause pain in the flanks or midback, or even breathlessness.

According to Ayurvedic therapeutics, the disease process can be addressed at any stage, but specific treatments are needed for specific stages. In these first two stages, one can reverse the process by oneself, using common sense to apply the principle of opposite qualities, and taking some home remedies. Once the disease process has gone beyond the gastrointestinal tract and entered the third phase, it is no longer under one's own control, and trained medical help is needed. (See sidebar on ama.)

3. SPREAD

The dosha begins to spread from its place of origin, overflowing into the bloodstream and the general circulation of the body, "looking" for a place to enter. Here the disease process has progressed to the point where eliminating the causal factor will not be enough. A *panchakarma* purification program (or a similar cleansing regimen) is needed in order to return the doshas to their respective sites in the gastrointestinal tract so they can be excreted from the body.

Ama, Agni, and the Disease Process

The body's biological fire, which governs the transformation of matter into energy, is of thirteen major types. The central fire, called *jatharagni,* governs the digestion and assimilation of food. The other agnis (the fire component in the cells, tissues, and organs) perform the local process of digestion and nutrition. When agni is robust and healthy, then whatever a person eats, the system digests, assimilates, and absorbs it, then eliminates the impurities. But when the doshas are aggravated because of poor diet, an unhealthy lifestyle, or negative emotions, they first affect agni, which becomes unbalanced. When agni becomes weakened or disturbed, food is not properly digested.

The undigested, unabsorbed food particles accumulate in the gastrointestinal tract and other subtle sites in the body and turn into a toxic, sticky, foul-smelling substance called *ama.* (Ama may also be formed by bacterial invasion and cellular metabolic waste.) In the third ("spread") stage of the disease process, ama overflows from its site of origin to other bodily channels such as the blood vessels, capillaries, and lymphatics, and clogs the channels and the cell membranes.

When these molecules of ama clog the channels, the cellular intelligence *(prana)* which is constantly flowing between the cells gets blocked, and some cells become isolated. An isolated cell is a lonely cell, and a lonely cell is a confused cell. Pathological changes begin to occur. But the root cause of cytopathological changes is the movement of these molecules of ama. So the ama has to be eliminated from the body by *panchakarma* or other means. (See "Techniques for Cleansing and Purification" in chapter 4.)

4. DEPOSITION OR INFILTRATION

The aggravated dosha enters an organ, tissue, or system that is weak or defective, due to previous trauma, genetic predisposition, accumulated emotional stress, repressed emotions, or other factors. These weak areas in the body can be described as negative locations, like potholes in the road. Smoking cigarettes, for example, creates weakness in the lungs; eating too much sugar creates weakness in the pancreas and blood tissue, and so on.

The newly arrived, aggravated humor (dosha) creates confusion within the cellular intelligence of the weaker tissue and overwhelms it, changing its normal qualities and functions. The quality of the aggravated dosha suppresses the normal qualities of the tissue and combines with it, creating an altered state, changed in structure and function. In this way, the "seeds" of disease begin to sprout.

Up to this point, the disease has not appeared on the surface, but it can be detected by a skilled physician or recognized by imbalances in the doshas such as those mentioned above. An alert person can feel subtle changes in the body. If the condition is not interrupted at this stage, it will erupt as a full-blown disease.

5. MANIFESTATION

In this stage, qualitative changes become apparent. The signs and symptoms of an actual disease appear on the surface; the person becomes sick. Whether in the lungs, kidneys, liver, joints, heart, brain, or wherever, the seeds of disease now sprout and begin to manifest in the area of the defective tissue.

6. CELLULAR DEFORMITY LEADING TO STRUCTURAL DISTORTION

Now the pathological process is fully developed and the disease completely manifested. Structural changes appear, and complications of other organs, tissues, or systems become evident. This is also the stage it which the disease, now fully developed, is therefore most difficult to treat.

In the fifth stage, for example, when aggravated pitta dosha is invading the wall of the stomach, it may manifest as an ulcer. But in the sixth stage, the pitta will perforate the ulcer and cause hemorrhaging, or it may provoke a tumor. Function begins to be disturbed in the fifth stage, but here the structure of the tissue is affected, as well as the surrounding tissues and systems.

Obviously, treatment—restoration of balance and normal functioning—is far easier at earlier stages. That is why prevention is emphasized so strongly in Ayurveda. It is much more effective to treat the illness in its seed stage, before it sprouts and grows.

Both health and disease are processes. Disease is a process of abnormal movement of the doshas, while health is a process of their normal functioning. The wise person understands that the normal rhythm and quality of the process can be reestablished by changing diet and lifestyle and avoiding the etiological factors that cause disease.

The key is awareness. The more you are alert to how your mind, body, and emotions are reacting to changing circumstances; the more you are aware of your constitution and the moment-to-moment choices you can make to maintain health, the less opportunity you create for becoming sick.

SAMPRAPTI (PATHOGENESIS): THE SIX STAGES OF THE DISEASE PROCESS

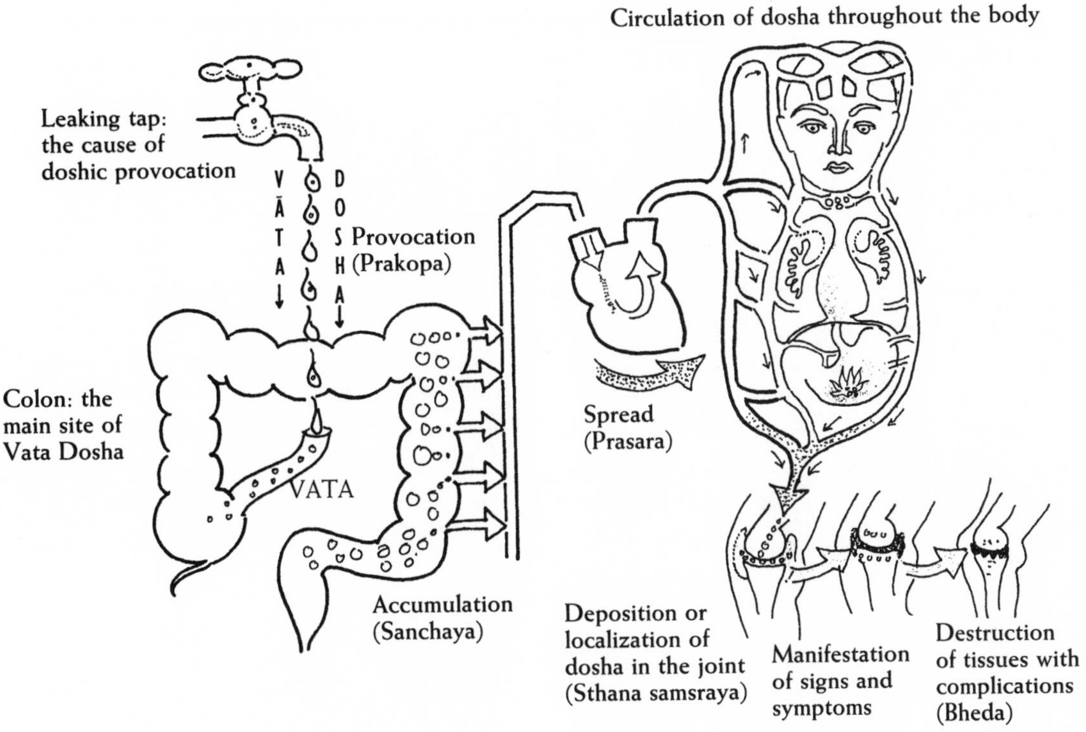

Circulation of dosha throughout the body

Leaking tap: the cause of doshic provocation

VĀTA

DOSHA

Provocation (Prakopa)

Colon: the main site of Vata Dosha

VATA

Accumulation (Sanchaya)

Spread (Prasara)

Deposition or localization of dosha in the joint (Sthana samsraya)

Manifestation of signs and symptoms

Destruction of tissues with complications (Bheda)

Part II

Putting Ayurveda to Work

Chapter 4

How We Can Stay Healthy

The goal of Ayurveda is to maintain the health of a healthy person and heal the illness of a sick person. Part III of this book contains hundreds of suggestions to help you if you have fallen ill. But staying well is far easier than curing an illness, especially once an imbalance has progressed through the later stages of the disease process. That is why prevention is so strongly emphasized in Ayurvedic medicine. In this chapter we will consider some of the fundamental principles and approaches recommended by Ayurveda for remaining healthy.

Awareness

The master key to remaining healthy is *awareness*. If you know your constitution, and you can remain alert to how your mind, body, and emotions respond to the changing conditions in your environment and the numerous facets of your daily life, such as the food you eat, you can make informed choices to maintain good health.

As we saw in chapter 3, the cause is the concealed effect and the effect is the revealed cause, as the seed contains the potential tree and the tree reveals the potency of the seed. To treat the cause is to treat the effect, to prevent it from coming to fruition. If a kapha person always has kapha problems in the spring season, such as hay fever, colds, congestion, sinus headaches, and weight gain, such a person should watch his diet and eliminate kapha-producing food like wheat, watermelon, cucumber, yogurt, cheese, candy, ice cream, and cold drinks. (Ice is not good for a kapha person; it will produce congestive disorders.)

The knowledge of the causes of disease, and the understanding that "like increases like" and "opposites balance," give us all the information we need to maintain or restore our health, simply through conscious attention, moment-to-moment awareness of our behavior.

If I am living consciously, I may observe that after I ate yogurt two weeks ago, I felt congested and a cold developed. Then it cleared up and I was okay for a few days. When yogurt comes my way again, the memory will come up and my body will say, "Hey, last time you ate yogurt, you got sick!" If I bring lively awareness and listen to my body, it will tell me, "I don't want yogurt." To listen to the body's wisdom, the body's intelligence, is to be aware, and this is one of the most effective ways to prevent disease.

Developing an awareness of the potential causes of imbalance, and of one's moment-to-moment state of well-being, is the necessary first step to maintaining health. The second step is taking action.

Taking Action to Modify the Cause

You can't control the weather, but you can dress properly, so that cold winds, or rain, or summer's heat will not aggravate the doshas. Changes in the weather are a potential cause of doshic imbalance. Windy, cold, dry weather will aggravate vata dosha; hot, sticky weather is sure to provoke pitta; cold, cloudy, wet weather will increase kapha dosha. Once we have knowledge and understanding, it is time to take action. Put on a hat, a scarf, a warm coat; stay out of direct sunlight. Modify the cause.

Potential causes of illness and imbalance are constantly arising, both within us and on the outside. The weather is changing, our surroundings are changing, our thoughts and feelings are changing, and stressful situations are coming and going. In response to these changes, we have to act skillfully. As the Bhagavad Gita says, "Skill in action is called *yoga*."

I have to be smart enough to know my previous history and to learn from it. When I eat garbanzos, I get a stomachache, so *this* time I should not eat them. Or if there is nothing to eat except garbanzos, then I can add cumin powder, ghee, and a little mustard seed, and it will be suitable for me to eat. The garbanzos' dry, light vatagenic effect will be modified by the moist, oily ghee and the warming spices.

A substantial part of the Ayurvedic pharmacy is the Ayurvedic art of cooking. Adding specific seasonings changes the property of food and can cause a "forbidden" food, one that might have provoked imbalance, to become acceptable. Some people, for example, are sensitive to potatoes. Potatoes give them gas and little aches and pains in the muscles and around the joints. But if they peel off the skin and sauté the potato with ghee and a little turmeric, mustard seed, cumin powder, and cilantro, it mitigates the vata-provoking property of the potato and the body can then handle it. One can take action to modify the cause; the body's response will be different, and that particular causative factor will not have an adverse effect.

This principle applies equally well to psychological factors. You may know that watching violent movies upsets you and gives you nightmares. The violent imagery disturbs your doshic balance, provoking anxiety and fear. You have observed this happening to you; the next time you are confronted with the "opportunity" to subject yourself to a violent movie, you can just say no.

It keeps coming down to the same central issue: consciousness, awareness, finding out, "What is my role in this situation? What do I know? What can I do?"

Restoring Balance

The first step in staying healthy is developing awareness of the potential causes of disease so you can avoid them or deal with them intelligently. The second step is taking action to modify causes you can't avoid or control (such as the weather). The next step is to restore balance once it begins to be lost. The main method for doing this is to apply the opposite quality or qualities.

If you're cold, have some hot soup or take something warm to drink. If you're agitated or upset (perhaps you watched that violent movie against your better judgment), sit down and do some meditation to calm your mind and emotions. If your pitta has been provoked and you're feeling hot under the collar, take a swim or have some sweet cooling fruit.

This principle seems so simple and makes such good sense that it is easy to overlook it in practical daily life. But it is extremely powerful and effective. If you apply it, you will find that you can quickly and effortlessly restore balance to your mind and body.

Techniques for Cleansing and Purification

Now we have to consider still another level of self-healing. What if you haven't taken the opportunity to develop awareness, to modify the cause, or to apply opposite qualities to restore balance, and you have begun to get sick? What to do now?

The principle of opposites is almost universally valid and helpful at any stage of disease. But once disease has begun to develop, it will not be sufficient. At this stage it becomes necessary to use techniques for cleansing and purifying your body of excess doshas and accumulated toxins.

As we have seen, when the doshas are aggravated because of poor diet, unhealthy lifestyle, negative emotions, or other factors, they first affect agni (the body's biological fire, which governs digestion and assimilation). When agni becomes weakened or disturbed, food is not properly digested. The undigested, unabsorbed food particles accumulate in the gastrointestinal tract and turn into the toxic, sticky substance called ama. In the third ("spread") stage of the disease process, ama clogs the intestines, overflows through other bodily channels such as the blood vessels, and infiltrates the bodily tissues, causing disease.

Ama is thus the root cause of disease. The presence of ama in the system can be felt as fatigue, or a feeling of heaviness. It may induce constipation, indigestion, gas, and diarrhea, or it may generate bad breath, a bad taste in the mouth, stiffness in the body, or mental confusion. Ama can most easily be detected as a thick coating on the tongue.

According to Ayurveda, disease is actually a crisis of ama, in which the body seeks to eliminate the accumulated toxicity. Thus the key to prevention of disease—once ama has begun to build up—is to help the body eliminate the toxins.

To remove ama from the system, Ayurveda employs many internal cleansing programs. One of these, most widely known in the West, is a five-procedure program known as *panchakarma* ("five actions"). The *panchakarma* programs used at Ayurvedic treatment centers include prepurification methods to prepare the body to let go of the toxins, followed by the purification methods themselves.

The first preparatory step is internal oleation. The patient is asked to drink a specific, small quantity of ghee (clarified butter) every day for several days. The ghee creates a thin film in the body's channels that lubricates them, allowing the ama lodged in the deep connective tissues to move freely, without sticking to the channels, to the gastrointestinal tract for elimination. Internal oleation is done for three to five days or even longer, depending on the individual circumstances.

This is followed by external oleation in the form of oil massage (*snehana*) and sweating (*swedana*). Oil is applied to the entire body with a particular kind of massage that helps the toxins move toward the gastrointestinal tract. The massage also softens both the superficial and deep tissues, helping to relieve stress and to nourish the nervous system. Then the individual is given a steam bath, which further loosens the toxins and increases their movement toward the gastrointestinal tract.

After three to seven days of these procedures, the doshas will have become well "ripened." At this point the physician will determine that the patient is ready to eliminate the aggravated doshas and accumulated ama. One of the five *karmas* or actions is selected as the most expedient route to eliminate the excess doshas. These procedures may include:

- therapeutic vomiting (*vamana*) to remove toxins and excess kapha from the stomach;
- purgation or laxative therapy (*virechana*) to help remove ama and excess pitta from the small intestines, colon, kidneys, stomach, liver, and spleen;
- medicated enema therapy (*basti*) to help remove excess vata from the colon. Aggravated vata is one of the main etiological factors in the manifestation of diseases. If we can control vata through the use of *bastis*, we have gone a long way toward eliminating the cause of the vast majority of diseases.
- *nasya* or nasal administration of medication, in which dry herbal powders or oils such as ghee are inserted into the nose to help remove accumulated doshas in the head, sinus, and throat areas, and to clear up breathing.
- *rakta moksha*, purification of the blood, which is traditionally done in one of two ways. Bloodletting, in which a small amount of blood is extracted from a vein, is one method, though it is illegal in the United States and is therefore not available here. The second way is to cleanse the blood using blood-purifying herbs such as burdock.

Panchakarma is not the only method used by Ayurveda to remove ama from the body. Depending on the individual's strength and the seriousness of the disease, one of two main approaches will be employed. If the person is weak and debilitated and the disease is strong, the preferred method is palliation and pacification (*shamanam*), which neutralizes ama through gentler methods of purification, including herbs. If the patient has more strength and energy and the illness is not so complicated or serious, then *panchakarma* is appropriate.

IMPORTANT NOTE: *Panchakarma* is a special, powerful procedure requiring guidance from a properly trained medical staff, not just someone with a modest amount of Ayurvedic training. It is performed individually for each person, with his or her specific constitution and medical condition in mind, and it requires close observation and supervision at every stage, including post-*panchakarma* support.

Should You Use Ghee?

The use of ghee for internal oleation is recommended for most people. However, *individuals with high blood levels of cholesterol, triglycerides, and sugar should not use it. So before you begin your home treatment, see a doctor and have your blood tested for these factors.*

If they are within the normal range, there is no problem. If they are high, then instead of ghee use flaxseed oil, which provides effective oleation and also contains fatty acids, which help to reduce cholesterol levels.

Take 2 tablespoons of the flaxseed oil three times a day for three days, fifteen minutes before eating.

A Simple Home Purification

Both for periodic prevention (to reverse any buildup of ama) and to deal with a specific health problem, *panchakarma* is a highly recommended art of cleansing and detoxification. If you are not near a center where *panchakarma* is available under the supervision of a trained Ayurvedic physician, you can do an effective purification program at home.

Begin your home detoxification program with internal oleation. For three days in a row, take about 2 ounces of warmed, liquefied ghee early in the morning. (See appendix 2 for instructions on making ghee.) For a vata person, take the ghee with a pinch of rock salt. For a pitta individual, take the 2 ounces of ghee plain. The kapha individual should add to the ghee just a pinch of *trikatu* (a mixture of equal amounts of ginger, black pepper, and *pippali,* or Indian long pepper).

The ghee provides internal oleation and lubrication, which is necessary so that the ama or toxins begin to come back from the deep tissue to the gastrointestinal tract for elimination.

After your three days of internal oleation, it is time for external oleation. For the next five to seven days, apply 7 to 8 ounces of warmed (not hot!) oil to your body from head to toe, rubbing it in well. The best oil for vata types is sesame, which is heavy and warming; pittas should use sunflower oil, which is less heating; kaphas do best with corn oil. You can do this oil massage for fifteen to twenty minutes.

After the oil is well rubbed in and absorbed, take a hot bath or shower. Then wash with some Ayurvedic herbal soap, such as *neem*. Let some of the oil remain on your skin.

The ancient Ayurvedic textbooks recommend rubbing some chickpea flour over the skin to absorb and help remove the oil. This works very well to remove the oil, but it is more suited to a culture in which individuals bathe outdoors. Today, if you use chickpea flour, be aware that oil, flour, and hot water combine into a formidable mass that can easily clog your plumbing. Flushing the drain with extra hot water immediately following your bath can help.

During your home purification, every night at least one hour after supper take ½ to 1 teaspoon of *triphala*. (For information on *triphala*, see appendix 2.) Add about half a cup of boiling water to the *triphala* powder, and let it steep ten minutes or until it has cooled down, then drink it. Along with its many healing and nourishing properties, *triphala* is a mild but effective laxative. It will provide the benefits of a more potent *virechana* or purgative treatment, but more gently and over a longer span of time. *Triphala* is safe and can be effectively used for months at a time.

To complete your home *panchakarma* treatment, on the last three days perform an Ayurvedic medicated enema, or *basti*, after your hot bath or shower. Use *dashamoola* tea for the enema. Boil 1 tablespoon of the herbal compound *dashamoola* in 1 pint of water for five minutes to make a tea. Cool it, strain it, and use the liquid as an enema. (See instructions for *basti* in appendix 3.) Retain the liquid as long as you comfortably can. And don't worry if little or no liquid comes out. For certain individuals, particularly vata types, the colon may be so dry and dehydrated that the liquid may all be absorbed. This is not harmful in any way.

This *snehana* (oleation both internal and external with ghee and oil), *swedana* (sweating using a hot shower or hot bath), and *virechana* (purgation) using triphala, followed by *basti* using *dashamoola* tea, constitute an effective *panchakarma* that you can easily do on your own at home.

During this entire time it is important to get plenty of rest, and to observe a light diet. From day four to day eight, eat only *kitchari* (equal amounts of basmati rice and mung dal cooked with cumin, mustard seed, and coriander, with about 2 teaspoons of ghee added to it). Kitchari is a wholesome, nourishing, balanced food that is an excellent protein combination. It is easy to digest and good for all three doshas, and it is also cleansing.

Be your own healer. Do this simple home purification, preferably at the junction between seasons. Take responsibility for your own healing. You will start to experience a great change in your thinking and in your feelings, and you will really fall in love with your life!

Schedule for Home Panchakarma

Here is an ideal schedule for your home *panchakarma* purification treatment:

DAY	INTERNAL OIL	EXTERNAL OIL & BATH	BASTI	DIET
1	X			Your doshic diet
2	X			"
3	X			"
4		X		Monodiet—kitchari with coriander/cumin/ fennel tea
5		X		"
6		X	X	"
7		X	X	"
8		X	X	"
9				Kitchari with steamed vegetables

Rejuvenation and Rebuilding

The purpose of *panchakarma* is not just to get well but to purify the body and strengthen it so that future diseases will not occur, and you can enjoy a long life in good health. In this regard the *panchakarma* purification can be seen as a preliminary to rejuvenation. If you want to dye your shirt, don't color it while it's dirty. Wash it first, then dye it. The washing is the *panchakarma* detoxification program, and the dyeing is the rejuvenation and revitalization.

Ayurvedic rejuvenatives (*rasayanas*) bring renewal and longevity to the cells, and when the cells live longer, the person lives longer. *Rasayanas* give strength, vitality, and longevity, strengthen tone, increase energy, and build immunity. The body's various agnis become more robust, so health becomes more robust.

For a vata individual, an excellent rejuvenative tonic is the herb *ashwagandha*. Take 1 teaspoon of *ashwagandha* in a cup of hot milk twice a day, morning and evening.

An excellent rejuvenative herb for pittas is *shatavari*. Take 1 teaspoon twice a day in a cup of warm milk. Kaphas can use *punarnava*, 1 teaspoon twice a day, but in a cup of warm water.

You can also use various herbal mixtures

Three Cautions About Home Panchakarma

1. *Panchakarma,* even in this gentle home program, has a powerful effect and should be done only by individuals of sufficient strength. If you are anemic, or feel weak and debilitated, even this home procedure is not for you.

2. Do not do *panchakarma* in a clinic, or even this home purification, if you are pregnant.

3. One result of *panchakarma,* even in this mild home version, is that the deep connective tissue may start releasing unresolved past emotions, such as grief, sadness, fear, or anger along with the built-up ama and excess doshas. If this happens, make yourself some Tranquillity Tea (see recipe on page 209), and meditate, using whatever method you have learned or the Empty Bowl meditation described in chapter 7. The releasing of emotions may happen weeks or even several months after you finish your home *panchakarma.*

designed to tonify the system, such as the traditional recipe *chyavanprash.*

To make your rejuvenation more effective, after completing your *panchakarma* purification program, set some time aside to build up your strength. Whether you take a weekend, a week, a month, or even more, use the time as a purposeful period of rest, relaxation, and rebuilding of body, mind, and spirit. Here are a few suggestions:

- Get plenty of rest.
- Observe celibacy so that you don't waste your vital energy.
- Eat carefully, according to the guidelines for your constitution.
- Meditate and do yoga postures regularly.

Quite a few more suggestions for rejuvenative herbs, foods, and tonics for all constitutional types are offered in Part III. See, for example, the recommendations under "Low Libido" and "Fatigue."

Self-Esteem

Self-esteem is at the core of healing. Because of the connectedness of mind and body, our sense of self-esteem is our cells' sense of self-esteem. This is because, according to Ayurveda, every cell is a center of intelligence and awareness. Every cell carries the sense of self for its own survival. It is the sense of self in the cell that maintains the size and shape of the cell. Self-esteem, self-confidence, and self-respect promote cellular intelligence, which is necessary for proper cell function and immunity.

Modern science is just now acknowledging the importance of the mind-body connection, but knowledge of it has been part of Ayurveda for five thousand years. Our sense of self, our attitudes and understandings, our feelings, are all psychobiological events.

Self-esteem is one such event, one that is strengthening to our cells and to all aspects of our bodies. A lack of self-confidence and self-love is detrimental.

Cancer is an example of this lack. Cancer cells have lost their intelligence and grow separate from the body. They are irregular and robust and have an isolated, selfish sense of self which is in conflict with the life of normal, healthy cells. When cancer occurs, it's as if a war is going on between the cancerous cells and the healthy cells. If the healthy cells are strong enough in self-esteem, they can conquer and kill the cancer cells. But if we do not have enough self-esteem and self-respect, then the cancer cells will win and will conquer the healthy cells.

Thus self-esteem is important for maintaining immunity. If you love yourself as you are, you will develop confidence, and that will heal disease. That is why cellular immunity, or natural resistance, depends upon self-esteem.

Chapter 5

Ayurvedic Lifestyle: The Ultimate Preventive Medicine

How you live your daily life is the key factor in determining your health and your quality of experience. It is also the factor over which you have the most control. You can't control the weather or your genetic makeup, but what you do every day either builds up your health, vitality, and resistance to disease, or wears you down. Your moment-to-moment choices—what to eat, how much to eat, how to respond to others, whether to exercise or not, how late to stay up at night, and so on—play a major role in your mental and physical health.

But how do you create your lifestyle, the rhythms of your daily living? Is it just pure habit, based on how your parents lived and how you grew up? Should the time you wake up be dictated by when you need to get to work, and should what you eat be determined by what's available at the fast-food shops? If you decide to take control of your lifestyle and structure new, healthier habits, what principles will guide you?

According to Ayurveda, you couldn't do better than to strive to live your life in harmony with Mother Nature.

In Tune with Nature

Ayurveda flourished in a civilization vastly different from life today, a world in which human life was intimately intertwined with the life of nature. The great rhythms and forces of nature—the alternation of day and night, the rhythmic cycle of seasons—all affect us, as do the inevitable seasons and cycles of human life, birth and growth, aging and death. Through the plants we eat for food, the water we drink, and the air we breathe in common with all beings, we are inextricably one with nature.

The sages of settled mind who unfolded the wisdom of Ayurveda saw this, and they saw that the master key to good health is to get ourselves into harmony with nature.

Thus the ideal Ayurvedic daily routine that follows is, as you will see, based on patterns of nature.

Being in tune with nature also means being in tune with *your* nature, your constitution or *prakruti* (which means nature). It means being true to your own nature, to how you are built, mentally and emotionally as well as physically. It means that your food and exercise requirements, how much you need to sleep, how much sexual activity is healthy for you, what kind of climate is beneficial, all revolve around your doshic makeup, your individual nature.

Living in accordance with nature and natural law means continually balancing our inner ecology by adjusting to our ever-changing environment.

Ayurvedic Daily Routine

A daily routine is essential for maintaining good health and for transforming our body, mind, and consciousness to a higher level of functioning. A regulated daily routine puts us in harmony with nature's rhythms. It establishes balance in our constitution and helps to regularize our biological clock. It indirectly aids in digestion, absorption, and assimilation of food, and it generates self-esteem, discipline, peace, happiness, and long life.

Waking up too early or too late, undisciplined eating, staying up too late, job stress, and untimely bowel movements are a few habits that can unsettle us. Regularity in sleeping, waking, eating, and eliminating, indeed following a regular daily routine, brings discipline to life and helps maintain the integrity of the doshas.

Our body is a clock. Or rather, it is several clocks at once. According to Ayurveda, every organ has a definite time of maximum functioning. Morning time is the lung time. Midday is stomach time, when we feel hungry. Afternoon is liver time, and late afternoon is when the colon and kidneys operate at their peak.

This biological clock works in conjunction with the doshic clock. Morning and evening (dawn and dusk) are the times when the influence of vata is greatest. In the early morning, from about 2 A.M. to sunrise, vata creates movement and people awaken and tend to excrete waste. Again in the late afternoon, from about 2 P.M. until sunset, the influence of vata makes one feel light and active.

Early morning and evening are kapha times. From sunrise until about 10 A.M., kapha makes one feel fresh but a little heavy. Then again in the evening, from about 6 P.M. until around 10, kapha ushers in a period of cooling air, inertia, and declining energy.

Midday and midnight are pitta times. At midmorning, kapha slowly merges into pitta, and by noon one feels hungry and ready for lunch. Again from 10 P.M. until around 2 A.M., pitta is at its peak, and food is digested.

Thus there is a daily cycle of vata–pitta–kapha:

6 A.M.–10 A.M. = kapha
10 A.M.–2 P.M. = pitta
2 P.M.–6 P.M. = vata
6 P.M.–10 P.M. = kapha
10 P.M.–2 A.M. = pitta
2 A.M.–6 A.M. = vata

So there is a doshic clock (when a particular dosha is operating at its peak) and a biological clock (when a particular organ is operating at its peak). Based on these clocks, the Ayurvedic sages developed the *dinacharya*, or daily routine. This daily routine is the art of bringing harmony between the biological and doshic clocks and chronological time. Here are its most salient features:

WAKE UP EARLY

It is beneficial to wake up before the sun rises. At this time of the morning, pure qualities are lively in nature, which can bring freshness to the doors of perception and peace of mind.

Ideally, vata people should get up at about 6 A.M., pitta people by 5:30, and kapha people by 4:30. This is the ideal: do the best you can. If you can wake up at 5:30, it will be very good.

Right after awakening, look at your hands for a few moments, then gently move them over your face, neck, and chest down to your waist. This will bring more alertness.

SAY A PRAYER

It is good to start the day by remembering the Divine Reality that is our life. You may do this in your own way, as your religion or personal experience dictates. Or you may use this simple prayer:

Dear God, you are inside of me
Within my very breath
Within each bird, each mighty mountain.
Your sweet touch reaches everything
and I am well protected.
Thank you God
for this beautiful day before me.
May joy, love, peace, and compassion
be part of my life
and all those around me on this day.
I am healing and I am healed.

WASH YOUR FACE, MOUTH, AND EYES

Splash your face with cold water a couple of times. Swish and rinse out your mouth. Then wash your eyes with cool water, and massage the eyelids by gently rubbing them. Blink your eyes seven times, and then rotate your eyes in all directions: side to side, up and down, diagonally, clockwise, and counterclockwise. All this will help you feel alert and fresh. (See "Eyes—Ayurvedic Care" in Part III for more on eye exercises and eye washes.)

DRINK A GLASS OF WATER

Drink a glass of room-temperature water, preferably from a pure copper cup or tumbler. (Fill the cup the night before and let it sit overnight.) If the water is too cold, it may provoke kapha disorders such as colds, coughs, and sore throat. For kapha and vata individuals, it is actually better to drink hot water, but for a pitta person, lukewarm is best.

This water will not be absorbed but will wash the gastrointestinal tract and flush the kidneys. It also stimulates peristalsis in the intestines, stimulates the descending colon and ileocecal valve, and helps with having a good bowel movement.

It is not a good idea to start the day with coffee or black tea. These drain kidney energy, overstimulate the adrenals, and promote constipation. They are also habit-forming.

EVACUATION

Sit (or better, squat) on the toilet, and have a bowel movement. Even if you don't have the urge, sit for a few minutes, without forcing. If you do this every day, following your glass of warm water, the habit will develop. (See "Constipation" for suggestions on promoting healthy bowel movements.)

After evacuation, wash the anal orifice with warm water, then wash your hands with a gentle soap.

CLEAN YOUR TEETH AND TONGUE

Use a soft toothbrush for your teeth, and an herbal powder made of astringent, pungent, and bitter herbs. (See "Teeth and Gums—Ayurvedic Care" for further suggestions.)

Scrape your tongue every morning. This is an important part of daily hygiene, from which you can learn a lot about your health and habits. Note how coated your tongue is, and how your breath smells. If you get the smell of last night's pizza, that means the food is not yet thoroughly digested. If there is a lot of coating on the tongue, that means there is much ama or toxicity in the system. Perhaps you ate too late, or your dinner was hard to digest.

If there is ama on the tongue and a bad smell on the breath, don't eat breakfast. Eating breakfast is not good if you have not digested last night's dinner.

You can see that this daily regimen brings more awareness. By following this routine, you come in contact with your body and observe the functioning of your system. You know exactly what is happening. This knowledge gives you the power to create better health by altering your behavior.

To scrape your tongue, use a stainless-steel tongue scraper. You can also use a spoon. Gently scrape from the back or base of the tongue forward, until you have scraped the whole surface (seven to fourteen strokes). In addition to removing bacteria from the tongue, scraping sends an indirect message to all the internal organs and stimulates gastric fire and digestive enzymes.

GARGLE

To strengthen the teeth, gums, and jaw, to improve the voice and remove wrinkles from the cheeks, gargle twice a day with warm sesame oil. Also, hold the oil in your mouth and swish it around vigorously. Then spit it out and gently massage the gums with your index finger.

NOSE DROPS *(NASYA)*

Now put 3 to 5 drops of warm ghee, *brahmi* ghee, or sesame oil into each nostril. This helps to clean the sinuses and also improves voice, vision, and mental clarity. In dry climates, and during cold winters when the house is heated with dry air, nose drops help to keep the nostrils lubricated. (For more on *nasya*, see appendix 3.)

The nose is the doorway to the brain. Use of nose drops nourishes *prana* and enlivens consciousness and intelligence.

OIL MASSAGE

Take 4 or 5 ounces of warm (not hot) oil, and rub it all over your head and body. Gently massaging the scalp with oil can bring happiness into your day, as well as help prevent headaches and slow balding and graying of your hair. If you oil your body again before going to bed, it will help induce sound sleep.

Oil massage improves circulation, calms the mind, and reduces excess vata. The skin of the entire body becomes soft, smooth, and brightened.

Best Oils by Body Type

For Ayurvedic oil massage, use one of the following oils, according to your constitutional type:

Vata = sesame oil
Pitta = sunflower oil
Kapha = corn oil

BATHING

Following your oil massage, take a bath or shower. Bathing is cleansing and refreshing. It removes fatigue, brings energy and alertness, and promotes long life. Bathing every day brings holiness into your life.

EXERCISE

Everyone should do some exercise every day. A walk in the fresh early-morning air and some yoga stretching are good enough for many people; some additional aerobic exercise may also be beneficial, depending on your *prakruti*.

Kapha individuals, with their stronger, heavier physiques, can do the most strenuous exercise, and they benefit from it. Jogging, bicycling, tennis, aerobics, hiking, and mountain climbing are great for kaphas (though they don't like such vigorous exercise!). Pittas do well with a moderate amount (swimming is especially helpful for cooling pitta), while vata individuals do best with quieter exercises like walking, easy swimming, or yoga *asanas*.

As a general rule, Ayurveda recommends exercising up to one half of one's capacity. A good gauge is to exercise until sweat forms on the forehead, under the arms, and along the spinal column. Straining is absolutely not recommended.

Yoga stretching is recommended for all body types. Postures particularly beneficial for vata individuals include the Sun Salutation (twelve cycles, done slowly). The most important seat of vata in the body is in the pelvic cavity, and any exercise that stretches the pelvic muscles helps to calm vata. These include the Forward Bend, Backward Bend, Spinal Twist, Shoulder Stand, Plow, Camel, Cobra, Locust, Cat, and Cow poses, and Leg Lifts. The Headstand, Half Wheel, and Yoga *Mudra* are also beneficial. (For illustrations of yoga postures see appendix 4.)

The major seat of pitta is the solar plexus,

so exercises that stretch the muscles around the solar plexus are especially beneficial for individuals with a pitta *prakruti* and will help to pacify pitta. These include the Fish, Boat, Camel, Locust, and Bow poses. Pittas should also do the Moon Salutation (sixteen cycles, moderately fast). Avoid the Headstand, Shoulder Stand, Plow, and other inverted poses.

The important seat of kapha is in the chest. Exercises that stretch the pulmonary cavity and increase circulation in the chest are effective for kaphas and will help relieve and prevent bronchial congestion, cough, and other kapha illnesses. Beneficial postures include the Sun Salutation (twelve cycles, done rapidly) and the Shoulder Stand, Plow, Locust, Bridge, Peacock, Palm Tree, and Lion postures. (Illustrations of yoga postures are found in appendix 4.)

PRANAYAMA

After finishing your exercises, sit quietly and do some deep breathing: twelve Alternate Nostril breaths for vata; sixteen Cooling (*shitali*) breaths for pitta; one hundred Breath of Fire (*bhastrika*) breaths for kapha. (Instructions for these breathing exercises appear in chapter 6.)

MEDITATION

End your *pranayama* by going right into your meditation. Whatever system or technique of meditation you do, do it now. If you don't presently do any meditation practice, try the Empty Bowl meditation explained in chapter 7. You will find that meditation brings peace and balance into your life.

BREAKFAST

Now it is time for you to enjoy your breakfast! Your meal should be fairly light in the hot months, and more substantial in cold weather. Vata and pitta persons should eat some breakfast; kaphas are usually better off if they don't eat, since eating during kapha time will increase kapha in the body. Follow the dietary guidelines for the three doshas which appear in chapter 8.

Mealtimes for Each Dosha

	VATA	PITTA	KAPHA
Breakfast	8 A.M.	7:30 A.M.	7 A.M.
Lunch	11 A.M.–Noon	Noon	Noon–1 P.M.
Supper	6 P.M.	6–7 P.M.	7–8 P.M. No Snacks!

OFF TO WORK

After breakfast go to work or to your studies if you are a student. While walking to work (or to and from your car, the train, or the bus), be aware of every step. Carry your meditative mind with you. When you look at your boss or colleague, at the same time look inside. Then your work will become a meditation. You will find yourself looking at others with compassion and greater awareness.

It is better not to drink tea or coffee at work. If you are thirsty, have some warm water or some fruit juice if you prefer.

LUNCHTIME

By around noon you will become quite hungry. Have a bowl of soup and some salad, or some rice and vegetables, following the guidelines for your constitution. And don't drink too much during your meal. Take a cup of water (preferably warm but definitely not iced), and just take a sip between two mouthfuls of food. Drinking a little water improves digestion.

One can drink a cup of water an hour before lunch or an hour after lunch, but not immediately afterward, as that slows down digestion and creates ama.

SIT STRAIGHT, WALK STRAIGHT

Maintain your vertebral column straight. When you keep the backbone straight, energy flows upward and you maintain your awareness. It is difficult to be aware when the spine is crunched.

TAKE A WALK

When you've finished your job for the day, go home and take a walk, alone, silently, in the woods, in the park, or on the bank of the river. Listen to the water, the birds, the rustle of leaves, the barking of a dog. In that listening, the meditative mind is regained.

In this way, every day becomes heavenly. Every day becomes a celebration, something new. That's why the routine is most important. The discipline of the routine leaves room for awareness, openness, and freshness.

SUPPER TIME

At around six o'clock (see "Mealtimes for Each Dosha" box) have your supper. If you like to cook, you can cook according to the *Ayurvedic Cookbook for Self-Healing* that I have written with my wife, Usha Lad (see the Reading List). Don't watch television while eating. Pay attention to the food. Eating food with attention becomes meditation. And when you are eating with awareness, you will not eat too much; you'll eat just a sufficient amount.

It is better to eat when the sun is up. Eating late at night will change the body chemistry, sleep will be disturbed, and you will not feel rested in the morning. If you eat supper around 6, by 9 the stomach will be empty and you will sleep soundly.

AFTER DINNER

Sing songs while you wash the dishes. Be happy. Keep smiling.

About an hour after dinner, if you are taking *triphala* (an herbal compound that is both strengthening and purifying), take 1/2 teaspoon with some warm water.

Then if you like, you can watch TV, perhaps some news. You should know what's happening in this world of ours. Or you can read a magazine or a book.

BEFORE GOING TO BED

Before you go to bed, some spiritual reading is important, even if only for a few minutes.

And don't forget to drink a cup of hot milk, with a little ginger, cardamom, and turmeric. Drinking milk at bedtime helps to induce sound sleep. According to Ayurveda, that milk also nourishes *shukra dhatu,* the body's highly refined reproductive tissue.

Rubbing a little oil on the soles of your feet and on the scalp is also soothing and promotes restful sleep.

Finally, before you go to bed, do a few minutes of meditation. Sit quietly and watch your breath. In the pauses between breaths, you'll meet with nothingness, and nothingness is energy and intelligence. Allow that intelligence to deal with your problems. In this way, you'll begin and end your day with meditation, and meditation will stay with you even during deep sleep.

BEDTIME

It is recommended that vatas go to bed by 10 P.M. and sleep on their left side. Pittas should sleep on the right side, retiring between 10 and 11 P.M. The best bedtime for kapha individuals is between 11 and midnight; they should sleep on their left side.

Kapha individuals generally like to sleep about nine hours, and they feel it is good for them. But this is an illusion. Sleeping this long will slow down their metabolism, and they will put on weight and become chubby. The best schedule for them is to stay up until about 11 P.M. or midnight, then to wake up early, around 4:30 or 5:00 A.M. and go out for a walk. That shorter sleep will help to induce a light quality in their body, and they will start losing weight.

SEX

Ayurveda has some definite suggestions about the proper role of sex in our lives. Sex is a tremendous creative force, and through

Ideal Wake-up and Bed Times

	VATA	PITTA	KAPHA
Wake Up	6:00	5:30	4:30
Go to Bed	10:00	10:00–11:00	11:00–midnight

sex people share their love and compassion and can derive great pleasure.

Sex is also correlated with constitutional type. The recommended frequency of sexual activity is quite different for the different types. Kaphas, with their strong constitutions, can make love two to three times a week, whereas the suggestion for vatas is once or at most twice a month. Pitta individuals are in the middle; every two weeks is recommended for them.

Too-frequent lovemaking reduces *ojas,* the body's vital energy, and leaves the person weak and open to diseases. It also aggravates vata dosha.

To restore strength and replenish *ojas,* after each time you make love a massage is helpful, as are nourishing drinks such as almond milk. (See recipe for almond milk on page 127.) The best time for lovemaking is between 10 and 11 P.M. Sex in the morning or in the daytime is not recommended.

This entire daily routine is very important.

> I set more store by a good regimen that maintains my humors in balance and procures me a sound sleep. Drink hot when it freezes, drink cool in the dog days; in everything, neither too much nor too little; digest, sleep, have pleasure, and snap your fingers at the rest of it.
>
> —*Voltaire*

Seasonal Routines

The seasons, like the times of day, are characterized by cycles of vata, pitta, and kapha. Maintaining good health during all four seasons requires living in harmony with these natural cycles, continually adjusting to the changes in the outer environment through the food we choose to eat, the type and amount of exercise we do, the clothes we wear, and so on. The suggestions in this section will help you be at your best all year round.

Please remember that you cannot determine the seasons just by dates on the calendar. Ayurveda is a system of natural medicine, which means that you have to see what is happening in nature! In different geographic areas the seasons come at different times and have varied characteristics. In addition, in just one day there may be four seasons: sunshine and singing birds creating a springlike air in the morning; warm summery breezes at midday; gusts of cool, dry autumnal wind in the afternoon; cold, cloudy, wintry weather after dark. So look at nature as it is, and apply the appropriate principles and practices.

GUIDELINES FOR SUMMER

Summer is hot, bright, and sharp, the season of pitta. Thus the main recommendation for everyone, especially for individuals whose *prakruti* is primarily pitta, is to keep cool and not allow pitta dosha to become aggravated.

- In the morning, as part of your daily routine, rub 5 to 6 ounces of coconut oil or sunflower oil on your body before bathing. Coconut oil is calming, cooling, and soothing to the skin.
- Wear cotton or silk clothing; it is cool-

ing, light, and allows the skin to breathe. Loose-fitting clothes are best; they permit the air to pass through and cool the body.

• The best colors to wear in hot weather are white, gray, blue, purple, and green. Avoid red, orange, dark yellow, and black, which absorb and retain heat and will aggravate pitta.

• Follow the pitta-pacifying diet from the food guidelines in chapter 8. Good fruits for summer include apples, pears, melons, plums, and prunes. Watermelon and lime juice are also good in summer. Try steamed asparagus, broccoli, brussels sprouts, cucumber raita, and basmati rice. Kitchari made of basmati rice and mung dal, with a little ghee and grated coconut, makes a delicious light meal. Avoid sour fruits, citrus fruits, and even beets and carrots, which are all heating. Garlic, onion, chili, tomato, sour cream, and salted cheeses are also not recommended. You can eat more salads in summer than at any other time, as they are cooling, but they are best eaten for lunch. If you eat meat, you can have some light meat—chicken, turkey, or shrimp—once a week. Avoid dark meats, which are heating.

• Don't drink hot water or hot drinks in the summer. Room-temperature or cool drinks are best. Ice and iced drinks, however, inhibit digestion and create toxins (ama) in the body; it is best never to drink them.

• A refreshing drink is cool lassi. Mix 1 part yogurt with 4 parts water, and blend 2 or 3 minutes until creamy. You can add 1/4 teaspoon roasted cumin seed before blending, or for a sweet-flavored drink, add 2 tablespoons Sucanat or other sweetener and 1 drop of rose water. The juice of 1/4 lime in a cup of cool water with a pinch of cumin powder is also refreshing.

• Working in a hot kitchen provokes pitta. If you cook, cook in the early morning or in the evening. If someone cooks three days in a row, on the fourth day you should treat that person to dinner in a restaurant. This will avoid conflicts in the relationship.

• If you customarily drink alcoholic beverages, avoid whiskey, brandy, rum, and red wine, which are heating. Some cool beer during hot days will be all right.

• This is a season of generalized low energy. Thus it is all right to take a short nap in the daytime.

• If you have to work outside, wear a wide-brimmed hat.

• Wear sunglasses outdoors during the brightest part of the day. Lenses should be smoky gray or green, not red or yellow and especially not blue or purple, which will damage the eyes.

• If you can, work indoors. Have some air conditioning in your car and in your room or office.

• Never lie in the sun in summer. If the weather is very hot, don't wear shorts or short sleeves, but wear loose-fitting clothing to protect your skin. No person having multiple moles should lie in the sun; it may provoke extreme pitta aggravation and lead to skin cancer.

• If you feel really hot, take a swim in a cool lake or pool, then drink a little lime juice in water.

• Avoid strenuous exercise. If you are accustomed to running or other vigorous aerobic exercise, do it early in the morning at the coolest part of the day.

• Do some mild yoga exercises and quiet meditation twice a day. Good postures for summer include the Fish, Camel, Boat, Cobra, Cow, and Palm Tree poses. Pitta individuals should not do inverted poses such as Headstand and Shoulder Stand, which can be pitta-provoking. Also, do the Moon Salutation. (See illustrations in appendix 4.)

• Perform *shitali pranayama,* a cooling breathing exercise described in chapter 6.

• Certain jewelry and gems will help cool pitta. These include a necklace of sandalwood beads, a jade or pearl necklace, amethyst crystals, moonstone, malachite crystals, and any silver jewelry.

• In the evening, after dinner, go for a walk in the moonlight. Dress in white clothes, with white flowers in your hair or a garland of white flowers around your neck.

• You can go to bed a little later on summer nights, around 11 P.M. or midnight. Rub some coconut oil on your scalp and the soles of your feet for a cooling effect before going to sleep. Sleep on your right side.

• Sandalwood, jasmine, and khus oils are cooling and are good fragrances to wear in the summer. Also, place a few drops of sandalwood oil on your pillow, and you will be sleeping with sandalwood perfume all night.

• Sex should be minimized in the summer, as it is heating and will provoke pitta. If you want to have sex, do it between 9 and 10 P.M., when it is cooler but not yet pitta time.

> During the summer, the sun evaporates the moisture of the earth and therefore induces hot, dry and sharp qualities in the atmosphere, resulting in pitta aggravation. In summer sweet, cold, liquid, and fatty food and drinks are beneficial. One should avoid or minimize excessive exercise and sex, alcohol, and diets which are salty, sour, pungent, or hot. In summer time one should enjoy forests, gardens, flowers, and cool water. During the night one should sleep on the open airy roof of the house, which is cooled by the rays of the moon.
>
> —*Charaka Samhita*

GUIDELINES FOR FALL

Autumn is dry, light, cold, windy, rough, and empty (trees drop their leaves). All these qualities provoke vata dosha. So naturally the guidelines for autumn revolve around pacifying vata.

• If you can, wake up early, around 5 A.M., when the air is calm and the birds are not yet out of bed. There is an extraordinary silence and peace at this time of day.

• Good yoga *asanas* for the autumn season include the Lotus pose, Forward Bend, Backward Bend, Vajrasana (Sitting on the Heels), Spinal Twist, Camel, Cobra, Cow, and Cat. Shoulder Stand and Headstand are all right in moderation. Also do the Sun Salutation a minimum of twelve cycles. As a maximum, you can do as many Sun Salutations as your age, but you have to build up to this through regular daily practice. Finish your yoga session with *savasana,* the relaxation pose.

• Gentle Alternate Nostril *pranayama* is good following yoga postures. Then meditate for at least ten to fifteen minutes.

• Every morning before your bath or shower, rub 6 to 9 ounces of warm sesame oil all over your body, from head to toe. Sesame oil is warming and heavy and will help to balance vata. Then take a nice warm shower. Leave a little of the oil on your skin.

• Good fall colors for pacifying vata are red, yellow, and orange. White is also helpful.

• After your yoga, meditation, and bath, have some breakfast. Try oatmeal, cream of rice, cream of wheat, tapioca, or any grain that will help to settle vata. (See the food recommendations for vata in chapter 8.) For lunch and supper, tortillas, chapatis, basmati rice, mung dal kitchari, and steamed vegetables are all good fall foods to balance vata. Salads are not recommended. Mushy, soft soups and stews are good, and be sure to use some ghee.

• Don't drink black tea or coffee after dinner. Try some herbal tea, such as cumin-coriander-fennel tea (equal proportions), or ginger-cinnamon-clove tea.

• Fasting is not good during the autumn season. It generates too much lightness and emptiness, which provoke vata.

• Be sure to keep warm. Dress warmly enough both indoors and out. On a windy, gusty day, cover your head and ears.

• Very active, vigorous exercise should be avoided, especially by individuals with a vata constitution.

• A short afternoon nap is acceptable for vatas.

• Try to be in bed by 10 P.M.

• Drinking a cup of warm milk at bedtime is good in the autumn season. It induces sound, natural sleep. Heat the milk until it begins to boil and rise up, then let it cool enough to drink comfortably. You might add a pinch each of ginger and cardamom and a small pinch of nutmeg. These herbs are warming and soothing and will help both with digesting the milk and with relaxation.

• At the junction between summer and fall, a *panchakarma* treatment will help remove excess vata from the system. (See chapter 4.) If you can't go to an Ayurvedic clinic, try the home purification treatment outlined in chapter 4. A crucial component of this treatment should be the *basti* or medicated enema, as follows:

1. Boil 2 tablespoons of *dashamoola* powder in 1 pint of water for 5 minutes.
2. Strain out the herbs, and to the liquid add 1/2 cup warm sesame oil.
3. When this mixture has cooled to a comfortable temperature, use it for the enema. Try to retain it for 30 minutes.
4. After half an hour or after a good bowel movement, add another 1/2 cup warm sesame oil to the rectum. Try to retain this oil for at least 10 minutes.

• This procedure will lubricate the colon, calm vata, and remove stress from the lower back and neck areas. You can do this *basti* once a week during the autumn season to keep vata in check.

• During this season, take particular care to avoid loud noise, loud music (such as rock), fast driving, and too much sexual activity. Avoid cold drafts and cold winds. These all aggravate vata.

• Excellent herbs for pacifying vata dosha in the autumn are *dashamoola* (actually a formula consisting of ten herbs), *ashwagandha*, *bala*, and *vidari*.

GUIDELINES FOR WINTER

In winter, the sky is cloudy, the weather is cold, damp, and heavy, and life in the cities moves slowly; it is generally a season of kapha. A kapha-pacifying regimen should be adopted, especially by kapha individuals. However, certain vata-provoking qualities, such as dry, cold, windy, and clear, are sometimes prominent on winter days, so vata individuals need to keep this in mind.

• In winter there is no need to get up early. The 5:00 rising time suggested for summer and autumn is not necessary now. Unless you have to get up earlier to go to work, you can get up around 7 A.M.

• After brushing your teeth and scraping your tongue (see the Daily Routine, page 59), do some yoga *asanas*, including the Sun Salutation. Beneficial postures for winter season include the Fish, Locust, Boat, Bow, Lion, and Camel poses, Shoulder Stand and Headstand. These postures help to open the chest, stretch the throat, drain the sinuses, and relieve congestion of the chest.

• Follow your yoga postures with some breathing exercises. *Bhastrika* (Breath of Fire) will cleanse kapha dosha. Follow this with a few minutes of Right Nostril breathing, which promotes circulation and heat. (See instructions in chapter 6.)

• Winter is a season of kapha. So, like slow and steady kapha, don't be in a rush. Be sure to follow your breathing exercises with some quiet meditation.

• After meditation apply some warm sesame oil to your entire body, then take a hot shower. Sesame oil, which is warming, is beneficial for all constitutional types in the winter.

• For a good winter breakfast, have some oatmeal, cornmeal, barley soup, tapioca, kitchari, or poha (cooked rice flakes). About an hour later, drink tea made of these herbs:

dry ginger	*1/2 teaspoon*
cinnamon	*1/2 teaspoon*
clove	*a pinch*

Boil these herbs in a cup of hot water for five minutes, and drink the tea. It will increase heat and pitta, improve circulation, and eliminate mucus from the system. However, if you have an ulcer, don't drink this tea; it will be too heating.

• Wear bright warming colors such as red and orange.

• Always wear a hat outdoors in winter. More than 60 percent of the body's heat is lost through the head. Also cover your neck and ears.

• For lunch, eat kapha-soothing food but not food that is vata-aggravating. Whole-wheat bread, steamed vegetables, and hot mushy soup with much ghee and some crunchy croutons would be just right.

• If you like to eat meat, Ayurveda says that winter is the time to eat it, because agni (digestive fire) is strong. Chicken and turkey are good choices.

• Although a nap may be acceptable in summer and autumn (especially for pitta and vata individuals, respectively), sleeping in the daytime is not recommended during winter because it will increase kapha, slow down metabolism, and reduce the gastric fire.

• Ayurveda recommends drinking a little

dry red wine—a few ounces at most—in the winter to improve digestion and circulation. *Draksha* (Ayurvedic herbal wine) is a good choice. Take 4 teaspoons of draksha with an equal amount of water before or after dinner.

• The winter season, when the sky is covered by clouds and it is gray outdoors, is conducive to loneliness and depression. Following the kapha-pacifying routine will definitely help. If possible, don't be away from your wife, husband, boyfriend, or girlfriend in the winter. When it is cold outside and inside there is no one to sleep with, you will definitely feel lonely. When you have your companion in the winter, you feel great!

• At the end of the day, rub a small amount of sesame oil on your scalp and on the soles of your feet.

• According to Ayurvedic tradition, winter is the season in which you can have sex more often.

• The best herbs for winter are *pippali*, licorice, ginger, *punarnava*, black pepper, and *kutki*. You can also use the herbal tonic *chyavanprash*.

• Some light fasting, for a day or two, is all right if your digestive fire is strong. You can drink some apple juice or pomegranate juice during your fast if you like.

• At the junction between autumn and winter, individuals who tend to get kapha problems in winter (colds, coughs, flu, sinus congestion, and the like) should receive *panchakarma* at an Ayurvedic clinic, under the care of an Ayurvedic physician, to remove excess kapha dosha. This will help give you a problem-free winter.

GUIDELINES FOR SPRING

Spring is the king of the seasons. In the Bhagavad Gita Lord Krishna reveals his predominant attributes in the eleventh chapter: "I am the Soul in the body, the Mind in the senses, the Eagle among birds, the Lion among animals. Among all the trees I am the sacred *Bodhi* tree, and of the seasons, I am Spring."

In spring Mother Earth wakes up and causes sprouting; energy moves up; everything is blooming and flowering, full of colors and greenery. People feel energetic and love to go outdoors. It is the season of celebration.

The qualities of spring are warm, moist, gentle, and unctuous. Due to the warmth, the accumulated snow and ice of winter begin to melt. Similarly, accumulated kapha in the body starts liquefying and running. That is why so many people get spring colds. In addition, as flowers shed their pollen, fragrance, and perfume, making vata and pitta people happy, many kapha individuals get hay fever and allergies.

As early winter carries some of the qualities of fall, so early spring is much like winter, and many of the recommendations are the same. For example, *panchakarma* is highly recommended, to clear the system of accumulated kapha dosha and help prevent allergies, hay fever, colds, and sinus congestion.

• Good herbs for spring include ginger, black pepper, *pippali*, and a tea made of cumin, coriander, and fennel in equal proportions. *Sitopaladi*, *punarnava*, and *sudarshan* are also beneficial.

• Strictly avoid heavy, oily food. Also, it is better not to eat sour, sweet, and salty foods, as they provoke kapha. Stay away from dairy products, especially in the morning. Avoid ice cream and cold drinks, which are especially kaphagenic.

• Favor bitter, pungent, and astringent foods. All legumes, such as yellow split peas, red lentils, and garbanzo and pinto beans, are recommended. Radishes, spinach, okra, onions, and garlic can be used, along with hot spices such as ginger, black pepper, cayenne pepper, and chili pepper. (But don't overdo these hot spices if your constitution is predominantly vata or especially if it is pitta.) After each meal, drink some tea made from ginger, black pepper, and cinnamon.

• Use less ghee and fewer dairy products, and use more honey, which is heating. A cup of hot water with a teaspoon of honey helps balance kapha during the spring season. (But never cook honey; it clogs the subtle channels and acts as a toxin in the system.) You can end your meal with a cup of freshly made lassi (see page 65 for recipe).

• For those who eat meat, chicken, turkey, rabbit, and venison are permissible; seafood, crab, lobster, and duck are not recommended during spring season.

• This is a good season to observe a juice fast of apple, pomegranate, or berry juice.

• Wake up early, and go for a morning walk. Also, do the Sun Salutation and kapha-reducing yoga postures, such as the Fish, Boat, Bow, Locust, Lion, and Camel poses, and the Headstand and/or Shoulder Stand. *Bhastrika* and Right Nostril breathing are also helpful (see chapter 6).

• Sleeping in the daytime aggravates kapha; hence it is not recommended during this season.

As spring advances and the weather heats up, you will want to change from a kapha-pacifying regimen to the pitta-pacifying guidelines suggested for summer. In fact, as the weather alternates between cold and hot, you will need to be alert day-to-day and use your common sense to remain in balance.

Chapter 6

Breathing Techniques

Prana is the bridge between body, mind, and consciousness. It is the constant movement of awareness. *Prana* carries awareness to the object of our perception; that movement of awareness through *prana* is called attention. The internal movement of *prana* is the movement of sensation, thought, feeling, and emotion. Thus *prana* and mind are deeply connected.

The physical manifestation of *prana* is breath. Breathing and mind are closely connected. Ayurveda says that breathing is the physical part of thinking and thinking is the psychological part of breathing. Every thought changes the rhythm of breath, and every breath changes the rhythm of thinking. When one is happy, blissful, and silent, breathing is rhythmic. If one is disturbed with anxiety, fear, or nervousness, the breathing is irregular and interrupted.

Ancient Vedic seers (*rishis*) discovered this intimate relationship between breathing and mental activity and uncovered the art of *pranayama*. *Pranayama* equals *prana* plus *ayam*. *Ayam* means "to control," *prana* is "breath." By controlling the breath, we can control mental activity.

The Secret of Pranayama

The *rishis* also found an intimate relationship between the right and the left breath cycle. You may have noticed that sometimes you breathe more easily through the left nostril, and sometimes your breathing shifts more to the right nostril. This shift happens about every 45 to 90 minutes. Just as the right side of our body is governed by the left side of the brain and vice versa, breathing better through the left nostril activates the right hemisphere of the brain, and breathing better through the right nostril activates the left brain.

The left brain is associated with male energy, the right with female energy. The left brain is for logical thinking, investigation, inquiry, aggressiveness, competition, and judgment. Whenever we are judging, investigating, and so on, our right breath cycle is dominant and our left brain hemisphere is operating. Exactly opposite, when the right hemisphere is acting and the left breath cycle is working, we have female energy, which is associated with love, compassion, intuition, art, poetry, and religion. So when an artist is drawing a picture or a poet writing a poem, he or she is using some part of the right brain. And when the scientist is working in the lab, investigating and solving a problem, at that time he or she is using some part of the left brain.

The secret of *pranayama* is the secret of handling the male and female energy operating in our nervous system. In Alternate Nostril *pranayama,* when we inhale through the left nostril, we charge the right brain. When we inhale through the right nostril, we charge our left brain. When yogis do Alternate Nostril breathing, their male and female energies become equally balanced. When these energies are balanced, the neutral energy is awakened and one experiences pure awareness, which is called *brahman.*

When we do *pranayama,* the *nadis* (subtle channels of the nervous system) become purified, the mind becomes controlled, and we can go beyond male and female energies to pure, choiceless, passive awareness.

This is the basis for *pranayama.* Then there are numerous types of *pranayama*: practices to heat or cool the body; Right Nostril breathing to awaken more male energy; Left Nostril breathing to awaken more female energy; and so on.

Six Breathing Techniques

ALTERNATE NOSTRIL *PRANAYAMA*

One of the simplest breathing practices, and one that is very effective, as we have discussed, is Alternate Nostril *pranayama.*

1. Sit comfortably on the floor in a cross-legged posture, keeping the spine straight. If you are not comfortable in this position, sit upright on the front edge of a chair with your feet flat on the floor.
2. Close the right nostril with your right thumb, and inhale through the left nostril. Inhale into the belly, not into the chest.
3. After inhaling, hold your breath for just a moment.
4. Exhale through your right nostril while closing the left with the ring and little finger of your right hand.
5. Repeat steps 1 to 3, but this time start by inhaling through the *right* nostril (while you close the left nostril with your ring and little finger).

You can do this breathing exercise for five to ten minutes.

NOTE: This *pranayama,* as well as the others in this book, is best learned under the guidance of an accomplished teacher.

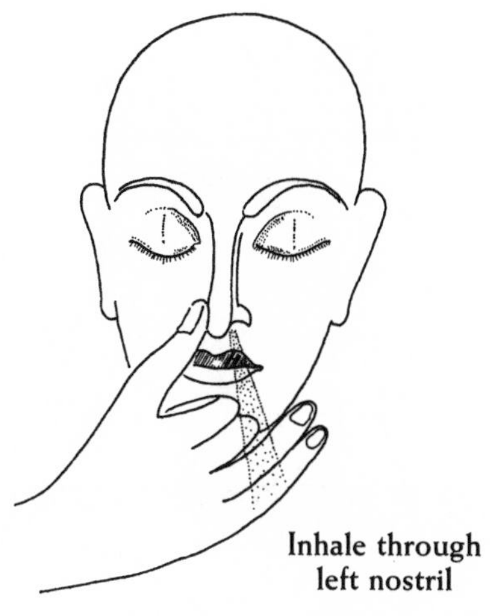

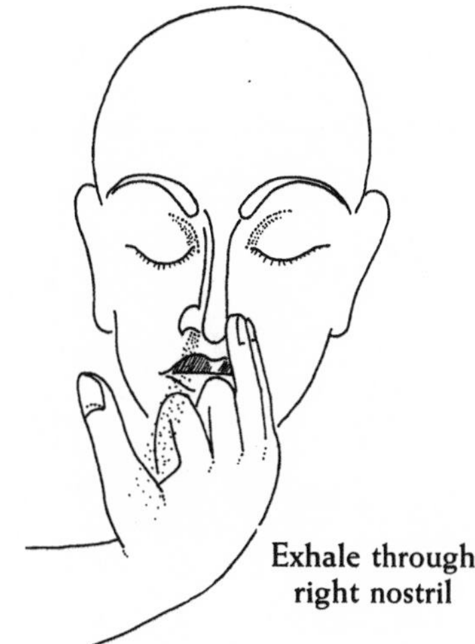

ALTERNATE NOSTRIL PRANAYAMA

SHITALI PRANAYAMA (COOLING BREATH)

Curl your tongue into a tube. Inhale slowly through the curled tongue, swallow, and then exhale normally through the nose, keeping the mouth closed. You will feel the incoming air cool your saliva, your tongue, and the oral mucous membranes.

This form of breathing is helpful for pacifying high pitta. It lowers the oral temperature, makes the saliva cool, helps to quench thirst, and improves digestion, absorption, and assimilation. *Shitali* is effective for high blood pressure, burning throat or tongue, and a burning sensation in the eyes. It cools the entire body.

If you can't curl your tongue into a tube, an alternative way to perform *shitali* is with your teeth lightly clenched together and your tongue pressed up against the teeth. The air is then inhaled through the teeth. Some people feel pain when cool air is drawn through the teeth; keeping your tongue against your teeth will provide warmth and prevent this discomfort.

BHASTRIKA PRANAYAMA (BREATH OF FIRE)

This breathing exercise increases the vital capacity of the lungs, relieves allergies and asthma, and helps make the lungs strong and healthy. It also heats the body.

Inhale passively (through the nose), but exhale actively and with *a little* force. Start slowly and increase the speed. Imagine a steam locomotive moving slowly and picking up speed. Do one round of 30 strokes or exhalations, then rest for one minute. You can do up to five such rounds of *bhastrika* in the morning and five in the evening.

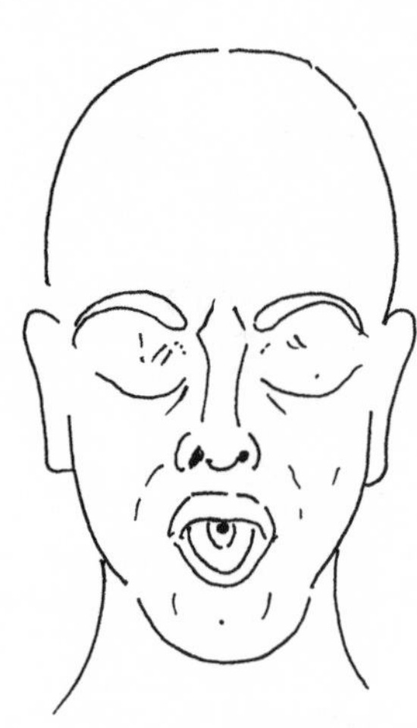

SHITALI PRANAYAMA
(COOLING BREATH)

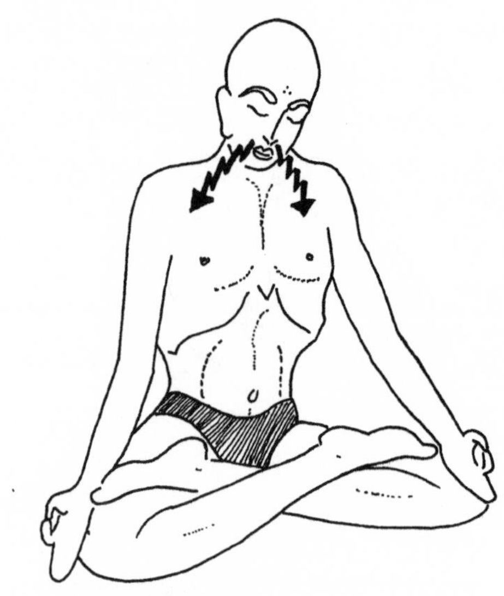

BHASTRIKA PRANAYAMA
(BREATH OF FIRE)

BHRAMARI PRANAYAMA (HUMMING BREATH)

On inhalation, constrict the epiglottis so as to create a humming sound. On exhalation, the sound is long and low. The inhalation, which is more high-pitched, is traditionally said to be like a female bee; the exhalation, which has a deeper sound, like a male bee.

If you find it difficult to make the humming sound on the inhalation, just inhale naturally, take a deep breath into the belly, and then do the humming on the exhalation.

When doing *bhramari,* touch the tip of your tongue lightly to the edge of the soft palate near the back of the roof of your mouth. Be sure the teeth are not clenched.

Bhramari improves the melodiousness of the voice. The humming vibrates the nervous system and is a form of sound therapy for the brain. It is also good for the thyroid, thymus, and parathyroid glands. Do ten cycles.

UJJAYI PRANAYAMA (BREATH OF VICTORY)

Sit in either Vajrasana or the Lotus posture, with your hands resting on your knees, palms up. Keep your head, neck, and chest in a straight line. Lower your head into a slight chin lock by moving your head in and down, toward your chest. Bring your awareness to the throat area.

Now comes the slightly tricky part. Without actually swallowing, start the action of swallowing, to raise the trachea upward. At the same time, while constricting your epiglottis, as in silently "saying" the letter *e,* slowly and deeply inhale into the belly. The inhaled air will create a soft, gentle whispering sound of rushing air as it brushes the throat, trachea, heart, and diaphragm.

After inhaling, swallow and hold your breath at the belly for a moment, then slowly exhale the air by again constricting the epiglottis—as if humming, but without producing any humming sound.

Ujjayi pranayama brings great joy. It calms the mind, relaxes the intercostal muscles, and really brings a sense of victory. *Ujjayi* is good for all three doshas and helps to reestablish constitutional balance. It promotes longevity. Do twelve cycles (repetitions) at a time.

SURYA BHEDI PRANAYAMA (RIGHT NOSTRIL BREATHING)

Put a cotton "plug" in your left nostril so that you will breathe through the right nostril, or block the left nostril by gently pressing with the ring and little finger of the right hand. Sit comfortably. Breathe in and out through the right nostril only. Repeat ten times.

Chapter 7

Meditation and Mental Discipline

Meditation is an art of bringing harmony to body, mind, and consciousness. Life with meditation is a flowering of bliss and beauty. Life without meditation is stress, confusion, and illusion.

During ancient times meditation was often considered a way of life. Truly, meditation is not separate from daily living, but as a discipline, we have to practice certain techniques, methods, and systems. Once we have practiced a form of meditation and mastered it, that discipline stays with us in every aspect of our lives. So whatever technique you do, whatever system you follow, according to the instruction given by your teacher, please do that.

But what is meditation, and what is not?

Meditation is not concentration. In concentration we narrow the mind, and a narrow mind is a limited mind. We need that limited, pointed, concentrated mind to probe into any subject, to solve problems, to learn a language, to fly an airplane. We need it. But not in meditation.

In concentration we build a wall of resistance, and in the effort to control the mind, we lose energy. Some people meditate that way for an hour, and when they're finished, they feel tired, because for that hour they were fighting and fighting, negating everything, saying no to all thoughts and perceptions, trying to focus the mind.

Concentration is all-exclusive, but meditation is all-inclusive. Meditation is open, choiceless awareness. Everything is welcome. Meditation says yes to everything, while concentration says no to everything.

Concentration is effort. Wherever there is effort, there is a maker of the effort. The maker of the effort is the ego. Concentration nourishes the ego, the maker of the effort. The more the concentration, the more ego.

In meditation, there is no effort and no

effort-maker. Therefore there is freedom. You are just sitting quietly and listening to everything, whether it is the call of a bird, the cry of a child, the rustle of the leaves. Every sound is welcome. Whatever the sound, allow it to come to you. When you listen to the sound, you become the center and the sound is peripheral, rushing toward you, to meet with you.

In listening to any kind of sound without judgment, without criticism, without liking or disliking, you become the center and all sounds rush toward you, to dissolve into you. Follow the sound. Allow it to pass through you. Don't resist. Then a magical phenomenon happens. You become empty. You become silent, pure existence.

When a breeze comes to you, allow that breeze to pass through you. No effort, no resistance. Remember, peace is not the opposite of sound. Every sound dissolves into peace. You are that peace, and sound comes to meet with you and dissolve into you.

Look at any object, a tree, a flower, even the wall. There is no choice in the looking, no judgment, just choiceless observation.

Awareness is the act of listening, the act of looking. No effort is required, no concentration. In awareness, in meditation, concentration happens naturally. It is given to you as a gift. But in concentration, in choosing, you miss meditation.

In expanded, empty consciousness, thinking stops, breathing becomes quiet, and one simply exists as pure awareness. In that state there is great joy, beauty, and love. Individual consciousness merges with Cosmic Consciousness, and one goes beyond time and thought.

In that state, whether the eyes are open or closed does not matter. It comes like a breeze without invitation, because this state is your true nature—love, bliss, beauty, and awareness. There is no fear, no depression, no anxiety, no worry, no stress. One becomes the witness of anxieties, worries, and stress. In that state, healing occurs.

This is what is called discipline. Discipline means learning, and one who is learning is called a disciple. So we have to learn the art of discipline. Discipline means putting everything in its right place. Thought has a right place, desire has a right place, job has a right place, duty has a right place. Discipline brings harmony in our life. Therefore discipline and meditation go together. There is no meditation without discipline, and no discipline without meditation. They are one. Mind in meditation is mind in discipline.

The so-called concentrated mind is a controlling mind. A confused mind controls. But a mind that is free, alert, and aware is blissful. That mind is a disciplined mind. And discipline is the perfume of life. Without that perfume, life never becomes celebration.

When you meditate, sit with your back straight. If you can, sit in the Lotus pose (or Half Lotus if that is more comfortable for you). If that is not comfortable, you can sit on a chair but keep your vertebral column erect.

With persistent practice, you can increase the time you spend in the Lotus to one, two, or even three hours. If one sits properly in a Lotus pose for three hours a day, enlightenment will soon come.

Sitting in the Lotus pose helps to open the heart. Breathing becomes quiet, and thinking automatically slows and stops. To go beyond thought is to go beyond suffering, because it is thought that creates suffering.

Empty Bowl Meditation

Sit comfortably and quietly with your palms up and open and placed on your knees, like empty bowls. Open your mouth slightly, and touch the tongue to the roof of the mouth, behind the front teeth.

Begin by paying attention to your breath. Let your lungs breathe with no effort on your part. Simply watch the movement of your breath. Inhale. Exhale.

During inhalation, air touches the inside of the nostrils. Be aware of that breath. During exhalation, again air touches the nostrils. The ingoing air feels cool, the outgoing air is warm. For a fraction of a second, enter into your nose! Sit in the nostril and watch your breath: ingoing, outgoing, ingoing, outgoing. Let your lungs do their job. You are simply sitting and watching.

After five minutes, follow the breath. When the lungs inhale, go with the air into the nose, to the back of the throat, the trachea, lungs, heart, diaphragm. Go deep down behind the belly button, where you will experience a natural stop. For a fraction of a second, the breath stops. Stay in that stop, then when the lungs exhale, again follow the breath as it reverses its course. Come up from the belly button to the diaphragm, heart, lungs, trachea, and throat, back to the nose, then out of the body.

During exhalation the air goes out of the body to about nine inches in front of the nose, where there is a second stop. Again, stay in that stop for a moment.

These two stops are very important. The first stop is behind the belly button, the second outside the body in space. As your awareness rests in these two stops, time stops, because time is the movement of breath. When breath stops, mind stops, because mind is the movement of breath. When the mind becomes quiet, you simply exist, without body, without mind, without breath.

In that stop, you become like an empty bowl, and when you become an empty bowl, divine lips will touch you. God will come to you, to pour out his love. You do not need to seek God, for God is seeking you. From ages past, God is seeking an empty bowl, to fill with his love. But all bowls are full of desire, ambition, business, competition, success and failure.

Just sit quietly and stay in the stop. That stop is a door. Simply enter the door and jump into the inner abyss. You will feel an extraordinary tranquillity and peace surrounding you.

Practice this meditation for 15 minutes in the morning and in the evening. Over the days, weeks, and months, you will find your time in the stops naturally increasing until, eventually, inner and outer will merge and everything will happen within you.

NOTE: If you are more comfortable, you may practice this meditation in a prone position.

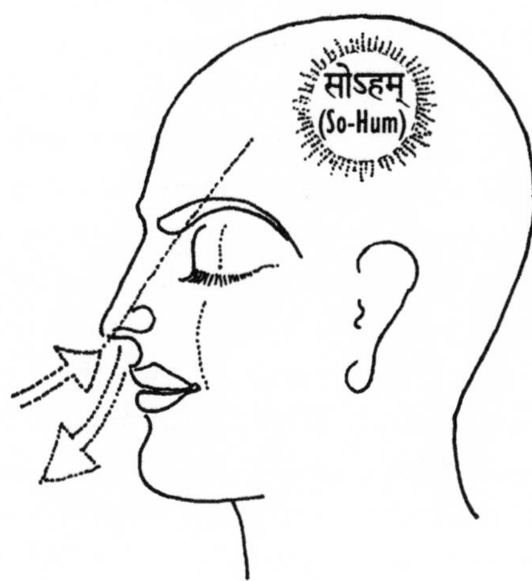

So-Hum Meditation

In *So-Hum* meditation we sit quietly and watch our breath, as in the Empty Bowl meditation, but we add the sound *So* on inhalation, *Hum* on exhalation. (Only silently; we don't speak the sounds aloud.)

When sound, breath, and awareness come together, it becomes light. We have seen that every atom radiates light and heat energy, which is a quantum wave. The moment we pay attention to our breath and start feeling *So-Hum, So-Hum* along with the breath, our breath becomes a quantum wave and radiates light. You may see that light of life at the third eye.

Inspiration (breathing in) is living; expiration (breathing out) is dying. When a child is born, with its first breath life expresses itself with inspiration. When someone dies, we say he has expired. The breath has gone out.

Hum means "I" or "individual ego"; *So* means "He, the Divine." So in the natural course of *So-Hum* meditation, when *So* goes in, life energy goes in and *Hum*, ego, our limited individuality, goes out. That is the significance of *So-Hum* meditation. When you inhale *So*, you are inhaling life. When you exhale *Hum*, you are exhaling ego and limitation.

So-Hum meditation properly practiced leads to the union of the individual with the universal Cosmic Consciousness. You will go beyond thought, beyond time and space, beyond cause and effect. Limitations will vanish. Your consciousness will empty itself, and in that emptying it will expand and peace and joy will descend as a benediction.

Double-Arrowed Attention (Witnessing)

In Vedic science, witnessing is called *samyag darshan*. This is a process of looking outward and inward simultaneously.

When we look at a tree, a star, a mountain, or a flower, something goes out from our eyes, touches the object, and comes back to us. That which goes out of our eyes in order to touch the object of perception, we call attention. Ayurveda says that attention happens when *prana* goes out and carries the vibration of awareness toward the object. Thus, attention is awareness plus *prana*, movement.

One arrow goes out and touches the object. At the same time, a second arrow of attention should go inside, toward the center of our heart, to observe the observer. At the time of looking, when you look at the object outside, at the same time, look at the looker; watch the watcher; observe the observer. What happens when the watcher is watched is that the watcher disappears. This simple watching, without a watcher, is called witnessing. In that witnessing, you develop intimacy, relationship, with the object of perception.

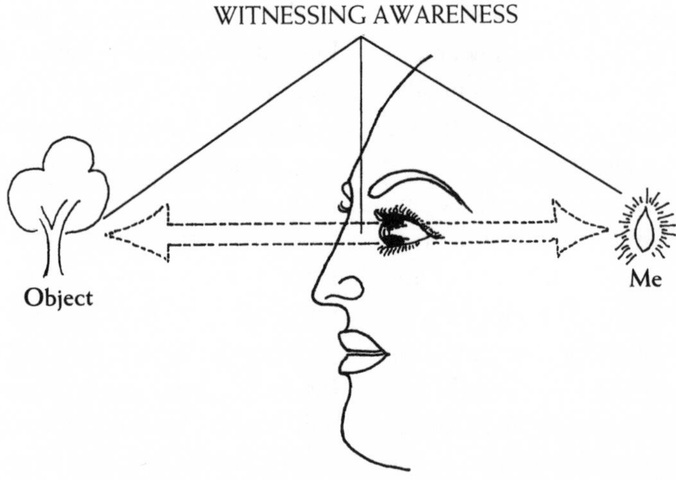

Chapter 8

Ayurvedic Dietary Guidelines

The purpose of this chapter is to help you choose a suitable diet for balance, harmony, and health in your life, based on Ayurvedic principles. Health-conscious people today are interested in the role good nourishment can play in their healing and in their health. Many have come to realize that proper food and diet can make a vital contribution to good health, while inappropriate eating is often responsible for poor health, lack of vitality, and susceptibility to disease.

The Ayurvedic tradition offers much insight into what food will suit and balance each individual, how to prepare and cook this food properly, how to avoid food combinations that will create toxins in the body, and what eating habits to cultivate—and which to avoid—in order to receive the most nourishment from what you eat. All these topics, except specific guidelines on how to prepare and cook the food, will be discussed in this chapter. (Interested readers may consult *Ayurvedic Cooking for Self-Healing* by Usha Lad and Dr. Vasant Lad, a complete reference guide to Ayurvedic cooking, including spices and herbs, healing qualities of common foods, menu planning, and dozens of delicious recipes.)

Food Guidelines for the Constitutional Types

What you eat should be suited to your individual constitution. Ideally, in deciding what to eat, you would know your constitution and understand its relationship to the qualities of various kinds of food, including whether each food would be helpful or aggravating to your unique doshic balance. You would have to take into account the taste of the food (we will discuss that issue later in this chapter), and whether its qualities are heavy or light, oily or dry, liquid or solid. You would also have to know whether the food is cooling or heating (*virya*), and its postdigestive effect (*vipaka*).

If you are interested, you can go more deeply into Ayurvedic theory in order to fully comprehend these factors (see the Reading List). Otherwise, the following charts take these factors into consideration in recommending what foods to eat or avoid.

The charts categorize foods according to their suitability for each doshic type. Here are a few points to remember:

• Foods marked "no" tend to aggravate that particular dosha, while foods marked "yes" pacify or balance that dosha. In planning your diet, choose foods that create balance, and avoid those that might provoke your predominant doshas or the dosha that is currently aggravated or increased.

• The recommendations are not meant to be absolute, but are guidelines. If a food is on your "no" list, that means you should avoid it most of the time, and if you eat it, eat a modest amount or do something to modify its effects. Apples, for example, are quite vata-provoking if eaten raw. But if you cook them and eat them warm, with a little ghee and warming spices such as cardamom or cinnamon, they are fine for vata individuals in modest amounts.

• Keep the seasons in mind. Summer, for example, is pitta season, and it is not good—especially for people with a predominantly pitta constitution—to eat too many hot, spicy foods, or pitta dosha will become aggravated. Similarly, during autumn, when the air is dry and cool and more vata is present in the atmosphere, everyone—but especially individuals with a vata constitution—should avoid dry fruit, salads, cold foods, and other vata-provoking items. In winter and early spring, the heavy, cold, moist season of kapha, one should make an extra effort to avoid cold food and drinks, ice cream, cheese, yogurt, melons, and other kapha-increasing foods.

• For individuals with a dual constitution (two doshas approximately equal), a little extra care is needed, but you can figure it out. For example, a vata–pitta individual needs to avoid vata-increasing foods in the fall and winter (but without increasing pitta too much) and minimize pitta-provoking foods in the summer (but without aggravating vata). Stated in positive terms, favor vata-balancing foods in the fall, pitta-pacifying foods in the summer.

Here are some general dietary guidelines for balancing the doshas:

Vata

- 50 percent whole grains—whole-grain cooked cereals, some breads and crackers
- 20 percent protein—eggs, high-quality dairy products, poultry, fish, seafood, beef, tofu, black and red lentils
- 20–30 percent fresh vegetables—with an optional 10 percent for fresh fruit

Pitta

- 50 percent whole grains—whole-wheat breads, cereals, cooked grains
- 20 percent protein—beans (except lentils), tofu, tempeh, cottage cheese,

FOOD GUIDELINES FOR THE BASIC CONSTITUTIONAL TYPES

Note: Guidelines provided in this table are general. Specific adjustments for individual requirements may need to be made, e.g., food allergies, strength of agni, season of the year, and degree of dosha predominance or aggravation. *okay in moderation; **okay rarely.

	Vata		Pitta		Kapha	
	NO	YES	NO	YES	NO	YES
FRUITS	*Generally most dried fruit*	*Generally most sweet fruit*	*Generally most sour fruit*	*Generally most sweet fruit*	*Generally most sweet & sour fruit*	*Generally most astringent fruit*
	Apples (raw)	Apples (cooked)	Apples (sour)	Apples (sweet)	Avocado	Apples
	Cranberries	Applesauce	Apricots (sour)	Applesauce	Bananas	Applesauce
	Dates (dry)	Apricots	Bananas	Apricots (sweet)	Coconut	Apricots
	Figs (dry)	Avocado	Berries (sour)	Avocado	Dates	Berries
	Pears	Bananas	Cherries (sour)	Berries (sweet)	Figs (fresh)	Cherries
	Persimmons	Berries	Cranberries	Cherries (sweet)	Grapefruit	Cranberries
	Pomegranates	Cherries	Grapefruit	Coconut	Kiwi	Figs (dry)*
	Prunes (dry)	Coconut	Grapes (green)	Dates	Mangoes**	Grapes*
	Raisins (dry)	Dates (fresh)	Kiwi**	Figs	Melons	Lemons*
	Watermelon	Figs (fresh)	Lemons	Grapes (red & purple)	Oranges	Limes*
		Grapefruit	Mangoes (green)	Limes*	Papaya	Peaches
		Grapes	Oranges (sour)	Mangoes (ripe)	Pineapple	Pears
		Kiwi	Peaches	Melons	Plums	Persimmons
		Lemons	Persimmons	Oranges (sweet)	Rhubarb	Pomegranates
		Limes	Pineapple (sour)	Papaya*	Tamarind	Prunes
		Mangoes	Plums (sour)	Pears	Watermelon	Raisins
		Melons	Rhubarb	Pineapple (sweet)		Strawberries*
		Oranges	Strawberries	Plums (sweet)		
		Papaya	Tamarind	Pomegranates		
		Peaches		Prunes		
		Pineapple				
		Plums				

Continued on next page

FOOD GUIDELINES FOR THE BASIC CONSTITUTIONAL TYPES *(Continued)*

	Vata		Pitta		Kapha	
	NO	YES	NO	YES	NO	YES
FRUITS *(Continued)*		Prunes (soaked)		Raisins		
		Raisins (soaked)		Watermelon		
		Rhubarb				
		Strawberries				
		Tamarind				
VEGETABLES	*Generally frozen, raw, or dried vegetables*	*In general, vegetables should be cooked*	*In general, pungent vegetables*	*In general, sweet & bitter vegetables*	*In general, sweet & juicy vegetables*	*In general, most pungent & bitter vegetables*
	Artichoke	Asparagus	Beet greens	Artichoke	Cucumber	Artichoke
	Beet greens**	Beets	Beets (raw)	Asparagus	Olives, black or green	Asparagus
	Bitter melon	Cabbage* (cooked)	Burdock root	Beets (cooked)	Parsnips**	Beet greens
	Broccoli	Carrots	Corn (fresh)**	Bitter melon	Potatoes, sweet	Beets
	Brussels sprouts	Cauliflower*	Daikon radish	Broccoli	Pumpkin	Bitter melon
	Burdock root	Cilantro	Eggplant**	Brussels sprouts	Squash, winter	Broccoli
	Cabbage (raw)	Cucumber	Garlic	Cabbage	Taro root	Brussels sprouts
	Cauliflower (raw)	Daikon radish*	Green chilies	Carrots (cooked)	Tomatoes (raw)	Burdock root
	Celery	Fennel (anise)	Horseradish	Carrots (raw)*	Zucchini	Cabbage
	Corn (fresh)**	Garlic	Kohlrabi**	Cauliflower		Carrots
	Dandelion greens	Green beans	Leeks (raw)	Celery		Cauliflower
	Eggplant	Green chilies	Mustard greens	Cilantro		Celery
	Horseradish**	Jerusalem artichoke*	Olives, green	Cucumber		Cilantro
	Kale	Leafy greens*	Onions (raw)	Dandelion greens		Corn
	Kohlrabi	Leeks	Peppers (hot)	Fennel (anise)		Daikon radish
	Mushrooms	Lettuce*	Prickly pear (fruit)	Green beans		Dandelion greens
			Radishes (raw)	Jerusalem artichoke		Eggplant

Olives, green
Onions (raw)
Peas (raw)
Peppers, sweet & hot
Potatoes, white
Prickly pear (fruit & leaves)
Radish (raw)
Tomatoes (cooked)**
Tomatoes (raw)
Turnips
Wheatgrass sprouts

Mustard greens*
Okra
Olives, black
Onions (cooked)*
Parsley*
Parsnip
Peas (cooked)
Potatoes, sweet
Pumpkin
Radishes (cooked)*
Rutabaga
Spaghetti squash*
Spinach (cooked)*
Spinach (raw)*
Sprouts*
Squash, summer & winter
Taro root
Turnip greens*
Watercress
Zucchini

Spinach (cooked)**
Spinach (raw)
Tomatoes
Turnip greens
Turnips

Kale
Leafy greens
Leeks (cooked)
Lettuce
Mushrooms
Okra
Olives, black
Onions (cooked)
Parsley
Parsnips
Peas
Peppers, sweet
Potatoes, sweet & white
Prickly pear (leaves)
Pumpkin
Radishes (cooked)
Rutabaga
Spaghetti squash
Sprouts (not spicy)
Squash, winter & summer
Taro root
Watercress*
Wheatgrass sprouts
Zucchini

Fennel (anise)
Garlic
Green beans
Green chilies
Horseradish
Jerusalem artichoke
Kale
Kohlrabi
Leafy greens
Leeks
Lettuce
Mushrooms
Mustard greens
Okra
Onions
Parsley
Peas
Peppers, sweet & hot
Potatoes, white
Prickly pear (fruit & leaves)
Radishes
Rutabaga
Spaghetti squash*
Spinach
Sprouts
Squash (summer)
Tomatoes (cooked)

Continued on next page

FOOD GUIDELINES FOR THE BASIC CONSTITUTIONAL TYPES *(Continued)*

	Vata		Pitta		Kapha	
	NO	YES	NO	YES	NO	YES
VEGETABLES *(Continued)*						Turnip greens Turnips Watercress Wheatgrass sprouts
GRAINS *Always use suitable grains when "generic" things are listed*	Barley Bread (with yeast) Buckwheat Cereals (cold, dry, or puffed) Corn Couscous Crackers Granola Millet Muesli Oat bran Oats (dry) Pasta** Polenta** Rice cakes** Rye Sago	Amaranth* Durham flour Oats (cooked) Pancakes Quinoa Rice (all kinds) Seitan (wheat meat) Sprouted wheat bread (Essene) Wheat	Bread (with yeast) Buckwheat Corn Millet Muesli** Oats (dry) Polenta** Quinoa Rice (brown)** Rye	Amaranth Barley Cereal, dry Couscous Crackers Durham flour Granola Oat bran Oats (cooked) Pancakes Pasta Rice (basmati, white, wild) Rice cakes Sago Seitan (wheat meat) Spelt Sprouted wheat bread (Essene)	Bread (with yeast) Oats (cooked) Pancakes Pasta** Rice (brown, white) Rice cakes** Wheat	Amaranth* Barley Buckwheat Cereal (cold, dry, or puffed) Corn Couscous Crackers Durham flour* Granola Millet Muesli Oat bran Oats (dry) Polenta Quinoa* Rice (basmati, wild)* Rye Sago

	Spelt Tapioca Wheat bran			Tapioca Wheat Wheat bran		Seitan (wheat meat) Sprouted wheat bread (Essene) Tapioca Wheat bran
LEGUMES	Adzuki beans Black beans Black-eyed peas Chickpeas (garbanzo beans) Kidney beans Lentils (brown) Lima beans Miso** Navy beans Peas (dried) Pinto beans Soybeans Soy flour Soy powder Split peas Tempeh White beans	Lentils (red)* Mung beans Mung dal Soy cheese* Soy milk* Soy sauce* Soy sausages* Tofu* Tur dal Urad dal	Miso Soy sauce Soy sausages Tur dal Urad dal	Adzuki beans Black beans Black-eyed peas Chickpeas (garbanzo beans) Kidney beans Lentils, brown & red Lima beans Mung beans Mung dal Navy beans Peas (dried) Pinto beans Soybeans Soy cheese Soy flour* Soy milk Soy powder* Split peas Tempeh Tofu White beans	Kidney beans Soybeans Soy cheese Soy flour Soy powder Soy sauce Tofu (cold) Urad dal Miso	Adzuki beans Black beans Black-eyed peas Chickpeas (garbanzo beans) Lentils (red & brown) Lima beans Mung beans* Mung dal* Navy beans Peas (dried) Pinto beans Soy milk Soy sausages Split peas Tempeh Tofu (hot)* Tur dal White beans

Continued on next page

FOOD GUIDELINES FOR THE BASIC CONSTITUTIONAL TYPES *(Continued)*

	Vata		Pitta		Kapha	
	NO	YES	NO	YES	NO	YES
DAIRY	Cow's milk (powdered) Goat's milk (powdered) Yogurt (plain, frozen, or w/fruit)	*Most dairy is good!* Butter Buttermilk Cheese (hard)* Cheese (soft) Cottage cheese Cow's milk Ghee Goat's cheese Goat's milk Ice cream* Sour cream* Yogurt (diluted & spiced)*	Butter (salted) Buttermilk Cheese (hard) Sour cream Yogurt (plain, or frozen, w/fruit)	Butter (unsalted) Cheese (soft, not aged, unsalted) Cottage cheese Cow's milk Ghee Goat's milk Goat's cheese (soft, unsalted) Ice cream Yogurt (freshly made & diluted)*	Butter (salted) Butter (unsalted)** Cheese (soft & hard) Cow's milk Ice cream Sour cream Yogurt (plain, frozen, or w/fruit)	Buttermilk* Cottage cheese (from skimmed goat's milk) Ghee* Goat's cheese (unsalted & not aged)* Goat's milk, skim Yogurt (diluted)
ANIMAL FOODS	Lamb Pork Rabbit Venison Turkey (white)	Beef Buffalo Chicken (dark) Chicken (white)* Duck Eggs Fish (freshwater or sea) Salmon Sardines Seafood Shrimp	Beef Chicken (dark) Duck Eggs (yolk) Fish (sea) Lamb Pork Salmon Sardines Seafood Tuna fish Turkey (dark)	Buffalo Chicken (white) Eggs (albumen or white only) Fish (freshwater) Rabbit Shrimp* Turkey (white) Venison	Beef Buffalo Chicken (dark) Duck Fish (sea) Lamb Pork Salmon Sardines Seafood Tuna fish Turkey (dark)	Chicken (white) Eggs Fish (freshwater) Rabbit Shrimp Turkey (white) Venison

		Tuna fish Turkey (dark)				
CONDIMENTS	Chocolate Horseradish	Black pepper* Chutney, mango (sweet or spicy) Chili peppers* Coriander leaves* Dulse Gomasio Hijiki Kelp Ketchup Kombu Lemon Lime Lime pickle Mango pickle Mayonnaise Mustard Pickles Salt Scallions Seaweed Soy sauce Sprouts* Tamari Vinegar	Chili pepper Chocolate Chutney, mango (spicy) Gomasio Horseradish Kelp Ketchup Mustard Lemon Lime pickle Mango pickle Mayonnaise Pickles Salt (in excess) Scallions Seaweed Soy sauce Vinegar	Black pepper* Chutney, mango (sweet) Coriander leaves Dulse* Hijiki* Kombu* Lime* Sprouts Tamari*	Chocolate Chutney, mango (sweet) Gomasio Kelp Ketchup** Lime Lime pickle Mango pickle Mayonnaise Pickles Salt Soy sauce Tamari Vinegar	Black pepper Chili peppers Chutney, mango (spicy) Coriander leaves Dulse* Hijiki* Horseradish Lemon* Mustard (without vinegar) Scallions Seaweed* Sprouts
NUTS	None	*In moderation:* Almonds Black walnuts	Almonds (with skin) Black walnuts	Almonds (soaked and peeled) Charole	Almonds (soaked & peeled)**	Charole

Continued on next page

FOOD GUIDELINES FOR THE BASIC CONSTITUTIONAL TYPES *(Continued)*

	Vata		Pitta		Kapha	
	NO	YES	NO	YES	NO	YES
NUTS *(Continued)*		Brazil nuts Cashews Charole Coconut Filberts Hazelnuts Macadamia nuts Peanuts Pecans Pine nuts Pistachios Walnuts	Brazil nuts Cashews Filberts Hazelnuts Macadamia nuts Peanuts Pecans Pine nuts Pistachios Walnuts	Coconut	Black walnuts Brazil nuts Cashews Coconut Filberts Hazelnuts Macadamia nuts Peanuts Pecans Pine nuts Pistachios Walnuts	
SEEDS	Popcorn Psyllium**	Chia Flax Halva Pumpkin Sesame Sunflower Tahini	Chia Sesame Tahini	Flax Halva Popcorn (no salt, buttered) Psyllium Pumpkin* Sunflower	Halva Psyllium** Sesame Tahini	Chia Flax* Popcorn (no salt, no butter) Pumpkin* Sunflower*
OILS	Flaxseed	*For internal & external use (most suitable at top of list):* Sesame	Almond Apricot Corn Safflower Sesame	*For internal & external use (most suitable at top of list):* Sunflower	Avocado Apricot Coconut Flaxseed** Olive	*For internal & external use in small amounts (most suitable at top of list):*

		Ghee Olive Most other oils *External use only:* Coconut Avocado		Ghee Canola Olive Soy Flaxseed Primrose Walnut *External use only:* Avocado Coconut	Primrose Safflower Sesame (internal) Soy Walnut	Corn Canola Sesame (external) Sunflower Ghee Almond
BEVERAGES	Apple juice Black tea Caffeinated beverages Carbonated drinks Chocolate milk Coffee Cold dairy drinks Cranberry juice Iced tea Icy cold drinks Mixed veg. juice Pear juice Pomegranate juice Prune juice**	Alcohol (beer or wine)* Almond milk Aloe vera juice Apple cider Apricot juice Berry juice (except for cranberry) Carob* Carrot juice Chai (hot, spiced milk) Cherry juice Grain "coffee" Grape juice Grapefruit juice Lemonade Mango juice Miso broth Orange juice Papaya juice	Alcohol (hard or wine) Apple cider Berry juice (sour) Caffeinated beverages Carbonated drinks Carrot juice Cherry juice (sour) Chocolate milk Coffee Cranberry juice Grapefruit juice Iced tea Icy cold drinks Lemonade Papaya juice Pineapple juice	Alcohol, beer* Almond milk Aloe vera juice Apple juice Apricot juice Berry juice (sweet) Black tea Carob Chai (hot, spiced milk)* Cherry juice (sweet) Cool dairy drinks Grain "coffee" Grape juice Mango juice Miso broth* Mixed veg. juice Orange juice* Peach nectar Pear juice	Alcohol (beer, hard, sweet wine) Almond milk Caffeinated beverages** Carbonated drinks Cherry juice (sour) Chocolate milk Coffee Cold dairy drinks Grapefruit juice Iced tea Icy cold drinks Lemonade Miso broth Orange juice	Alcohol (dry wine, red or white) Aloe vera juice Apple cider Apple juice* Apricot juice Berry juice Black tea (spiced) Carob Carrot juice Chai (hot, spiced milk)* Cherry juice (sweet) Cranberry juice Grain "coffee" Grape juice Mango juice Peach nectar

Continued on next page

FOOD GUIDELINES FOR THE BASIC CONSTITUTIONAL TYPES *(Continued)*

	Vata NO	Vata YES	Pitta NO	Pitta YES	Kapha NO	Kapha YES
BEVERAGES *(Continued)*	Soy milk (cold)	Peach nectar	Sour juices	Pomegranate juice	Papaya juice	Pear juice
	Tomato juice**	Pineapple juice	Tomato juice	Prune juice	Rice milk	Pineapple juice*
	V-8 juice	Rice milk	V-8 juice	Rice milk	Sour juices	Pomegranate juice
	Vegetable bouillon	Sour juices		Soy milk	Soy milk (cold)	Prune juice
		Soy milk (hot & well-spiced)*		Vegetable bouillon	Tomato juice	Soy milk (hot & well-spiced)
					V-8 juice	
	Herb Teas:	*Herb Teas:*	*Herb Teas:*	*Herb Teas:*	*Herb Teas:*	*Herb Teas:*
	Alfalfa**	Ajwan	Ajwan	Alfalfa	Marshmallow	Alfalfa
	Barley**	Bancha	Basil**	Bancha	Red Zinger	Bancha
	Basil**	Catnip*	Cinnamon*	Barley	Rosehip**	Barley
	Blackberry	Chamomile	Clove	Blackberry		Blackberry
	Borage**	Chicory	Eucalyptus	Borage		Burdock
	Burdock	Chrysanthemum*	Fenugreek	Burdock		Chamomile
	Cinnamon**	Clove	Ginger (dry)	Catnip		Chicory
	Cornsilk	Comfrey	Ginseng	Chamomile		Cinnamon
	Dandelion	Elder Flower	Hawthorn	Chicory		Clove
	Ginseng	Eucalyptus	Hyssop	Comfrey		Comfrey*
	Hibiscus	Fennel	Juniper berry	Dandelion		Dandelion
	Hops**	Fenugreek	Mormon tea	Fennel		Fenugreek
	Jasmine**	Ginger (fresh)	Pennyroyal	Ginger (fresh)		Ginger
	Lemon balm**	Hawthorn	Red Zinger	Hibiscus		Ginseng*
	Mormon tea	Juniper berry	Rosehip**	Hops		Hibiscus
	Nettle**	Kukicha*	Sage	Jasmine		Hyssop
	Passion flower**	Lavender	Sassafras	Kukicha		Jasmine
	Red clover**	Lemongrass	Yerba maté	Lavender		Juniper berry
		Licorice		Lemon balm		Kukicha

	Red Zinger** Violet** Yarrow Yerba maté**	Marshmallow Oat straw Orange peel Pennyroyal Peppermint Raspberry* Rosehips Saffron Sage Sarsaparilla Sassafras Spearmint Strawberry* Wintergreen*		Lemongrass Licorice Marshmallow Nettle Oat Straw Passion flower Peppermint Raspberry Red clover Sarsaparilla Spearmint Strawberry Violet Wintergreen Yarrow		Lavender Licorice* Lemon balm Lemongrass Mormon tea Nettle Passion flower Peppermint Raspberry Red clover Sarsaparilla* Sassafras Spearmint Strawberry Wintergreen Yarrow Yerba maté
SPICES	Caraway	*All other spices are good!* Ajwan Allspice Almond extract Anise Asafoetida (hing) Basil Bay leaf Black pepper Cardamom Cayenne* Cinnamon Cloves	Ajwan Allspice Almond extract Anise Asafoetida (hing) Basil (dry) Bay leaf Cayenne Cloves Fenugreek Garlic Ginger (dry) Mace	Basil (fresh) Black pepper* Caraway* Cardamom* Cinnamon Coriander Cumin Curry leaves Dill Fennel Ginger (fresh) Mint Neem leaves* Orange peel*	Salt	*All spices are good!* Ajwan Allspice Almond extract Anise Asafoetida (hing) Basil Bay leaf Black pepper Caraway Cardamom Cayenne

Continued on next page

FOOD GUIDELINES FOR THE BASIC CONSTITUTIONAL TYPES *(Continued)*

	Vata		Pitta		Kapha	
	NO	YES	NO	YES	NO	YES
SPICES *(Continued)*		Coriander	Marjoram	Parsley*		Cloves
		Cumin	Mustard seeds	Peppermint		Cinnamon
		Curry leaves	Nutmeg	Saffron		Coriander
		Dill	Oregano	Spearmint		Cumin
		Fennel	Paprika	Tarragon*		Curry leaves
		Fenugreek*	Pippali	Turmeric		Dill
		Garlic	Poppy seeds	Vanilla*		Fennel*
		Ginger	Rosemary	Wintergreen		Fenugreek
		Mace	Sage			Garlic
		Marjoram	Salt			Ginger
		Mint	Savory			Mace
		Mustard seeds	Star anise			Marjoram
		Nutmeg	Thyme			Mint
		Orange peel				Mustard seeds
		Oregano				Neem leaves
		Paprika				Nutmeg
		Parsley				Orange peel
		Peppermint				Oregano
		Pippali				Paprika
		Poppy seeds				Parsley
		Rosemary				Peppermint
		Saffron				Pippali
		Salt				Poppy seeds
		Savory				Rosemary
		Spearmint				Saffron
		Star anise				Sage
		Tarragon				Savory
		Thyme				Spearmint

		Turmeric Vanilla Wintergreen				Star anise Tarragon Thyme Turmeric Vanilla* Wintergreen
SWEETENERS	Maple syrup** White sugar	Barley malt Fructose Fruit juice concentrates Honey (raw & not processed) Jaggary Molasses Rice syrup Sucanat Turbinado	Honey** (raw & not processed) White sugar** jaggary Molasses	Barley malt Fructose Fruit juice concentrates Maple syrup Rice syrup Sucanat Turbinado	Barley malt Fructose Jaggary Maple syrup Molasses Rice syrup Sucanat Turbinado White sugar	Fruit juice concentrates Honey (raw & not processed)
FOOD SUPPLEMENTS	Barley green Brewer's yeast	Aloe vera juice* Bee pollen Amino acids *Minerals:* calcium, copper, iron, magnesium, zinc Royal jelly Spirulina Blue-green algae Vitamins A, B complex, B_{12}, C, D, & E	Amino acids Bee pollen** Royal jelly** *Minerals:* copper, iron Vitamins A, B complex, B_{12} & C	Aloe vera juice Barley green Brewer's yeast *Minerals:* calcium, magnesium, zinc Spirulina Blue-green algae Vitamins D & E	*Minerals:* potassium	Aloe vera juice Amino acids Barley green Bee pollen Brewer's yeast *Minerals:* copper, calcium, iron, magnesium, zinc Royal jelly Spirulina Blue-green algae Vitamins A, B complex, B_{12}, C, D, & E

ricotta cheese, raw milk, egg white, chicken and turkey (white meat only), shrimp, rabbit, venison
- 20–30 percent vegetables—with an optional 10 percent for fresh fruit

Kapha

- 30–40 percent whole grains—rye crackers, dry cereals, cooked grains
- 20 percent protein—chicken, turkey, boiled and poached eggs, small amount of goat's milk, and most beans (including garbanzos, adzukis, pintos, black beans, red lentils, navy and white beans, split peas, and black-eyed peas)
- 40–50 percent fresh vegetables—with an optional 10 percent for fresh or dried fruit. A daily salad is good.

The Six Tastes

Taste is important and has a direct effect on bodily doshas. According to Ayurveda, each food substance (and also each medicinal herb) has a specific taste. When the tastes are used in the proper amounts, individually and collectively, they bring about balance of our bodily systems.

The taste buds on our tongue are organized in six groups, corresponding to the six tastes recognized by Ayurveda: sweet, sour, salty, bitter, pungent, and astringent. These six basic tastes are derived from the five elements:

Earth + Water = Sweet
Earth + Fire = Sour
Water + Fire = Salty
Fire + Air = Pungent (Spicy)
Air + Space = Bitter
Air + Earth = Astringent

Different groups of taste buds on the tongue perceive taste and send a signal to the brain; from there, messages go out which not only directly influence digestion but also affect the doshas and all the body's cells, tissues, organs, and systems.

SWEET

The sweet taste is present in foods such as rice, sugar, milk, wheat, dates, and maple syrup. The qualities of sweet foods are usually oily, cooling, and heavy. The sweet taste increases the vital essence of life. When used moderately, it is wholesome to the body and promotes growth of all seven *dhatus* (plasma, blood, muscles, fat, bones, marrow and nerve tissue, and reproductive fluids). Proper use gives strength and longevity. It encourages the senses, improves complexion, and promotes healthy skin, hair, and a good voice. Sweet taste can relieve thirst and burning sensations and can be invigorating. It promotes stability.

Despite all these good qualities, excessive use of the sweet taste can produce many disorders. Sweet foods aggravate kapha and cause colds, cough, congestion, heaviness, loss of appetite, laziness, and obesity. They may also provoke lymphatic congestion, tumors, edema, diabetes, and fibrocystic changes in the breast.

SOUR

The sour taste is found in foods such as citrus fruits, sour cream, yogurt, vinegar, cheese, lemon, green grapes, and fermented food. Sour substances are liquid, light, heating, and oily in nature. When used in moderation, they are refreshing and delicious, stimulate appetite and salivation, improve digestion, energize the body, nourish the heart, and enlighten the mind.

If one uses the sour taste in excess, it can cause excessive thirst, hyperacidity, heartburn, acid indigestion, ulcers, and sensitive teeth. As it has a fermenting action, it may be toxic to the blood and can cause skin conditions such as dermatitis, acne, eczema, boils, and psoriasis. The hot quality may lead to an acid pH in the body and may cause burning in the throat, chest, heart, bladder, and urethra.

SALTY

Sea salt, rock salt, and kelp are examples of the salty taste. Salt is heating, heavy, and oily. Used moderately, it relieves vata and increases pitta and kapha. Due to its water element, it is laxative, and due to its fire element, it lessens spasm and pain of the colon. In moderation it promotes growth and maintains water electrolyte balance. It stimulates salivation, improves the flavor of food, and aids in digestion, absorption, and the elimination of wastes.

Too much salt in the diet may cause aggravation of pitta and kapha. It makes the blood thick and viscous, causes hypertension, and worsens skin conditions. Feeling hot, fainting, skin wrinkling, and baldness may be due to excessive use of the salty taste. Salt may also induce water retention and edema. Patchy hair loss, ulcers, bleeding disorders, skin eruptions, and hyperacidity may all result from overuse of the salty taste.

PUNGENT

The pungent taste is present in various hot peppers (cayenne, chili, black), as well as in onions, radishes, garlic, mustard, and ginger. It is light, drying, and heating in nature. Used in moderation, it improves digestion and absorption and cleans the mouth. It clears the sinuses by stimulating nasal secretions and tearing of the eyes. The pungent taste aids circulation, breaks up clots, helps in the elimination of waste products, and kills germs and parasites. It brings clarity of perception.

On the other hand, overuse of the pungent taste in the daily diet may cause negative reactions. It can kill sperm and ova, causing sexual debility in both sexes. It may induce burning, choking, fainting, and fatigue with feelings of heat and thirst. By aggravating pitta, it can cause diarrhea, heartburn, and nausea. Pungency can also aggravate vata (it is derived from both the fire and air elements), resulting in giddiness, tremors, insomnia, or pain in the leg muscles. Peptic ulcers, asthma, colitis, and skin conditions may result from excessive use.

BITTER

This taste is found in coffee, bitter melon, aloe vera, rhubarb, and the herbs yellow dock, fenugreek, turmeric root, dandelion root, and sandalwood. Bitter is the taste most lacking in the North American diet. It is cool, light, and dry in nature, increases vata, and decreases pitta and kapha. Though bitter is not delicious in itself, it promotes the flavor of other tastes. It is antitoxic and kills germs. It helps to relieve burning sensations, itching, fainting, and obstinate skin disorders. It reduces fever and stimulates firmness of the skin and muscles. In a small dose it can relieve intestinal gas and works as a digestive tonic. It is drying to the system and causes a reduction in fat, bone marrow, urine, and feces.

Overuse of the bitter taste may deplete plasma, blood, muscles, fat, bone marrow, and semen and may result in sexual debility. Extreme dryness and roughness, emaciation, and weariness may be the result of excessive eating of the bitter taste. It may at times induce dizziness and unconsciousness.

ASTRINGENT

The astringent taste is present in unripe bananas, pomegranates, chickpeas, green beans, yellow split peas, okra, alfalfa sprouts, and the herbs goldenseal, turmeric, lotus seed, arjuna, and alum. It is cooling, drying, and heavy in nature and produces a dry, choking sensation in the throat. Taken in moderation, the astringent taste calms pitta and kapha but excites vata. It helps in the healing of ulcers and stops bleeding by promoting clotting.

Excess use may cause dryness in the mouth, difficulty in speech, and constipation, as well as abdominal distention, heart spasms, and stagnation of circulation. It may affect the sex drive and lead to depletion of sperm. It can give rise to emaciation, convulsions, Bell's palsy, stroke paralysis, and other neuromuscular vata disorders.

EFFECTS OF TASTES ON THE DOSHAS

The tastes have the following effects upon the doshas:

VATA. People of vata constitution should avoid bitter, pungent, and astringent substances in excess, because they increase air

How the Tastes Affect the Doshas

TASTE	VATA	PITTA	KAPHA
Sweet	↓	↓	↑
Sour	↓	↑	↑
Salty	↓	↑	↑
Pungent	↑	↑	↓
Bitter	↑	↓	↓
Astringent	↑	↓	↓

Herbs and the Six Tastes

The taste of an herb is not incidental but is directly related—indeed, directly responsible—for much of its therapeutic value. That is why Ayurvedic herbs are generally taken in a form that requires tasting them, rather than concealing the taste in a capsule.

There is no problem in taking an herb that has a sweet, pungent, or otherwise tempting taste. But most people, particularly in Western culture, don't like the bitter or astringent tastes, and if they have to take an herb with either of these tastes, they want to put the herb into a capsule and swallow it without tasting it. Since the stomach has no taste buds, when the herb is taken this way, the effects and benefits derived from the taste are lessened, because they are not perceived. When we eat food, we don't lose the effect of the tastes because we have to chew; when we use capsules, we miss the taste of the herb.

One of the reasons the Ayurvedic physician prescribes an herb is to balance whatever taste is lacking in the body. The herb transmits that taste and its effects into *rasa dhatu* (plasma). *Triphala,* for example, provides all the tastes except salty, but it tends to yield the predominant taste that is lacking in the body, which for most Westerners is the bitter taste. That's why for many people *triphala* tastes bitter for some time. Later, after regular use, the bitter taste will have been received into the *rasa dhatu,* and *triphala* may taste sour or sweet.

In Ayurvedic medicine, most herbs are classified according to their predominant taste, secondary aftertaste, and "potential" taste. The main taste acts on *rasa dhatu,* the aftertaste acts on the nervous system, and the third taste has either a heating or a cooling effect.

This explains why it is important to have the effect of taste on the tongue when taking Ayurvedic medications.

and have a tendency to cause gas. Foods and herbs containing sweet, sour, and salty tastes are good for individuals of vata constitution.

PITTA. Pitta individuals should avoid sour, salty, and pungent substances, which aggravate bodily fire. However, sweet, bitter, and astringent tastes are beneficial for pittas.

KAPHA. Kapha individuals should avoid foods containing the sweet, sour, and salty tastes, for they increase bodily water. Better for them are foods with pungent, bitter, and astringent tastes.

Healthy and Unhealthy Eating Habits

How you eat is as important as what you eat. Here are some suggestions for healthy eating, followed by a list of habits to avoid.

EATING HABITS TO CULTIVATE

- Choose foods according to your constitution. They will nourish you and not aggravate your doshas.
- Choose foods according to the season.
- Eat fresh, *sattvic* food of the best quality you can afford.
- Do not eat unless you feel hungry.
- Do not drink unless you feel thirsty. If you are hungry and you drink instead of eating, the liquid will dissolve the digestive enzymes and reduce your gastric fire.
- Sit, don't stand, to eat.
- When eating, eat. That is, don't read, watch TV, or be distracted by too much conversation. Focus on the food.
- Chew well, at least 32 times per mouthful. This enables the digestive enzymes in the mouth to do their work properly.
- Eat at a moderate speed. Don't gobble your food.
- Fill one-third of your stomach with food, one-third with water, and leave one-third empty.
- Don't eat more at a meal than the amount of food you can hold in two cupped hands. Overeating expands the stomach so that you will feel the need for additional food. Overeating also creates toxins in the digestive tract.
- During meals, don't drink iced drinks or fruit juice; sip a little warm water between mouthfuls of food.
- Honey should never be cooked. If it is cooked, the molecules become like a glue that adheres to mucous membranes and clogs the subtle channels, producing toxins.

UNHEALTHY EATING HABITS

- Overeating
- Eating too soon after a full meal
- Drinking too much water, or no water, during a meal
- Drinking very chilled water during a meal, or indeed at any time
- Eating when constipated
- Eating at the wrong time of day, either too early or too late (see "Ayurvedic Daily Routine," starting page 57)
- Eating too much heavy food or too little light food
- Eating fruit or drinking fruit juice with a meal
- Eating without real hunger
- Emotional eating
- Eating incompatible food combinations (see chart on page 101)
- Munching between meals

Incompatible Food Combinations

The shelves of pharmacies and health food stores these days are lined with digestive aids and pills for indigestion and gas. It is likely that most of these gastrointestinal problems begin with poor food combining.

According to Ayurveda, certain food combinations disturb the normal functioning of the gastric fire and upset the balance of the doshas. Combining foods improperly can produce indigestion, fermentation, putrefaction, and gas formation. If such a situation in your stomach and intestines is frequent or prolonged, it can lead to disease. As just one example, eating bananas with milk can diminish agni (gastric fire) and change the intestinal flora, resulting in toxins and causing sinus congestion, cold, cough, allergies, hives, and rash. Such disturbances generate ama, the toxic substance that is the root cause of most ailments.

The following table lists some (but far from all) of the incompatible food combinations worth avoiding. You can alleviate some of the ill effects of these combinations by using spices and herbs in your cooking. A strong digestive fire can be the most powerful means of dealing with these combina-

NAME OF FOOD	INCOMPATIBLE WITH
MILK	BANANAS Fish, Melons, Yogurt, Sour Fruits, Kitchari (mung dal and basmati rice), Bread made with yeast
YOGURT	MILK Sour fruits, Melons, Hot drinks—including coffee and tea—Fish, Mango (thus mango lassi is not a good idea), Starches, Cheese, Banana
MELONS "Eat them alone or leave them alone"	EVERYTHING, especially: Grains, Starches, Fried foods, Cheese
EGGS	MILK Yogurt, Melons, Cheese, Fruits, Potatoes
STARCHES	BANANAS Eggs, Milk, Dates
HONEY (never cook honey)	GHEE in equal proportions (by weight) Grains
CORN	Dates, Raisins, Bananas
LEMONS	Yogurt, Milk, Cucumber, Tomato
NIGHTSHADES (Potato, tomato, eggplant)	Yogurt, Milk, Melon, Cucumber

Particularly to be avoided are such concoctions as banana milkshakes and "fruit smoothies" made with milk. Mixed fruit salads are also incompatible. Some blended fruit drinks made with all fruit may be all right, but check this chart first.

Recommendations Regarding Milk and Milk Products

In Ayurveda, milk and dairy products such as ghee and freshly made yogurt are considered highly important to the diet. However, the process of pasteurization, which kills bacteria and other potentially harmful microorganisms, may also destroy the enzymes necessary for proper digestion. If the milk is heated for a fairly long period of time, such as fifteen or twenty minutes, the enzymes will definitely be destroyed, and calcium and other nutrients may not be absorbed.

When milk is heated just until it reaches the boiling point, its enzymes are not destroyed, and it becomes less kaphagenic. So if you can obtain organic, unpasteurized milk from certified dairies and heat it just to the boiling point, that would be best.

Nevertheless, pasteurized milk from the supermarket, and dairy products made from that milk, are still better than no dairy products at all.

tions. Chew a bit of fresh ginger (sprinkled with salt and lime juice if you like) before meals to stimulate digestion.

Note that for each food in capital letters on the left, the food in capitals on the right is the most incompatible; foods in small letters are less incompatible.

Food and the Three Gunas

The Ayurvedic tradition teaches that food is not only for nutrition, to nourish the body, but also affects the mind and consciousness. As we have a physical constitution (vata–pitta–kapha), we also have a mental constitution characterized by the three *gunas*: *sattva, rajas,* and *tamas.*

According to the Sankhya philosophy of creation, *sattva, rajas,* and *tamas* are universal qualities necessary for the creation of the universe (see page 9). They are equally necessary for maintaining our psychobiological functions.

Because of *sattva,* we remain conscious and reawaken every morning. Because of *rajas,* our thoughts, feelings, and emotions move in a creative way. Because of *tamas,* we become tired, exhausted, and heavy; without *tamas* there is no sleep. Another way to look at it is that *sattva* brings clarity, *rajas* brings perception, and *tamas* gives solid, concrete experience.

These three qualities are also necessary for the functioning of every cell. *Satva* is potential energy, *rajas* is kinetic energy, and *tamas* is inertia. The potential energy in the cell is awareness; it becomes active due to the kinetic energy of *rajas;* then the cell becomes inert because of the *tamasic* quality. Thus these three qualities are absolutely nec-

Psychological Constitutions

Indian philosophy classifies human temperaments into three basic types: *sattvic, rajasic,* and *tamasic.* These types all differ in psychological and moral disposition, as well as in their reactions to social, cultural, and physical conditions, as is described in the classical texts of Ayurveda.

Sattvic qualities imply essence, reality, consciousness, purity, and clarity of perception. People in whom *sattvic* qualities predominate are loving, compassionate, religious, and pure-minded, following truth and righteousness. They tend to have good manners and positive behavior, and they do not easily become upset or angry. Although they work hard mentally, they do not get mental fatigue, so they need only four to five hours of sleep at night. They look fresh, alert, aware, and full of luster and are recognized for their wisdom, happiness, and joy. They are creative, humble, and respectful of their teachers. Worshiping God and humanity, they love all. They care for people, birds, animals, and trees and are respectful of every life and existence.

Rajasic individuals are loving, calm, and patient—so long as their own interests are served! All their activities are self-centered and egotistical. They are kind, friendly, and faithful only to those who are helpful to them.

All movement and activity is due to *rajas,* which leads to the life of sensual enjoyment, pleasure and pain, effort and restlessness. People in whom *rajasic* qualities predominate tend to be egoistic, ambitious, aggressive, proud, and competitive and have a tendency to control others. They like power, prestige, and position and are perfectionists. They are hard-working people but may be lacking in proper planning and direction. Emotionally they tend to be angry, jealous, and ambitious and to have few moments of joy. They suffer from a fear of failure, are subject to stress, and are quickly drained of mental energy. They require eight hours of sleep.

Tamas is darkness, inertia, heaviness, and a tendency toward materialism. Individuals dominated by *tamas* are often less intelligent. They tend toward depression, laziness, and excess sleep, even during the day. A little mental work tires them easily. They like jobs with less responsibility, and they love to eat, drink, sleep, and have sex. They tend to be greedy, possessive, attached, irritable, and uncaring toward others. They are willing to harm others for their own self-interest.

There is a constant interplay of these three *gunas* in everyone's consciousness, but the relative predominance of either *sattva, rajas,* or *tamas* is responsible for an individual's psychological constitution.

essary for the psychobiological activities of the human body.

In the Ayurvedic literature, food is classified as *sattvic, rajasic,* or *tamasic* according to the mental qualities it promotes. In brief, *sattvic* food is light, healthy food that increases clarity of mind, *rajasic* food is tempting food that increases activity and agitation, and *tamasic* food is heavy, dulling food that creates depression and heaviness and leads to many disorders.

Sattvic food is light and easy to digest. It brings clarity of perception, unfolds love and compassion, and promotes the qualities of forgiveness and austerity. *Sattvic* foods include fruit, steamed vegetables, and fresh vegetable juice. Milk and ghee are *sattvic* foods that build up *ojas* and give vitality to *prana.*

Rajasic foods are hot, spicy, and salty. They are irritants and stimulants, and they are tempting foods (once your hand goes into the bag, you cannot stop eating them), such as salty crackers and potato chips. *Rajasic* foods also include certain heavily spiced foods, such as hot pickles and chutneys, which stimulate the senses. These foods make the mind more agitated and susceptible to temptation. Gradually, from eating these foods, the mind becomes more *rajasic,* which means it tends toward anger, hate, and manipulation.

Tamasic food is heavy, dull, and depressing and induces deep sleep. Under that category comes any dark meat, lamb, pork, and beef, as well as thick cheese. Old and stale food is also *tamasic.*

However, the heavy, dulling effect of *tamasic* food occurs only when it is eaten in excess. In moderation, *tamasic* food is grounding and promotes stability. If, for example, an individual has an excess of the *rajasic* quality—the mind is hyper and ungrounded and there is insomnia—some *tamasic* food eaten in moderation will help the person become more grounded and get some sleep.

We can classify food into categories of *sattvic, rajasic,* or *tamasic* according to the table on the facing page.

RELATIONSHIP OF THE *GUNAS* AND THE DOSHAS

Students of Ayurveda frequently ask whether there is a relationship between the three *gunas* and the three doshas. There is not a direct correspondence, but there is a relationship.

Sattva is present in the doshas in this order:

1. in pitta as knowledge and understanding
2. in vata as clarity and lightness
3. in kapha as forgiveness and love

Tamas is present in the doshas in this order:

1. It is heavy, dull, and sleepy in kapha.
2. In pitta, it expresses as aggressiveness and competitiveness.
3. There is very little of it in vata, but it is represented as confusion.

Rajas, active and hyper, is present in vata and in pitta but is virtually absent from kapha.

Vata is approximately 75 percent *rajas,* 20

Food Categories of Tamasic, Rajasic and Sattvic

	TAMASIC	RAJASIC	SATTVIC
FRUIT	Avocado Watermelon Plums Apricots	Sour fruits Apples Bananas Guava	Mango Pomegranate Coconut Figs Peaches Pears
GRAINS	Wheat Brown Rice	Millet Corn Buckwheat	Rice Tapioca Blue corn
VEGETABLES	Mushrooms Garlic Onion Pumpkin	Potato Nightshades Cauliflower Broccoli Spinach Tamarind Pickles Winter squash	Sweet potato Lettuce Parsley Sprouts Yellow squash
BEANS	Urad dal Black Pinto Pink	Red lentils Toor dal Adzuki	Mung Yellow lentils Kidney Lima
DAIRY	Cheese (hard, aged)	Old, sour milk Sour cream	Milk Fresh homemade yogurt or cheese
MEAT	Beef Lamb Pork	Fish Shrimp Chicken	None

percent *sattva,* and 5 percent *tamas.* Pitta is 50 percent or more *sattva,* 45 percent *rajas,* and up to 5 percent *tamas.* Kapha is maybe 75 percent *tamas* and 15 to 20 percent *sattva,* with very little *rajas.* Here is another way we can see these relationships:

	SATTVA	RAJAS	TAMAS
VATA	Clarity Creativity Lightness	Hyperactivity Nervousness Fear Anxiety Ungroundedness	Confusion Lack of direction Indecisiveness Sadness Grief
PITTA	Knowledge Understanding Comprehension Recognition	Aggressiveness Competitiveness Power Prestige	Anger Hatred Envy Jealousy
KAPHA	Love Compassion Forgiveness	Attachment Greed Possessiveness	Deep confusion Unconsciousness Coma Depression

Now you have more than enough background information to benefit from the remedies and recommendations made in Part III. I hope you have enjoyed this introduction to Ayurveda and that you will incorporate its principles and practices into your life. If you do, I know your health will improve and your life will blossom physically, mentally, emotionally, and spiritually.

Part III

Secrets of Ayurvedic Self-healing: An Encyclopedia of Illnesses and Remedies

How to Use the Encyclopedia

The ancient Ayurvedic art of healing deals with every individual's life as a whole. To the Ayurvedic *vaidya* (physician), every individual is an indivisible, complete, unique being. At the same time, Vedic philosophy teaches that there is a concurrent and inherent relationship between the macrocosm (the universe) and the microcosm (the individual). The individual is constantly exposed to environmental changes, seasonal changes, changes in diet, lifestyle, emotions, job, financial status, and relationships. These changes are constantly bombarding every human being. To remain healthy or to regain health, all these factors have to be taken into consideration.

As you have learned, when the body's doshic balance of vata–pitta–kapha is disturbed, illness may result. The purpose of Ayurvedic healing is not just to relieve the symptoms of a specific illness but to bring the out-of-balance factors back into harmony.

Thus, the purpose of Ayurvedic remedies, whether they be herbal medications, dietary and nutritional changes, yoga postures, cleansing procedures, or breathing exercises, is to eradicate the underlying causes of the disease, not merely to remove the symptoms. Of course one must deal directly with emergency or life-threatening symptoms, such as wheezing in asthma, heart pain in heart conditions, or high fever in infections. But if the fundamental causes of the illness are not dealt with, the problem will manifest again in the same or another form.

Components of Ayurvedic Healing

The Ayurvedic approach to restoring health is known as *chikitsa* (disease management) and traditionally consists of eight components. If you glance at the accompanying box, you will note that *chikitsa* is a complete healing program that begins with identifying and eliminating the underlying cause of the illness, proceeds by purifying the body and reestablishing balance, and ends with strengthening and revitalizing the affected organs, tissues, and systems so that the disease will not recur.

If you become sick, your illness is not likely to become completely healed unless you change the behaviors that gave rise to it. Dietary indiscretions, a stressful lifestyle, unresolved emotions, insufficient exercise—these are some of the factors that are at the root of most illness. Identifying and eliminating these causal factors are essential components of the healing process. If you take some of the recommended herbal formulas but allow unhealthy lifestyle habits to continue unabated, it's not likely that you will experience lasting or significant improvement.

That is why, for each condition, I have suggested not only medications but numerous other measures you can use for healing, such as specific yoga postures and breathing exercises, foods to favor or avoid, massage oils, teas, healing pastes, and many other ways to promote healing. In addition, Part II of the book provides suggestions for your diet and daily routine that can get you established in a healthy way of living in harmony with nature. Please make use of these recommendations as part of your own personal holistic program for creating and supporting health.

Your body's innate healing mechanisms

Ayurvedic Disease Management (Chikitsa)

The traditional Ayurvedic program of healing has eight essential components:

1. Find out the person's *prakruti* (constitution).
2. Find out the *vikruti* (the present altered state of the doshas in the body).
3. Find out the cause or causes of the illness, such as diet, lifestyle, emotional patterns, quality of relationships, genetic predisposition, and so on.
4. As the first line of treatment, remove the cause.
5. Provide the proper regimen (diet, exercise, *pranayama*, etc.), according to the person's *prakruti*, *vikruti*, seasons, climate, age, and so on.
6. Provide a detoxification procedure: either palliation *(shamana)* or elimination *(shodana*, such as *panchakarma)*.
7. Provide rejuvenation *(rasayana)* for the body in general, to increase immunity and to strengthen specific organs and tissues.
8. Provide therapies that are (a) antagonistic to the provoked dosha and (b) antagonistic to the disease, based on the principle that opposite qualities balance.

are always at work, striving to maintain or restore total health and balance. The recommendations offered here will support the body in its natural process of healing.

The following points will help you to make best use of this encyclopedia of Ayurvedic healing.

Diagnosis and Treatment

Ayurvedic first-aid treatments are effective if you first do a careful, discriminating diagnosis to determine whether the condition is vata, pitta, or kapha in nature. A specific treatment, for a specific type of condition, will be beneficial.

On the other hand, if you do not take the time to diagnose carefully, the treatment may not be appropriate, and consequently you will not get the desired result. So before deciding on an Ayurvedic line of treatment, look carefully at the physical signs and symptoms that will help you determine whether it is a vata, pitta, or kapha illness or condition. Then choose the recommended treatment.

On the few occasions when it is not mentioned whether a condition is vata, pitta, or kapha, you can feel comfortable using any general treatment suggestions made for that condition.

A NOTE ABOUT HERBAL MEDICATIONS. The pharmacopoeia of Ayurveda is vast, including literally thousands of medicines, many of them herbal preparations. For each condition listed here, I have tried to include several very simple remedies, utilizing common kitchen herbs or household strategies such as taking a warm bath. I also recommend some common Ayurvedic herbs, most of which are easily obtained from various sources (see Resources). For guidelines on how to prepare your own herbal formulas, how to take herbs, how to make ghee, and other important information, please see appendix 2.

SEE WHAT WORKS. For each condition, several suggestions are made. No one expects you to use all of them. Try what sounds good to you, and observe how it works. If it solves the problem, you don't need to try any others. If it doesn't seem to work, then try a different approach. Each person is different and will react differently to these remedies.

DON'T BE DISCOURAGED IF A REMEDY DOESN'T WORK. In self-treatment using Ayurvedic principles and remedies, keep in mind a fundamental therapeutic guideline. If you diagnose your problem to be, for example, a vata disorder and embark on a treatment to reduce vata, then find that the treatment is not working or appears to be exacerbating the problem, this indicates that your diagnosis was not entirely correct.

This does not mean you should give up on Ayurvedic remedies! Simply try using the treatment recommended for either pitta or kapha, whichever makes more sense to you considering your symptoms. If you are untrained in Ayurvedic diagnosis, you may simply have made a mistake. So use your best judgment and try again.

Sometimes the effect of the first remedy can give you a clue for a more beneficial treatment. For example, perhaps you thought your condition was due to excess kapha, and you decided to use a heating herb such as ginger, pepper, or *trikatu* to treat it. If the condition worsens and you develop symptoms of aggravated pitta, such as irritability or a skin rash, you can infer that perhaps the problem was actually related to excess pitta. Reassess the situation, and take the next step.

BE SURE TO TREAT YOUR ACTUAL CONDITION. Most imbalances and illnesses are related to constitution. As it is often said, "*Prakruti* indicates disease proneness." Vata individuals are likely to have vata-related problems, pitta individuals will have primarily pitta conditions, and kaphas will have kapha illnesses.

However, in a small percentage of cases, your illness or condition may not coincide with your own constitutional type. For example, you may be predominantly a pitta type, but you may have a vata condition such as insomnia or constipation. It may be the result of any combination of vata-aggravating factors in your life, such as a vata diet, a cold dry climate, or irregular hours. So when remedies are suggested, be careful to choose options that fit the symptoms of your *condition*, not necessarily your body type.

HOW LONG TO TAKE A REMEDY. In general, remedies should be used until your symptoms disappear. This may be a few days, a few weeks, or a few months, depending on several important factors, such as: How severe is the disease or condition? How long have you had it? How motivated are you to get well?

First, assess your desire to get well. If you have a strong desire and are motivated to get results, the first thing you need is diligence in following the prescribed Ayurvedic regimen. Because of the law of *karma* (cause and effect), to a great extent you will derive benefits according to your own actions. So in addition to taking your herbs two or three times a day as recommended (no skipping, no forgetting them at home...), you also need to address the underlying causes of your condition by rethinking your diet, daily routine, exercise program, etc. Chances are that the herbal remedies alone, without some changes in your lifestyle, will not be powerful enough to override the very behavior patterns that caused the illness in the first place.

If your condition is serious, and you are diligent with your remedies and make appropriate lifestyle changes and still the symptoms persist, you need to see your doctor for help. On the other hand, if the condition is chronic, it is unrealistic to expect that something that has persisted for years is going to disappear in a week or a month.

So in deciding how long to use the recommended remedies, use your common sense. And do your best right from the start: If you don't, and you end up not getting the results you would like, it's human nature that you will question whether you could have done better.

Every disease process in the body, and every process of healing, has its own momentum, speed, and duration. You cannot make the mango ripen quickly; it ripens of its own accord. So in order to eradicate the disease completely, allow sufficient time, and have patience. Ayurveda is not a quick fix. Anything that is quickly fixed does not resolve the problem totally.

Cautions

CONSULT YOUR DOCTOR. Some of the conditions in this book are serious medical conditions which require the supervision of a medical doctor. Mild or preclinical cases may sometimes be completely healed using these Ayurvedic recommendations, but these remedies are not a substitute for consulting with a physician.

If you are already under a doctor's care for a specific illness or condition, the Ayurvedic remedies suggested here may be used in conjunction with the regimen outlined by your physician. But it is only fair and proper to do so with his or her knowledge and supervision.

Ask your doctor to carefully monitor your progress. As time goes by, you may be able to minimize or eliminate your dependence on strong medications if your body's balance can be brought to a point at which diet, exercise, herbs, and other Ayurvedic methods are sufficient to control or eliminate the condition.

DETERMINE THE SEVERITY OF THE DISEASE. The vast majority of minor injuries and illnesses can be treated at home, with such natural means as lifestyle changes, diet, herbs, and simple yoga stretching exercises. But sometimes it is absolutely crucial to get medical attention from a qualified physician or even from a trained hospital staff. This is extremely important and must always be remembered.

For example, diarrhea that lasts for a day or even a couple of days can be effectively treated at home (see "Diarrhea"). But suppose a person has profuse diarrhea that goes on for some time, so that he or she becomes severely dehydrated. This is a serious condition that requires hospitalization. It cannot be treated at home or even in the outpatient department; it needs admission to a hospital so that intravenous feeding can begin immediately.

Or suppose someone has a high fever, perhaps 104 or 105 degrees Fahrenheit, and is babbling incoherently, appears delirious, and is losing consciousness. This is a serious situation and one has to act promptly to get help.

So always be alert to the severity, intensity, persistence, or recurrence of any disease condition, and be sure to treat it properly. And remember: If you are not a trained medical professional, you may not always know. When in doubt, see a doctor.

A WORD ABOUT LICORICE TEA. On several occasions I recommend the use of licorice tea. Individuals with hypertension (high blood pressure) may use this tea for emergencies (such as to relieve an asthma attack—see "Asthma"), but they should not use it on a regular basis; it promotes sodium retention, which may increase blood pressure.

Illnesses and Remedies, A–Z

Abdominal Cramps

See "Muscle Cramps and Spasms"

Acne

See also "Skin—Ayurvedic Care"

Acne is the result of high pitta moving under the skin and breaking out in pimples. Ayurveda recommends several natural approaches that, taken together, can effectively control acne.

The possible pitta-provoking causes are numerous. They include emotional stress, premenstrual hormonal changes, and exposure to chemicals or too much sunlight. The problem might also be a bacterial infection. It is important to find out the cause, so it can be properly treated or, in the case of exposure to chemicals or sunlight, simply avoided.

FOLLOW THE PITTA-PACIFYING DIET. Because acne is a pitta condition, the first step is to follow the pitta-pacifying diet detailed in chapter 8. Avoid spicy and fermented foods, salt, fried foods, and citrus fruits. Favor blander foods such as rice, oatmeal, and applesauce.

USE THESE HERBS TO BALANCE PITTA. The following formula is excellent for pacifying the excess pitta that causes acne:

kutki
guduchi
shatavari

Make a mixture of equal proportions of these three herbs (you might start with 1 teaspoon of each), and take 1/4 teaspoon of your mixture 2 or 3 times a day. After meals, place the powder on your tongue and wash it down with warm water.

• A helpful tea, made from common household herbs, is cumin-coriander-fennel tea. After each meal, steep 1/3 teaspoon of each of these three seeds in hot water for 10 minutes, strain, and drink. Use this tea 3 times a day.

DRINK BLUE WATER. Fill a clear glass bottle or jar with water, and cover it with some translucent blue paper (such as blue cellophane, available at art supply and some grocery stores). Put the bottle in the sun for about 2 hours. Drink 1 to 3 cups of the water

Healing Pastes for Your Skin

Here are three pastes you can make at home and apply to your skin. They can be effective in reducing acne.

1. Mix 1 teaspoon of chickpea flour (available at Indian grocery stores and natural food stores) with enough water to make a paste, and wash your face with this mixture. Rinse off, then apply either of the following:
2. Mix almond powder with a little water, and apply the paste to your face. Let it dry and remain on your skin for up to half an hour, then rinse it off. (You can easily make the almond powder yourself in a coffee or nut grinder.)
3. A paste of sandalwood and turmeric powders mixed in goat's milk is healing for the skin. Take 1/4 teaspoon turmeric and 1/2 teaspoon sandalwood powder, mix them together, and add sufficient goat's milk to make a paste. Apply this mixture to your face. *Note:* Your face will look yellow for some time—up to 5 days—but this formula is quite effective in alleviating acne.

each day. This will have a cooling, soothing effect. Believe it or not, it works!

DRINK ALOE VERA JUICE. You might try drinking half a cup of pure aloe vera juice twice a day.

KEEP YOUR COLON CLEAN. Keeping your colon clean is important, in order to remove toxins from the body. You can easily accomplish this by taking the herb *amalaki,* 1/2 to 1 teaspoon daily, as a powder on the tongue. Take it before bedtime, and wash it down with warm water.

APPLY MELON. Rub some melon on the skin at bedtime, and leave it on overnight. Its cooling, anti-pitta quality will help heal acne. It also makes the skin soft.

YOGA POSTURES. Recommended yoga *asanas* for acne are the Lion Pose and the sequence of postures called the Moon Salutation. (See appendix 4 for illustrations.)

BREATHING EXERCISE. Breathing through the left nostril only, for 5 to 10 minutes, will help to reduce pitta. (This is called the Moon Breath and is said to be cooling; breathing through the right nostril is called the Sun Breath and is heating.) Simply cover the right nostril with your thumb, and breathe normally through the left side. If the nostril is blocked, don't force it; try again later.

RELAX YOUR FACE. Rub your hands together vigorously to create a bit of warmth, and place both hands over your face for a couple of minutes. This will relax the facial muscles and increase the blood supply.

You can also rub your hands until the palms become warm, then gently touch just the heart of the palm to the eyelashes. Our eyelashes are intensely electrically charged; they take that warmth and relieve the pitta under the skin that is coming out in the form of acne.

VISUALIZATION. The root cause of acne is emotional stress. One effective way to relieve that stress is visualization. Close your eyes and visualize that the acne is clearing up and going away—as if you are communicating with the tissues in your skin that are bursting out in acne. This works.

A final suggestion: Avoid frequent looking in the mirror and feeling bad about the acne.

Addictions

See also "Smoking"

Why are people addicted? In the majority of cases (excluding tragic situations such as babies who are born addicted because of their mother's addiction), people who are addicted start out simply seeking more pleasure and joy in their life. Their life is difficult and unhappy, their relationships may be painful and unfulfilling, they may be dissatisfied and stressed at work, and they simply don't know how to deal with the situation. So they escape from the reality of their circumstances into drugs or alcohol.

Whether the addictive substance is tobacco, marijuana, alcohol, or something else, it soon goes beyond being a psychological escape and becomes a chemical dependency. Then, unless a certain level of the addictive substance is present in the blood, the person's brain doesn't function properly.

Treatment depends on how serious and long-standing the addiction is. For milder addictions, such as a recent smoking habit, the person may simply be able to stop. But if a chronic alcoholic suddenly stops drinking, it creates alcohol withdrawal syndrome that is difficult to deal with.

CLEANSING. To effectively handle the problem of addiction, it is important to do *panchakarma,* an effective Ayurvedic cleansing and detox program. See chapter 4 for a description of *panchakarma* treatments you can receive at an Ayurvedic clinic, and a home *panchakarma* program you can do for yourself.

DOSE REDUCTION. Along with this cleansing program, slowly decrease the dose of the addictive substance. According to Ayurveda, unless some strong medications are available to deal with withdrawal, it is not good to completely stop using the addictive substance all at once, or a stressful withdrawal syndrome will probably occur.

• With nicotine toxicity (which affects the lungs and cardiovascular system) and alcohol toxicity (which affects the liver) we have to strengthen the affected organs. For alcohol toxicity, use this formula:

chitrak 3 parts
kutki 3 parts

Take 1/2 teaspoon of these herbs, with 2 tablespoons of aloe vera juice, 3 times a day.

• Ayurveda suggests a bitter wine made of aloe vera juice. (It is called *kumari asava.*) In place of hard liquor or other alcoholic drinks, the person who is addicted to alcohol can take small amounts of this light, dry wine. Try 4 teaspoons diluted with an equal amount of water. Then gradually reduce the amount of herbal wine in the dose, while at the same time using the above herbal formula to strengthen the damaged liver.

• The same applies to tobacco. For a person who is addicted to nicotine, remove one-third to one-half of the tobacco from each cigarette (at the end you light), and fill the paper with a mixture of rose petals, *brahmi,* and *jatamamsi* (equal proportions). Smoke it until the tobacco starts burning. The moment the tobacco starts, put out the cigarette and discard it.

NASAL MEDICINE. Doing *nasya* with *brahmi* ghee will also reduce the toxicity of nicotine (see appendix 3).

EXERCISE. Most of the time, whenever there is the desire to drink or to smoke, the person should go out for a walk in the fresh air, or do some other exercise, or go for a swim.

TIME TO SEE THE DOCTOR

If there is strong alcohol addiction and the person experiences a headache, tremors, drowsiness, depression, or other alcohol withdrawal symptoms when he or she stops drinking, see a doctor right away: Medical help is needed.

APPETITE STIMULATION. Some people drink because they have a low appetite. Unless they have a drink, they never feel hungry. In such cases, instead of alcohol, they can have some ginger tea to stimulate their appetite (see also "Appetite, Low"). Or try this recipe for a tea to stimulate agni, the digestive fire:

Agni Tea

1 quart water
1/8 pinch cayenne pepper
1/2 handful minced ginger root
2 tablespoons Sucanat or other sweetener
1/8 to 1/2 teaspoon rock salt

Put all the above ingredients in a pot and boil for 20 minutes.

Take the pot off the burner, cool for a few minutes, then add the juice of half a lime. Do not boil the lime juice.

YOGA *ASANAS.* Some yoga exercises will also be beneficial. Sun Salutations Should be included, and some Alternate Nostril breathing. *So-Hum* Meditation will also be helpful. (See chapters 6 and 7.)

Allergies

See also "Food Allergies"

According to Ayurvedic *samprapti* (pathogenesis), allergies are a doshic reaction to a specific allergen, such as pollen, dust, chemicals on a rug, ragweed, or any strong chemical smell. These allergic reactions are classified as vata type, pitta type, and kapha type.

• *Vata-type allergies* are characterized by bloating of the stomach, gastric discomfort, or even intestinal colic. A vata allergy may lead to sudden wheezing, sneezing, headache, ringing in the ears, or insomnia. For example, some individuals, when exposed to dust or pollen, suddenly start wheezing. The wheezing is due to narrowing of the bronchial tree due to vata dosha. That person may also experience insomnia and other vata-type symptoms.

• *In a pitta type of allergy,* pitta dosha is already present under the skin. If the person comes in contact with an allergen, such as chemicals, ragweed, or certain synthetic fibers, then the pitta penetrates through the capillaries due to its hot and sharp qualities and creates a rash, itching, hives, urticaria, allergic dermatitis, or eczema—all pitta-type allergic reactions.

• *Kapha allergies* are often experienced during spring season, when plants and trees shed their pollens into the atmosphere. When the pollens, such as juniper or any other flower pollen, are inhaled, they enter the nasal-respiratory passage, and in some people they irritate the delicate mucous membrane, leading to hay fever, colds, congestion, a cough, sinus infection, and even asthma.

In order to treat allergies effectively, first we have to find out whether it is vata, pitta, or kapha type. Then we can determine the specific line of treatment.

In most cases, perhaps 80 percent, your *prakruti* (constitution) predicts your allergy proneness. That is, there is usually a correspondence between a person's constitution and the type of allergic reaction. A person of pitta *prakruti* is more likely to have a pitta allergic reaction, especially when the *vikruti* or current status of the system shows a pitta imbalance. But it may also happen that due to diet, environmental conditions, emotional factors, or other causes, a kapha person may have a vata imbalance, and so forth.

TREATMENT FOR VATA-TYPE ALLERGIES

BASTI. One of the most effective remedies for vata-type allergies is a *dashamoola* tea *basti* (enema). Boil 1 tablespoon of the herbal compound *dashamoola* in 1 pint of water for 5 minutes to make a tea. Cool it, strain it, and use the liquid as an enema. (See appendix 3 for complete directions.) Vata symptoms, such as wheezing, sneezing, dryness of the throat, dryness of the colon leading to distension, constipation, and abdominal discomfort, can be immediately corrected by this *dashamoola* tea *basti*.

HERBAL REMEDIES. Use this herbal formula:

ashwagandha 1 part
bala 1 part
vidari 1 part

Mix these herbs in equal proportion, and take 1/4 teaspoon of the powder 3 times a day, washed down with warm water, to relieve vata allergies.

• To soothe an extreme wheezing condition, make one cup of either ginger or licorice tea, boiling 1 teaspoon of the herb for about 3 minutes in 1 cup of water. Then add 5 to 10 drops of *mahanarayan* oil, mix thoroughly, and take 1 sip every 10 to 15 minutes. (If you do not have *mahanarayan* oil, you can substitute 1/2 teaspoon of plain ghee.)

TREATMENT FOR PITTA-TYPE ALLERGIES

HERBAL REMEDIES. This herbal formula is effective to pacify pitta:

shatavari 8 parts
kama dudha 1/2 part
guduchi 1 part
shanka bhasma 1/4 part

Take 1/2 teaspoon of this mixture 2 or 3 times a day after meals, with a little warm water.

• For hives, rash, urticaria, dermatitis, or eczema, apply *neem* oil or *tikta ghrita* (bitter ghee) on the skin.

BLOOD PURIFICATION. Traditionally, Ayurveda has suggested that individuals with high pitta, who are prone to developing pitta-type problems such as sunburn in the summer season, do *rakta moksha,* or bloodletting, before the onset of the summer. Although this practice is currently not very well respected in the West, it is still used widely in India, as it has proven to be an effective preventive and healing measure. To make use of it today, you might consider donating about 1/2 pint or 100 cc. of blood to a blood bank. That will help to defuse pitta conditions such as allergic dermatitis and allergic eczema.

• To produce a similar effect, you can use a blood-cleansing herbal combination. For example, mix the herbs *manjistha* and *neem* in equal amounts.

manjistha 1 part
neem 1 part

Take 1/2 teaspoon of this mixture 3 times a day with warm water after meals. It will cleanse the blood and help to heal pitta-type allergies.

• The common Western herb burdock is also an effective blood purifier; you can make a tea from 1/2 teaspoon burdock per cup of boiling water and drink it 2 or 3 times a day.

TREATMENT FOR KAPHA-TYPE ALLERGIES

HERBAL REMEDIES. Kapha allergies generally take the form of respiratory-pulmonary congestion, cough, cold, asthma, or hay fever. For relief from these conditions, use the following herbal formula:

sitopaladi 4 parts
yashti madhu 4 parts
abrak bhasma 1/8 part

Take about 1/4 teaspoon of this mixture 3 times a day with honey.

PURGATION THERAPY. Kapha-type allergies occur when excess kapha collects in the stomach and lungs. One way to relieve this congestion is purgation therapy (*virechana*).

Use flaxseed oil (available in most natural food stores), and take 1 teaspoon 2 or 3 times a day for 2 or 3 days. This will be quite effective. Or you can use *triphala* (see below).

VOMITING THERAPY. The Ayurvedic therapy that is particularly effective for removing excess kapha from the stomach and respiratory tract is *vamana,* or vomiting therapy. I have noticed, however, that people in the West have a strong cultural bias against vomiting, and many seem particularly uncomfortable with this procedure. It not only seems physically repugnant but may be emotionally difficult as well, as some emotional purification may arise as a result of the physical purification. So if you tend to have strong emotions or have trouble dealing with them, it might be better for you not to try *vamana.*

If you want to try it—and I want to emphasize that it is very effective for eliminating excess kapha—the procedure is to drink a stomach full of licorice tea and salt water and then to regurgitate it, emptying the stomach. Start by drinking several cups of licorice tea, followed by a pint of water with about 1 teaspoon of salt mixed in. Drink enough to fill your stomach, then rub the back of the tongue and vomit it out.

> IMPORTANT CAUTION: If you have high blood pressure, low blood pressure, hiatal hernia, or a history of heart problems, do not do *vaman* therapy.

HEALING GUIDELINES FOR ALL TYPES OF ALLERGIES

USE TRIPHALA. For all three types of allergies, one can take 1/2 to 1 teaspoon of *triphala* at night. (See appendix 2 for instructions for preparing *triphala.*) *Triphala* acts as both a laxative and a purgative. It consists of three herbs: *amalaki, bibhitaki,* and *haritaki. Haritaki* works on vata dosha, *amalaki* on pitta dosha, and *bibhitaki* on kapha dosha.

DIETARY CHANGES. For vata allergy, follow a vata-soothing diet; for pitta type of allergy, the pitta-pacifying diet; and for kapha allergy, the kapha-reducing diet. (Diet guidelines may be found in chapter 8.)

WATCH YOUR FOOD COMBINATIONS. It is important for individuals with allergies not to eat incompatible food combinations, such as milk and yogurt, meat and dairy, poultry and dairy, melon and grains, or fruits and grains. Avoid such things as banana milk shakes and "fruit smoothies" made with milk. For a more complete list of food incompatibilities, please turn to page 101.

AVOID THE CAUSE. For most allergies, one should try to avoid the immediate cause: the allergen. People who are allergic to cats, dogs, hair, pollen, mold, and so on should simply try to avoid them. Also try to stay away from synthetic fibers such as polyester and rayon, which can cause pitta-type skin allergies. It is best to wear cotton clothing. Because of the large quantity of pesticides routinely sprayed on cotton, you might consider using only organic cotton products, though they tend to be more expensive.

BLOCK THE ALLERGENS. Generally, the respiratory passage is open to dust and other allergens. One way to minimize the effect of allergens that you can't avoid is to lubricate the nasal mucous membrane with ghee. This prevents direct contact of the allergen with the mucous membrane.

USE *NEEM* OIL. Another way to reduce or avoid the effect of environmental allergens is to apply *neem* oil to the exposed part of the body. The presence of the oil on the skin, as well as the disinfectant properties of *neem*, will minimize contact with the allergen.

> NOTE: Use *neem* herbalized oil—that is, *neem* leaves cooked in a base of sesame or another oil. Pure *neem* extract will be too strong. If you find that even this herbalized *neem* oil is too strong and creates an itching or burning sensation, mix it half and half with coconut oil.

MEDITATE FOR STRESS REDUCTION. Most allergies are stress related. Because of stress, imbalance is created in mind and body. The practice known as Empty Bowl meditation helps to restore balance and thus helps take care of stress-related allergies. (See chapter 7 for guidelines.)

YOGA POSTURES. The most helpful yoga *asana* for kapha and vata allergies is the Sun Salutation. For pitta allergies, do the Moon Salutation. For help with yoga *asanas*, see appendix 4.

BREATHING EXERCISES. Alternate Nostril breathing is effective for respiratory allergies such as hay fever, wheezing, and sneezing. *Bhastrika* (Breath of Fire) is good for kapha-type congestive allergies (see chapter 6). Also, *ujjayi pranayama* helps to improve immunity and is beneficial for all types of allergies.

Anemia

Modern medicine has delineated several types of anemia: iron-deficiency anemia, pernicious anemia, sickle-cell anemia, and hypoproteinemic anemia (lack of protein in the blood), as well as certain vitamin-deficiency anemias, such as B-12 and folic acid–deficiency anemia. Certain bleeding disorders, such as profuse menstrual bleeding, bleeding hemorrhoids, or bleeding gums, can lead to anemia because of blood loss. Whenever modern medicine deals with the problem of anemia, it considers all these etiological factors.

Ayurveda looks at anemia quite differently. Ayurvedic classification of anemia falls under three basic doshic conditions: vata type, pitta type, and kapha type. It doesn't matter whether a person has iron deficiency or folic acid deficiency; what is important is how the anemia is expressing itself through a particular individual. As it turns out (see box page 123), there is also a correspondence between the Ayurvedic interpretation and the understanding according to modern medicine.

TYPES OF ANEMIA

• In vata-type anemia, the person looks thin, with dry, rough, scaly skin, and has cracking of the joints. He or she looks emaciated and pale, may suffer from breathlessness and constipation, and may pass tarry black stool.

• In pitta-type anemia, the eyes are slightly yellowish, the person may get high-colored urine, and the stools are dark brown or have a slightly yellowish tinge. There may be nausea or pain in the liver and/or spleen area. Dizziness or vertigo may be experienced, and the person may become easily irritated by light.

• In kapha-type anemia, there is often swelling (edema), and the person's skin feels cold and clammy and looks shiny. Because of the edema, the skin gets stretched so much that you can often see the reflection of the window on it.

By careful observation one can tell whether the anemia is vata, pitta, or kapha type. By treating that dosha, one treats the root cause and can alleviate the anemia.

TREATMENT

FOR VATA-TYPE ANEMIA. For vata anemia, Ayurveda suggests taking *tikta ghrita,* which is bitter ghee (see appendix 2). One teaspoon of *tikta ghrita* 5 to 10 minutes before breakfast, lunch, and dinner will help to improve the blood volume.

• One can also use a mixture of

kaishore guggulu 2 parts
abrak bhasma 1/8 part
ashwagandha 5 parts
dashamoola 5 parts

Take 1/2 teaspoon of this mixture 3 times a day with warm milk to help correct vata-type anemia.

• A specific formula is given in Vedic literature for a cleansing, detoxifying herbal remedy for vata-type anemia. It is called *gandharva haritaki,* which is *haritaki* powder roasted in castor oil in an iron pan. Place 1 tablespoon castor oil in an iron pan and heat on the stove; when the oil is warm enough, sauté 1 ounce of the herb *haritaki.* The *haritaki* will become thick and will turn slightly brown. (You have to stir it.) Take 1/2 teaspoon of *gandharva haritaki* at bedtime, washed down with warm water. Take it for 2 months or until the blood returns to normal.

NOTE: This mixture may cause loose stools; if this happens, reduce your dosage until comfortable.

FOR PITTA-TYPE ANEMIA. For pitta anemia, Ayurveda suggests *shatavari* ghee. (The *shatavari* and the ghee are cooked together. Directions for preparing herbalized and medicated ghees and oils appear in appendix 2.) Take 1 teaspoon of *shatavari* ghee 3 times a day, before breakfast, lunch, and dinner.

• One can also use this herbal formula:

shatavari 5 parts
brahmi 3 parts
neem 2 parts
loha bhasma 1/8 part

Mix these herbs, and take 1/2 teaspoon of the mixture 3 times a day with 2 tablespoons of aloe vera gel. This combination will be quite effective in treating pitta-type anemia.

FOR KAPHA-TYPE ANEMIA. Where there is swelling, use:

punarnava 5 parts
gokshura 3 parts
kutki 2 parts

Take 1/2 teaspoon of this herbal mixture twice a day with a few sips of warm water. Or you can mix it with a little honey and then wash it down with water.

FOR ALL TYPES OF ANEMIA

EAT IRON-RICH FOODS. Iron is a good blood builder, so foods rich in iron, such as beets, carrots, grapes, raisins, and currants, are used in the Ayurvedic treatment of most anemias. Figs, dates, and date sugar are also good sources of iron. Pomegranate juice and cranberry juice can be used as blood builders, as can a combination of beet and carrot juice. (Add a pinch of cumin to your carrot/beet juice for maximum effect.) Chlorophyll is also a good source of iron, and many times Ayurveda does suggest using chlorophyll, generally in the form of spinach, chard, and other fresh green vegetables.

YOGURT AND TURMERIC. Eat a cup of plain yogurt with up to 1 teaspoon turmeric on an empty stomach, morning and afternoon. Do not eat this after sunset. If kapha is unbalanced, eat this at noon only.

BLUE-GREEN ALGAE. Blue-green algae can also be effectively used, but primarily for pitta anemia. Because it is a rich source of *prana*, it is not good for vata individuals, as it will make them quite hyper. Kapha types may also find it beneficial.

COPPER WATER. Vata and kapha individuals may find copper water effective. Fill a genuine copper glass or cup with water and let it stand overnight, then drink it in the morning (see appendix 1).

DIET AND LIFESTYLE CHOICES. These choices should follow the general guidelines (diet, exercise, and so on) for each doshic

Correlation of Ayurvedic and Western Types of Anemia

Clinical observation has shown that the various types of anemia classified by modern medicine can be correlated with the types of anemia delineated by Ayurveda. For example, pitta-type anemia has been associated with mononucleosis and hepatitis and may lead to problems with the liver. Cobalamine (vitamin B-12)-deficiency anemia is also associated with pitta. Kapha-type anemia may lead to hypo-proteinemic anemia and swelling, while vata-type anemia may be associated with iron deficiency and folic acid–deficiency anemia. By treating the vata–pitta–kapha types of anemia, Ayurveda can at the same time treat the types of anemia categorized by modern medicine.

constitutional type. For vata problems, follow the anti-vata guidelines; for pitta anemia follow the pitta-soothing diet and other guidelines; and for kapha-type anemia, follow the kapha-reducing guidelines.

YOGA *ASANAS*. Yoga postures good for anemia of both the vata and kapha varieties include the Locust pose, Lotus pose, and inverted poses (Shoulder Stand, Plow pose, Headstand), which bring the blood supply to the vital organs such as the thyroid, thymus, and brain. Headstand will not be good for pitta-type anemia, but the Sun Salutation, as well as the Boat, Bow, and Bridge poses, will be effective.

BREATHING EXERCISE. For all anemic conditions, *surya pranayama* (Right Nostril breathing) is recommended. Block your left nostril with your right ring finger and breathe only through the right nostril. Right Nostril breathing stimulates the liver, which plays an important role in building the blood.

Anger and Hostility

Anger and hostility are signs of aggravated pitta in the nervous system. Pitta is necessary for right understanding and judgment, but when it gets disturbed or out of balance, it creates misunderstanding and wrong judgment, leading to anger and hostility. The aim is to bring the pitta back to its normal constitutional function.

Here are several simple home remedies to cool down that hot pitta and keep tempers under control.

DIET. Perhaps most important, a person who becomes angry easily or often should follow the pitta-pacifying diet (see chapter 8), especially avoiding hot, spicy and fermented foods, citrus fruit, and sour fruit. Favor simple, bland foods and cool drinks, and avoid alcohol and drinks with caffeine.

KEEP COOL. It's also not recommended for people with a pitta body type to take saunas or steam baths, to get overheated from exercise or sports, or to be in too much direct sun. In other words: keep cool.

OIL MASSAGE. Rub some *bhringaraj* oil or coconut oil on your scalp and on the soles of the feet. That will help to bring down the excess pitta. (See instructions for preparing herbalized ghees and oils in appendix 2.) You can do this every night before getting in bed to regularly moderate pitta. Be sure to wear some old socks and a hat, or put a towel on your pillow, to prevent the oil from staining.

USE SANDALWOOD OIL. Another simple and effective way to help balance your emotions is to place a drop of sandalwood essential oil on the "third eye" area between your eyebrows, as well as on the throat, breastbone, navel, temples, and wrists. Just a small amount of oil is sufficient.

HERBAL TEAS. Drink chamomile-tulsi-rose tea.

chamomile 1 part
tulsi (holy basil) 1 part
rose petal powder 2 parts

Steep 1/2 teaspoon of this mixture in 1 cup of hot water, cool it, and then drink. You can drink it 3 times a day, after each meal.

• You can use an even simpler formula. Take 1/2 teaspoon of chamomile and 1 teaspoon of fresh, finely chopped cilantro leaves, and steep them in 1 cup hot water for about 10 minutes. Allow this tea to cool before you drink it.

HAVE A PITTA-PACIFYING DRINK. Into 1 cup of grape juice, add 1/2 teaspoon cumin, 1/2 teaspoon fennel, and 1/2 teaspoon sandalwood powder. This cooling, pitta-pacifying drink will help to settle angry feelings and other pitta symptoms such as burning in the stomach.

GHEE NASYA. Dip your little finger into a jar of *brahmi* ghee (or plain ghee if you haven't made *brahmi* ghee), and lubricate the inside of your nostrils with a small amount. (Make sure your nails are trimmed so you don't scratch yourself.) Then gently inhale the ghee upward. This sends a calming message to the brain. You will become quite tranquil; anger and hostility will dissolve like a cloud in the sky.

DO BREATHING EXERCISES. A cooling *pranayama* to help dissipate anger is *shitali pranayama*. Make a tube of your tongue; breathe deeply through your mouth down into your belly; hold the breath for a few seconds; exhale through your nose. Do about 12 repetitions. (See the illustration in chapter 6.)

YOGA POSTURES. Good yoga *asanas* for pitta include the Camel, Cobra, Cow, Boat, Goat, and Bridge poses. (See appendix 4 for illustrations of yoga postures.) Avoid the Headstand or other inverted poses such as the Plow and Shoulder Stand. Do not perform the Sun Salutation; do the Moon Salutation instead.

MEDITATE. There is an ancient method of meditation that involves watching your every emotion come and go, without either naming it or trying to tame it. As the feelings arise, breathe deeply, and exhale the emotions out.

Angina

Angina, or to give it its full name, angina pectoris (chest pain), is a condition created by kapha dosha. Accumulated kapha blocks the flow of *prana* vata into the coronary artery, so that the heart muscles do not receive sufficient blood and oxygen supply. It is a kind of local anemia, resulting in pain that can be severe and frightening. Typically, the pain starts from the breastbone in the center of the chest, goes to the left shoulder, and passes along the inner side of the upper arm to the tip of the little finger.

HERBAL REMEDIES. To heal angina, the following herbal remedy is effective:

shringa bhasma 1/8 part
musta 3 parts
arjuna 3 parts

Take 1/2 teaspoon of this mixture 2 or 3 times a day with warm water.

Another effective remedy is to boil $^1/_2$ cup each of milk and water, add $^1/_2$ teaspoon of *arjuna* and 2 pinches of saffron, and take twice or 3 times a day. You may find this remedy beneficial for both chest pain and heart palpitations.

SPECIAL HERBS. In India, angina is often directly dealt with by taking certain powerful herbs sublingually (under the tongue) to produce immediate relief, as nitroglycerin tablets are often used in modern medicine. Ask your Ayurvedic physician about these herbs.

A HEALING PASTE. Topically, one can apply a paste to the chest. Make the paste of ginger powder (1 teaspoon) and *shringa bhasma* (just a pinch). Add sufficient warm water, and apply.

DEER HORN. Try to get hold of some deer horn. (Indian groceries and Chinese herb stores are possible sources.) Using a mortar and pestle or another kind of grinding stone, rub the deer horn on the rough stone until a little paste is formed. Applying a little of that paste on the chest can instantaneously relieve angina pain.

> TIME TO SEE THE DOCTOR
>
> The heart is a precious, vital organ. Any symptom related to the heart could be a sign of heart disease or a signal that heart disease is developing. So if you have any chest pain that could be due to your heart, please consult your doctor. Especially—but not exclusively—if you get chest pain from less exertion than usual, or if your chest pain lasts longer than a few minutes, treat it as a medical emergency.

GOLD WATER. Taking 1 teaspoon of gold water 2 or 3 times a day before food is also effective. (See appendix 1 for instructions on making gold water.)

YOGA POSTURES. If there is no acute angina pain, you can improve coronary circulation by doing some gentle yoga stretching. Beneficial postures include the Camel pose, Boat pose, Locust pose, gentle Spinal Twist, and Cobra pose. These postures stretch the coronary arteries and increase blood supply to the heart.

Anxiety

Anxiety, which often is associated with insomnia and feelings of fear, is due primarily to aggravation of vata dosha in the nervous system. So to heal anxiety, we have to balance vata.

Here are several effective Ayurvedic remedies to pacify vata, heal anxiety and fear, and improve your sleep.

CALMING TEA. Make a tea of the following herbs:

tagar or valerian 1 part
musta 1 part

Steep $^1/_2$ teaspoon of these herbs in 1 cup hot water for 5 to 10 minutes, and drink.

Time to See the Doctor

Everyone experiences worry and anxiety from time to time. But if severe anxiety continues for a long time or becomes overwhelming and interferes with your social or occupational functioning, medical attention is required. Here are three reasons to see a doctor:

1. You chronically experience severe symptoms such as shortness of breath, chest pressure or pain, and dizziness, along with extreme worry and tension.
2. You have panic attacks—short, unexplained periods of intense fear.
3. You avoid people, places, or situations in order to avoid feeling anxious.

This formula effectively pacifies vata and reduces anxiety. You can drink this tea twice a day.

RELAXING BATH. A warm bath of ginger and baking soda will help you pacify anxiety. Use $^1/_3$ cup ginger and $^1/_3$ cup baking soda in a tubful of water. Soak for 10 to 15 minutes.

ALMOND MILK. Almond milk helps to eliminate anxiety. Soak about 10 raw (not toasted) almonds overnight in water. Peel off the skins, and put the almonds in the blender. Add 1 cup warm milk. While blending, add a pinch of ginger and a small pinch of nutmeg and saffron.

ORANGE JUICE. For anxiety accompanied by a fast heart rate, a cup of orange juice with 1 teaspoon of honey and a pinch of nutmeg powder can be effective.

CALMING PRESSURE POINT. Make a fist with your left hand, so that the fingers rest in the middle of the palm. Locate the point where the middle finger ends, in the "heart" of the palm. Then, with the thumb of your right hand, press firmly on this point in the center of your left hand. Press for 1 minute. This

Ayurvedic Oil Massage

Giving yourself a full-body oil massage will greatly help to reduce anxiety. Vatas should use sesame oil; pittas, sunflower or coconut oil; kaphas, corn oil. Use 6 or 7 ounces of warmed-up *(not hot)* oil, and rub it over your whole body from head to toes. Ordinarily this massage is done before the morning bath, but if you have high anxiety or insomnia, you can also do it before going to bed.

A minimassage is also effective: Using the appropriate oil for your constitution, rub some on your scalp and spend a few minutes rubbing the bottom of your feet.

will calm down the agitation of *prana,* which causes anxiety.

RELAXATION POSE. Lie down on your back in the yoga posture known as *savasana,* the "Corpse" or Relaxation pose, arms by your sides.

MEDITATE TO RELAX. Sitting quietly, focus your attention on the top of your head while doing the *So-Hum* meditation (described in chapter 7).

Appetite, Low

Poor appetite is a condition of low *jatharagni* (digestive fire). Low agni may be due to slow metabolism, or slow metabolism caused by low agni; each affects the other. Low agni creates not only poor appetite but also indigestion, bloating, ama (toxins) in the gastrointestinal tract, coating on the tongue, and bad breath. Lack of energy is also common.

The most effective treatment for this situation may surprise you: Don't eat. A short fast will help to kindle the digestive fire. Skip breakfast, and don't nibble anything. By noon your appetite will probably return, and you will be hungry and ready to eat.

Lack of appetite is often due to continual munching, combined with drinking cold drinks, which depress agni. For the sake of good digestion and long-term health, as well as reviving your appetite, both of these bad habits have to be stopped.

If you are not hungry even by lunchtime, take some fresh ginger, chop a little into small pieces, add some lime juice and a pinch of rock salt, and chew it up. That will kindle agni and stimulate the appetite.

Low appetite may also be due to emotional factors. If that is the case, make a tea of ginger, *brahmi,* and chamomile in equal proportions. Use 1 teaspoon of this mixture per cup of water, steep for 5 to 10 minutes, and drink.

Also, take $^1/_2$ teaspoon of *triphala* in a cup of warm water every night before going to bed. Pour boiling water into the *triphala,* and let it cool until it's comfortable to drink.

These few simple measures should be enough to help you regain a healthy appetite. If you try them and still don't feel like eating, see your doctor, as lack of appetite can be a symptom of a more serious illness.

Arthritis

Ayurveda distinguishes three categories of arthritis, corresponding to vata, pitta, and kapha. To treat this condition properly, it is vital to carefully diagnose which type you have.

TYPES OF ARTHRITIS

• *If arthritis is due to vata,* your joints will crack and pop. They become dry and are not swollen as they may be if excess vata is not the cause. The joints may also feel cold to the touch. They are painful mostly upon movement, and there is usually one particular tender spot. Jogging, jumping, trampolining, or any strenuous exercise tends to aggravate the pain.

• *Pitta-type arthritis* is characterized by inflammation; the joint becomes swollen and is painful even without movement. It often looks red and feels hot to the touch.

• *In kapha-type arthritis,* the joint also becomes stiff and swollen, but it feels cold and clammy rather than hot. A little movement, rather than aggravating the pain, tends to relieve it. The pain is greater in the morning, and as the person starts moving around, the pain diminishes.

FOR ALL TYPES OF ARTHRITIS

Treatment for each type of arthritis is unique, as we shall see in a moment. But for all cases, it is important to know that arthritis begins in the colon.

Depending on the person's lifestyle, diet, and emotional pattern, either vata, pitta, or kapha goes out of balance. Then that particular dosha slows down agni (digestive fire), resulting in the toxic, sticky by-product of inadequate digestion known as ama.

Vata, the main active dosha, brings the ama into the colon, and from there it travels through the system and lodges in the *asthi dhatu* (bone tissue) and in the joints, giving rise to the stiffness and pain characteristic of arthritis.

So our aim in treating arthritis is to remove the ama from the joint and bring it back to the colon, and then to eliminate it.

This is why, to relieve arthritis, it is important to keep the colon clean. To accomplish this, if you do not know positively whether it is vata, pitta, or kapha arthritis, taking *triphala* at night (1 teaspoon) with some warm water (1/2 to 1 cup) will be effective for all types. Alternatively, if you know positively which type it is, you can use *haritaki* for vata-type arthritis, *amalaki* for pitta-type, and *bibhitaki* for kapha-type arthritis (1/2 to 1 teaspoon with warm water in all cases).

Now for the complete treatments.

FOR VATA-TYPE ARTHRITIS

• Follow the vata-pacifying diet (chapter 8). Favor warm, easy-to-digest foods, and avoid cold foods and drinks, including salads. Avoid beans, drying grains such as barley and corn, and the nightshades: tomato, potato, and eggplant.

• Take *yogaraj guggulu,* 1 tablet 3 times per day.

• Apply *mahanarayan* oil on the affected joint, followed by application of local moist heat. For example, say you have an arthritic ankle. Apply the *mahanarayan* oil, rub it into the skin, and then soak your foot in warm to bearably hot water. Add a "teabag" of brown mustard seeds to the water. You can make the bag by wrapping 2 tablespoons of mustard seeds in a handkerchief or cheesecloth.

• Helpful yoga postures include Forward Bend (don't strain), the Chest-Knee pose, Maha Mudra, and the Half Bridge pose. (For illustrations of yoga postures, see appendix 4.)

FOR PITTA-TYPE ARTHRITIS

Pitta arthritis often has more pain and inflammation associated with it than other types.

• Follow the pitta-pacifying diet (chapter 8). Particularly avoid hot, spicy foods, pickles, spinach, and tomatoes.

• These Ayurvedic herbal formulas will help you. Take 1 tablet of *kaishore guggulu* (350 mg.) 3 times a day, and 1/2 teaspoon *sudarshan* twice a day, washed down with warm water.

• Externally, apply cool castor oil or coconut oil to the painful area.

• Application of a cooling substance, such as sandalwood powder paste, is soothing. Make the paste by taking 1 teaspoon of sandalwood powder and adding sufficient water to make a paste. Rub it gently onto the joint.

• If the joint is hot and inflamed, you can put an icebag on it. This will help to ease the pain and inflammation.

• Helpful yoga postures include the Boat, Bow, Camel, Cow, and Locust poses, as well as the series of postures known as the Moon Salutation. (See appendix 4 for illustrations of yoga postures.)

• You can also perform *shitali pranayama*, as follows: Make a tube of your tongue. Breathe deeply through your mouth down into your belly. Hold the breath for a few seconds, then exhale through your nose. Do about 12 repetitions. (See illustration in chapter 6.)

FOR KAPHA-TYPE ARTHRITIS

Arthritis is classified as kapha when the joint is painful, swollen, stiff, and feels cold and clammy to the touch.

• Follow the kapha-reducing diet (chapter 8). Especially, take no dairy products and no cold drinks.

• A potent herbal formula to help with this type of arthritis is *punarnava guggulu* tablets (250 mg.). Take 1 tablet 3 times a day.

• Externally, you can apply a paste of *vacha* (calamus root) powder. Add sufficient warm water to 1 teaspoon of powder to make a paste, and apply to the joint.

• When there is an effusion (when the joint fills with fluid), you can make an effective paste of equal amounts of *punarnava* powder and ginger powder. Mix 1 teaspoon of each with enough warm water to form a paste, and apply.

• Yoga postures that are helpful for kapha-type arthritis include the Tree, Triangle, Forward Bend, and Spinal Twist. (Illustrations of yoga postures appear in appendix 4.)

RHEUMATOID AND OSTEOARTHRITIS

In addition to the vata–pitta–kapha method of classifying arthritis, this condition can also be classified as either rheumatoid arthritis or osteoarthritis. If you are sure which condition you have, the following guidelines will add more specificity to your treatment.

FOR RHEUMATOID ARTHRITIS. Take 1 *simhanada guggulu* tablet (350 mg.) 3 times a day, and 1 *chitrak-adhivati* (200 mg.) tablet twice a day.

• A quarter teaspoon of *yogaraj guggulu* washed down with a little warm water 3 times a day is also recommended.

• You can also drink 1 cup of ginger tea with 2 teaspoons of castor oil added. Castor oil contains natural precursors of steroids, which help to heal the inflammatory condition of rheumatoid arthritis. Take this tea before going to bed. Expect some laxative effect from the castor oil.

FOR OSTEOARTHRITIS. Take 1 tablet of *yogaraj guggulu* twice a day. At night, take 1/2 teaspoon *gandharva haritaki* (*haritaki* sautéed in castor oil) with warm water. If you don't have *gandharva haritaki*, use ginger tea with castor oil, as described above.

Asthma and Wheezing

Bronchial asthma is characterized by sudden attacks of short, gasping breaths accompanied by wheezing. If the attack is not stopped, the person may have increasing difficulty breathing.

The underlying cause of all asthmatic conditions is increased kapha dosha in the stomach. From there it moves into the lungs, trachea, and bronchi. The increased kapha blocks the natural flow of air, creating spasm in the bronchial tree and resulting in asthma and wheezing.

Ayurvedic treatment for asthma aims to bring the kapha lodged in the lungs and bronchi back to the stomach, from which it can be eliminated.

Asthma may be brought on by allergies, a

To Immediately Stop Wheezing

Boil 1 teaspoon of licorice root (*yashti madhu*) in a cup of water for a couple of minutes to make a licorice tea. Just before drinking the tea, add 5 to 10 drops of *mahanarayan* oil if you have some, or use 1/2 teaspoon of plain ghee. Take one sip of this tea every 5 to 10 minutes.

In some instances, the licorice tea may induce vomiting. This is beneficial: It eliminates kapha and relieves the spasm of the bronchial tubes, and the person usually feels better immediately.

You can use this licorice tea not only for emergencies but, if you are prone to develop asthma, every day as a preventive. The only exception is that individuals with hypertension should not use much licorice tea, as it makes the body retain sodium. They may take it as an emergency measure to avert an asthma attack, but they should not drink it regularly.

NOTE: Prepare the tea as soon as you begin to feel an attack coming on, when there is tightness in the chest, some difficulty breathing, or whatever warning bell symptoms you recognize from past experiences. Don't wait until you are already having serious problems breathing.

Once you prepare the tea, it can last for 72 hours and not lose its effectiveness.

cold, congestion, cough, or hay fever. It can be instigated by pollen, dust, animal hair, or various foods, or an increase of kapha internally. Regardless of the cause, during an asthmatic attack it is important to immediately relieve the difficult breathing and asthmatic wheezing.

HERBAL REMEDIES

The following herbal remedies can be taken on a regular basis for long-term prevention of asthma.

• Mix 1 teaspoon cinnamon and 1/4 teaspoon *trikatu* into a cup of boiling water. Let it steep for 10 minutes, and add 1 teaspoon of honey before drinking. You can take this tea twice a day.

• A tea made of half licorice and half ginger is also beneficial for asthma prevention. Use half a teaspoon of the combined herbs per cupful of water.

• Also try 1/2 teaspoon bay leaf and 1/4 teaspoon *pippali* mixed into 1 teaspoon honey, taken 2 or 3 times a day.

• Another remedy that can relieve congestion and alleviate breathlessness is 1/4 cup onion juice with 1 teaspoon honey and 1/8 teaspoon black pepper. This remedy will also be effective for immediate relief of asthma.

• This herbal formula is helpful both for prevention and immediate relief:

sitopaladi 1/2 *teaspoon*
punarnava 1/2 *teaspoon*
pippali *pinch*
abrak bhasma *pinch*

For immediate relief, take this entire mixture with honey, a little bit at a time. For long-term usage, take it once a day.

• You may also find 1/3 cup spinach juice with a pinch of *pippali* effective. Drink this twice a day.

THREE MUSTARD SEED REMEDIES

Mustard seeds are effective in healing the bronchial system. Here are three ways to take advantage of their heating and healing power:

1. Rubbing a little brown mustard oil onto your chest will give some relief.
2. Make a tea by mixing ground mustard seeds and *pippali* (or black pepper if you don't have *pippali*). Steep 1/4 teaspoon of each for 10 minutes in 1 cup hot water, then add 1 to 2 teaspoons honey. Drink 2 or 3 times a day, or for better results sip it every 15 minutes throughout the day.
3. Mix 1 teaspoon of brown mustard oil with 1 teaspoon natural organic sugar. Take 2 or 3 times a day on an empty stomach.

OTHER APPROACHES

IF YOU HAVE AN INFECTION. In some people, the underlying cause of asthmatic wheezing may be an infection descending from the nose and sinuses. If this is the case, putting 5 to 10 drops of warm ghee in each nostril will help.

TRY TO AVOID ALLERGENS. If your asthma and wheezing are due to a food allergy, then avoid the problematic food. Similarly, avoid any object that may provoke your condition, such as dusty books, moldy basements, and some chemicals.

FOODS TO AVOID. Avoid most dairy products, including all cheeses. Avoid fermented foods and all hydrophilic food substances such as salty items, cucumber, and tuna fish. Some people need to avoid mushrooms, peanuts, walnuts and other nuts, and yeast. The reaction may be immediate, for people extremely sensitive to these substances, or it may take several hours to develop.

FOR CHRONIC BRONCHIAL ASTHMA. If you have chronic bronchial asthma, try this remedy. Insert about 7 cloves into a peeled banana, and keep it overnight. Next morning eat the banana and the cloves. Don't eat anything for an hour, then drink 1 cup of hot water with 1 teaspoon of honey. This will energize the lungs and should reduce asthmatic wheezing.

YOGA FOR ASTHMA. Effective yoga *asanas* to help relieve asthma are the Bow and Cobra poses, sitting in the Vajrasana, and the inverted poses including Shoulder Stand and Plow. (Illustrations of yoga postures appear in appendix 4.)

> **TIME TO SEE THE DOCTOR**
>
> Asthma can ordinarily be controlled using these Ayurvedic remedies. However, if you find that medicines that ordinarily help you breathe more comfortably no longer seem to be working, or if, along with your difficulty breathing, you have chest pain, swollen feet, and profuse sweating, and you have a history of heart problems, you need to seek immediate medical attention.

Athlete's Foot

People with kapha–pitta constitutions, who sweat a lot, are most prone to get athlete's foot. This is an itchy, inflammatory condition between the toes, often accompanied by sweating on the soles of the feet.

Athlete's foot can be effectively treated with Ayurvedic remedies. Begin by cleaning the problem area with some tea tree oil on a cotton swab. This natural antiseptic oil is widely available in natural food stores and elsewhere.

Then apply a mixture of aloe vera gel and turmeric. Mix 1 teaspoon of aloe vera gel with 1/2 teaspoon turmeric, and apply some of the mixture to the affected areas. But be a little careful: This mixture will turn your skin and socks yellow! If you use it at night, it will stain your sheets, so you might wear a pair of old socks to prevent the discoloration. Continue with this treatment twice a day for at least 2 weeks

An alternative treatment is to wash your feet with *neem* soap. Then dry thoroughly with a hair drier or soft towel, and apply some *neem* oil (about 1/4 teaspoon) mixed with about 10 drops of tea tree oil. Apply that mixture topically to the affected area with a cotton swab.

If you have athlete's foot or are prone to get it, avoid fermented food and sugar.

Backache

Backache is uncommonly common these days. It has become an occupational hazard in many different kinds of work. People may pull or strain their back muscles while lifting a heavy load or while sitting at a desk in front of a computer. Emotional factors can also lead to back pain, as can injuries, such as from a car accident. Some people may even have a slipped disk, which can lead to severe back pain. Whatever the cause of your backache, the following natural Ayurvedic home remedies will be helpful.

HERBAL REMEDIES. Take *yogaraj guggulu,* 1 tablet 3 times a day, or 1 tablet of *kaishore guggulu* 2 or 3 times a day. Both of these special Ayurvedic formulas are available from most sources of Ayurvedic herbs (see Resources).

- Backache can also be relieved by the use of the herb *musta,* which is a muscle painkiller. Take 1/4 to 1/2 teaspoon 2 or 3 times a day with warm water.
- The herbs *tagara* and valerian are muscle relaxants. Taking 1/2 teaspoon of either with some warm water will relax the muscles that may be causing back pain. It will also help induce restful sleep.

Most back pain can be effectively treated with these herbs, but a ruptured or slipped disk often requires intensive medical care.

RUB IN SOME OIL. Rubbing the painful area of the back with *mahanarayan* oil is also effective for relieving the pain. Vata and pitta types should just rub the oil on the surface, while kapha types should give a deeper massage to the area for some time.

Alternatively, try this procedure: Apply a paste made of ginger powder mixed with sufficient water to the affected area. Leave it on for 10 to 15 minutes, wash it off, and then rub the back with some eucalyptus oil.

(Unless your back pain is in the neck or shoulder area, these back rubs will have to be done by a friend!)

TAKE A HOT HERBALIZED BATH. For extra healing and muscle relaxation, apply the *mahanarayan* oil on your back and then follow with a hot bath in which you put some ginger powder and baking soda (1/3 cup of each). Soak in the tub for 10 to 15 minutes. You may repeat this bath 2 or 3 times a week, perhaps on Tuesday, Thursday, and Saturday.

AN ENEMA CAN HELP. Individuals who suffer from backache often get constipated, and it may be difficult to tell which is the effect and which is the cause. The backache may be due to chronic constipation, or the spasming muscles and anxiety caused by the back pain may induce constipation. In either case, a simple enema of *dashamoola* tea will help.

Boil 1 tablespoon of *dashamoola* powder in a pint of water for about 5 minutes, cool it down, and add 1/2 cup sesame oil. When it is cool enough, use it as an enema, retaining the liquid for 5 to 10 minutes if you can. A *dashamoola*–sesame oil enema is soothing to vata and will help relieve both the constipation and the pain. (See appendix 3 for enema guidelines.)

GENTLE STRETCHES. Some gentle yoga exercises can help with back pain.

> IMPORTANT: All yoga postures should be learned with a trained yoga teacher, but especially when you have a backache, you should not do any yoga postures without expert guidance. This is especially true if your pain comes from a slipped disk.

In general, the following postures may be helpful:

Camel pose	Lotus pose
Cow pose	Forward Bend
Spinal Twist	Palm Tree pose
Locust pose	gentle, modified Fish pose

All these postures may be used both as a preventive measure and to help remedy back pain. But again, be sure to get advice from a trained teacher. (Illustrations of yoga postures appear in appendix 4.)

MORE TIPS TO HELP HEAL BACKACHE

- Backache is often due to excess vata, so it is helpful to reduce your consumption of vata-increasing foods. Avoid most beans, including black beans, pinto beans, adzuki beans, and garbanzo beans. Avoid raw, cold salads. (See chapter 8 for more on the vata-pacifying diet.)
- Avoid exposure to cold weather or cold winds.
- Sit quietly and meditate, or observe your breathing. This will help relax tense muscles. (For help with meditation, see chapter 7.)
- Don't walk in high-heeled shoes.
- Don't try to do jogging, jumping, or other strenuous exercise; rather, do some gentle yoga stretching as mentioned above.
- Sexual activity should be minimized.

Following these guidelines will help you heal your aching back as well as avoid back pain in the future.

Bad Breath

Bad breath is often a sign of systemic toxicity, either in the colon, intestine, or mouth. It can also be due to chronic indigestion or malabsorption. When digestion is weak or sluggish, the food you eat undergoes fermentation and putrefaction in the gastrointestinal tract, leading to the formation of ama, which has a foul smell.

Stand in front of a mirror, and stick out your tongue. If the back portion of the tongue is coated, that is the sign of ama, which is responsible for the bad breath.

The primary Ayurvedic aim in treating bad breath is to kindle gastric fire (agni), which in turn burns ama and alleviates the root cause of the condition. Here are several effective home remedies to prevent and treat bad breath.

DIETARY AND HERBAL REMEDIES

- First monitor your diet. It's important not to eat heavy meals, and to stay away from cold drinks, ice cream, cheese, and yogurt, all of which reduce the gastric fire and slow down digestion, with a likely increase of ama.

• Then, after each meal (generally after lunch and dinner), chew about 1 teaspoon of roasted fennel and cumin seeds (mixed half and half). This will improve digestion, which indirectly helps to detoxify the colon. The licorice-flavored fennel seeds alone would be delicious and helpful, but this mixture will have a better effect.

• Drink 1/2 cup of aloe vera juice twice a day until freshness is restored to the breath.

• Slowly chewing one or two cardamom seeds also helps to minimize bad breath. Cardamom aids digestion and helps to reduce ama.

• After each meal, drink a cup of cumin-coriander-fennel tea (equal proportions) as a digestive aid. Steep about 1/4 to 1/2 teaspoon of each herb per cup of hot water.

OTHER REMEDIES

TAKE CARE OF YOUR TEETH AND GUMS. Another cause of bad breath is poor oral hygiene. It's important to clean the teeth after each meal. Use an Ayurvedic toothpaste containing *neem* or an herbal formula. Also use dental floss every day. Applying some tea tree oil mixed half and half with *neem* oil to the gums and gently massaging will help prevent receding gums. Be sure to spit out the residue rather than swallowing. (See "Teeth and Gums—Ayurvedic Care.")

YOGA POSTURES. The yoga posture known as Yoga Mudra, the Lion pose, and sitting in the Lotus posture with a Forward Bend are good *asanas* for combating bad breath (see appendix 4).

BREATHING EXERCISE. You can also do the *pranayama* known as *shitali* (see instructions in chapter 6).

If you follow these guidelines, you can say good-bye to bad breath.

Baldness

See also "Hair Care Secrets"

Hair loss is a subtle metabolic disorder. It may be related to disease—I have seen hair loss in persons with diabetes, for example, or following typhoid infection. It may be due to some fungal infection on the scalp, or to hormonal imbalance. A deficiency of calcium, magnesium, and zinc may affect the nourishment of the hair enough that the hair starts to fall out. And there is a definite hereditary factor, in which genes appear to trigger hair loss at a certain age.

According to Ayurveda, early hair loss is often related to body type and the balance of the doshas. Pitta individuals, and those who have excess pitta in their system, are more likely than the other body types to lose their hair early in life, or to find that their hair becomes prematurely thin or gray. Excess pitta in the sebaceous gland, at the root of the hair, or folliculitis (inflammation of the hair follicles) can make the person start losing hair.

ALOE VERA. To reduce pitta and preserve the health of your hair, drink aloe vera juice (1/3 cup) or take some aloe vera gel (1 tablespoon with a pinch of cumin) 3 times a day for about 3 months.

OIL MASSAGE. Another effective way to pacify pitta is to rub some coconut oil on your scalp and on the soles of your feet at bedtime. Wear some old socks, and to preserve the health of your pillow, wear a loose woolen cap or cover the pillow with a towel so it won't get damaged by the oil.

• Massaging the scalp with *brahmi* oil or *bhringaraj* oil at bedtime can help to prevent hair loss. In addition to the qualities of the oil, the massage itself will improve circulation at the root of the hair, thus bringing more nutrients to support hair growth.

• Massaging the hair with vitamin E oil may also be effective in preventing or slowing hair loss.

FOOD FOR YOUR HAIR. Healthy hair depends upon a nourishing diet. Dairy products such as cheese, milk, and yogurt are beneficial for the hair (assuming you digest them well), as are white radish and daikon. Coconut, cooked apples, and cabbage are also useful.

• Eat a handful of white sesame seeds every morning. One handful of these small seeds contains about 1,200 mg. of calcium and magnesium and is a good source of nourishment for your hair.

HERBS FOR YOUR HAIR. Certain herbs are useful for nourishing the hair. Try this beneficial formula:

dashamoola	*5 parts*
bhringaraj	*4 parts*
jatamamsi	*3 parts*

At bedtime, add ½ teaspoon of this mixture to 1 cup of goat's milk, heat to boiling, and drink. This will build up the bones and nourish the hair.

MINERAL SUPPLEMENTS. You may also be able to improve the condition of your hair by taking mineral supplements to be sure you have enough calcium, magnesium, and zinc. Take a supplement containing approximately the following daily dose of minerals:

calcium	1,200 mg.
magnesium	600 mg.
zinc	60 mg.

Take these supplements at bedtime.

MASSAGE. Stress, stiffness in the neck, and whiplash from a car accident can also contribute to hair loss. To soften the neck muscles, relieve pain, and reduce stress, massage your neck and shoulder muscles before showering.

NECK EXERCISES. You can also do some simple neck exercises, such as turning your head to the left 3 times, to the right 3 times, lifting it up 3 times, moving it down toward your chest 3 times, and then rolling it gently in a circle 3 times in each direction.

ANTISTRESS TEA. To help you deal with stress, make a tea of equal proportions of *jatamamsi* and *brahmi*. Steep 1 teaspoon of the mix in 1 cup of hot water, and drink 2 or 3 times a day.

YOGA POSTURES. Yoga postures can help to relieve tension in your neck and indirectly aid in keeping hair healthy. Recommended postures include the Shoulder Stand, Camel pose, Cobra pose, and Cow pose. (Illustrations appear in appendix 4.)

MEDITATE FOR RELAXATION. You will also find meditation an effective means for reducing stress and tension. Try sitting quietly and observing your breathing. Or try the Empty Bowl meditation (described in chapter 7).

Bites and Stings

Any bite or sting of an insect can trigger a local irritation of pitta under the skin. As long as the venom of the insect remains there, it may keep on creating periodic allergic reactions, or may even create sting-bite nephritis, a serious condition involving generalized edema (swelling) and breathlessness, and the person can choke. So stings and bites, though usually quite innocuous, may occasionally be very serious; one has to be watchful.

CILANTRO. As soon as possible after receiving a sting or bite, take some cilantro juice. Place a handful of cilantro in a blender with about 1/3 cup water, blend thoroughly, and strain it. Drink the juice (use 2 teaspoons 3 times a day), and apply the pulp locally to the skin at the affected area. It will instantaneously pacify the itching, burning, and hives or rash created by the sting or bite.

DRINK COCONUT WATER. One can drink 1/3 cup of coconut water (the "juice" inside the coconut) with about 1/8 teaspoon *kama dudha* added. Drinking this mixture 2 or 3 times will help heal the reaction to the sting bite.

COCONUT ASH. Here is another simple and fascinating remedy. Take a piece of dried coconut, and set fire to it. It will catch fire like wax. Let it burn for about 1/2 inch and then blow it out. There will be a little smoke, and when the smoke disappears, a tarry black residue will remain. Apply that residue directly to the bite for instant relief.

Why does this work? Because coconut is a good source both for antihistamines and for natural steroids.

You may do the same thing with the ash from burning some of the outer coconut shell.

APPLY *NEEM* OIL OR *NEEM* PASTE. At the site of the bite, you can also apply *neem* oil or a *neem* paste. *Neem* is an antidote to most poisonous insect venoms. To make a paste, take a little *neem* powder and mix it with a little water. Apply it to the skin and leave it on for 10 to 20 minutes, then rinse it off. Do not use pure *neem* extract; instead use an herbalized oil made by boiling *neem* leaves in a sesame oil base. This is generally available in natural food stores or Indian groceries.

A HEALING PASTE. You will also find a paste made from 1/2 teaspoon of sandalwood powder plus 1/2 teaspoon turmeric soothing and healing. Mix the two herbs together with sufficient water to make a paste, and apply topically to the site of the bite.

PREVENTION. *Neem* oil is a much-used insect repellent in India and around the world. It contains a natural chemical compound that repels insects. Rub a little onto exposed skin before going outdoors.

Bladder Problems

See also "Urinary Incontinence"

Problems with the bladder and urination

may indicate cystitis, an inflammation of the bladder that causes a burning sensation when passing urine. Other bladder problems include frequent urination, or its opposite, stagnation or retention of urine in the bladder, leading to bladder distension. There may be pain in the bladder area while urinating, a condition called strangury. Let's look at each of these.

RETENTION OF URINE IN THE BLADDER

In this condition the bladder is distended but the person doesn't pass urine. It may be due to constriction of the urethra, enlargement of the prostate gland, or perhaps a stone in the urethra. The causes may be many, but the cure is simple:

- Take two towels or sponges, one dipped in hot water, the other dipped in cool water. About every minute, alternate placing them in the bladder area. This alternation of hot and cold stimulates the bladder, and the person easily passes urine.
- If alternating hot and cold compresses isn't completely successful, apply *punarnava* paste (*punarnava* powder with sufficient water to make a paste) to the skin directly above the distended bladder. Leave it on for about half an hour.
- If the retention is due to stricture (narrowing) in the urethra or enlargement of the prostate gland, then use this formula:

punarnava guggulu 4 parts
shilajit 1 part

Taking $1/2$ teaspoon of this mixture 3 times a day with warm water will help to dilate the stricture or relax the prostate gland and help to restore the easy flow of the urine.

CYSTITIS

Cystitis causes a burning sensation while urinating. To relieve this condition, drink coriander tea, cumin tea, or fennel tea. Or make a tea of equal proportions of these three herbs. Cumin-coriander-fennel tea is widely used in Ayurveda to relieve irritation of the bladder while passing urine.

You may also find this mixture effective for cystitis:

punarnava 5 parts
gokshura 4 parts
musta 3 parts

Take $1/2$ teaspoon of this herbal mixture 2 or 3 times a day with warm water.

BLADDER ATONIA

This is a condition in which the bladder's sphincter loses its tone or strength, and the bladder leaks urine. It is more common among women. A woman may sneeze or cough and inadvertently passes some urine. For this condition, take one handful of white sesame seeds along with 1 teaspoon of jaggery or natural, unrefined brown sugar, and chew it well, followed by half a cup of water to wash it down. This is a very simple remedy to bring tone back to the bladder. Take it once or twice a day until your condition is better.

For further discussion and suggestions, see "Urinary Incontinence" and "Prostate Problems."

Bleeding, External

Generally, within 5 to 6 minutes after getting a cut, the bleeding will stop by itself. The blood will clot, the bleeding will stop, and the cut will be sealed. In such cases—the vast majority—there is nothing much to do unless the cut is severe and bleeding is excessive.

Some people, however, bleed for a longer time, because the blood does not cooperate and clot quickly enough. When a person continues to bleed, it basically means that the blood is too thin. Although the problem usually has a relatively simple and benign cause, failure of the blood to clot—or gums, cuts, or wounds that start to bleed—may also be an early sign of blood cancer, leukemia, or hemophilia purpura, a pitta disorder that causes profuse bleeding under the skin.

From the Ayurvedic perspective, blood that fails to clot in a timely manner is due to a pitta imbalance. Excess pitta in the blood makes the blood hot, sharp, and penetrating and doesn't allow natural coagulation and clotting to occur. The basic prescription, then, is to follow a pitta-soothing diet, use pitta-soothing herbs, and take specifically hemostatic herbs, herbs that directly help to stop bleeding.

APPLY COLD. To stop external bleeding, start by applying cold. Use some ice (plain or wrapped in a cloth), which helps to constrict the blood vessels and stop bleeding. A bag of frozen vegetables from the freezer will do the job in an emergency.

APPLY PRESSURE. Other simple ways to stop bleeding, well known to most people, are

1. tying a tourniquet
2. applying pressure directly over the bleeding area
3. if the bleeding is in an extremity, raising the arm or leg higher than the rest of the body.

ALOE. Another effective approach is to apply some aloe. A pinch of aloe powder mixed into a paste with a pinch of turmeric powder will immediately stop most bleeding. Aloe vera gel will also be effective.

ASTRINGENT HERBS. Other astringent herbs are also effective. The Ayurvedic herbs *lodhra, kushtha,* and *bilva* are effective to stop bleeding, either alone or mixed in equal proportions into a paste that can be applied directly. They are also effective taken internally for continuing problems with bleeding; use 1/2 teaspoon 2 or 3 times a day.

COTTON ASH. For external bleeding, you will find this ancient, simple remedy effective. Take a small ball of sterilized cotton, and burn it. (Be sure it is real cotton, not the synthetic material often found these days, which will be totally ineffective.) When the cotton turns to black ash, wait for it to cool down, and then apply it to the bleeding wound and press. The ash will stick to the bleeding point and stop the bleeding instantaneously. Within a couple of days a scab will form, and the wound will completely heal.

NOTE: Don't remove the ash; leave it on the wound to form a scab. Otherwise you will open the cut again.

DRINK COLD WATER. Many times just drinking some cold water will stop the bleeding, as coolness constricts blood vessels.

Bleeding, Internal

See also "Rectal Bleeding"

Cases of internal bleeding include peptic ulcer, hematoma (a blood-filled swelling), and bleeding through the urethra. To help put a stop to the bleeding, make an herbal compound out of these Ayurvedic herbs:

lodhra
kushtha
bilva

Mix these herbs in equal amounts, and take 1/2 teaspoon 2 or 3 times a day. Each of these herbs helps to stop bleeding, so you can use just one if that's all you can locate, though the mixture will be most effective.

Pitta people bruise more easily; their blood vessels are thin and are more easily ruptured. People with pitta constitutions can help prevent internal bleeding by taking the same three Ayurvedic herbs, *lodhra, kushtha,* and *bilva.* Mix the three herbs in equal amounts, and take 1/2 teaspoon of the mixture 2 or 3 times a day with warm water, for as long as the condition lasts.

> **TIME TO SEE THE DOCTOR**
>
> The appearance of blood in the urine or stools can be a sign of serious illness such as kidney problems or cancer, and it should be investigated more deeply in consultation with your physician.

TURMERIC PASTE. When a person has been injured, the blood vessels sometimes rupture, causing a large bruise and a blood-filled swelling known as a hematoma. To stop the internal bleeding and pacify the hematomalike swelling, apply a paste made of 1 teaspoon turmeric powder, 1 teaspoon sandalwood powder, and a pinch of alum powder. (Mix the powders together with a little water to make a paste.) When the paste is on the skin, apply some pressure on the hematoma.

SAFFRON MILK. Another aid to stopping internal bleeding is to drink a cup of warm milk, to which 1/2 teaspoon of turmeric powder and a pinch of saffron have been added.

JUICES. Drinking cranberry or pomegranate juice is also helpful to stop internal bleeding.

Boils

Boils—painful, pus-filled inflammations of the skin and subcutaneous tissue—have many causes. They may be due to chronic constipation, or to high pitta in the blood. A toxic liver can also create boils. Repeated boils may be a sign of diabetes, so if you get boils repeatedly, check on your blood sugar.

NEEM POWDER PASTE. At the site of the boil, apply a paste of *neem* powder (preferably) or some *neem* oil. To make the paste, simply mix a little *neem* powder with warm water.

TRIPHALA WASH. Wash the affected area with *triphala* tea. Boil 1 teaspoon *triphala* in 1 cup of water. Cool, and wash your face or other affected area with the tea. Let it dry on the skin. (For information about *triphala*, see appendix 2.)

FOR DIABETES. If there is a history of diabetes in the family and you get repeated boils, use this formula:

neem 1 part
turmeric 1 part
kutki 1/2 part

Taking 1/2 teaspoon of this mixture 2 or 3 times a day with warm water will help take care of the root cause of the boil. Continue taking it until the boil disappears.

FOR CHRONIC CONSTIPATION. If the boil appears to be due to chronic constipation, do a *basti* (enema) using *dashamoola* tea. Boil 1 tablespoon of the herb *dashamoola* in a pint of water for 5 minutes. Let the liquid cool, strain it, and use it for an enema.

In addition, take 1/2 teaspoon of *amalaki* or the herbal compound *triphala* at night. Steep the *triphala* in a cup of hot water for 5 to 10 minutes and then drink. This purgation will help to remove excess pitta from the hematopoietic (blood-building) system, which is the cause of the boil. You may continue taking the *triphala* or *amalaki* indefinitely, even after the boil is healed, as a preventive and general health tonic.

COOLING, HEALING PASTE. Apply a paste of red sandalwood and turmeric powder locally. Use 1/2 teaspoon of each powder, and mix them together in warm water to make a paste.

BRING THE BOIL TO A HEAD. Apply cooked onions as a poultice, or apply a paste of ginger powder and turmeric (1/2 teaspoon of each) directly to the boil, to bring it to a head.

LIVER CLEANSERS. A boil may develop into an abscess, if the boil is due to an infection of the sebaceous glands (a pitta condition). It becomes inflamed, raised, and red. If you use a formula to help cleanse the liver, the condition will be improved.

A simple and effective liver cleanser is aloe vera gel. Take 2 tablespoons 3 times a day.

Or you may try this Ayurvedic formula:

shanka pushpi 3 parts
kutki 2 parts
gulwel sattva 1/8 part

Take 1/2 teaspoon of this mixture 3 times a day with warm water.

Breastfeeding Problems

There are several types of breastfeeding problems. Let's take them one at a time.

THE CHILD HAS NO APPETITE

In this case, the mother is producing a lot of milk, but the child has no appetite. Here are a number of effective, natural ways to help.

DRINK FENNEL TEA. Make a tea by steeping 1 teaspoon of fennel seeds in a cupful of boiled water. When the tea cools, give the baby 1 teaspoonful every 10 to 15 minutes.

Childhood is the kapha stage of life, when the body is building. It is also the time when many kapha disorders occur (such as colds and runny noses) and when kapha may stagnate in the stomach, slowing down the appetite. Giving this fennel tea will help to wash out the kapha and in a gentle way stimulate the secretion of digestive enzymes.

MAKE *GHRITA MADHU*. Mix a pinch of *pippali* in 1/2 teaspoon of honey combined with 1/2 teaspoon ghee. Give it to your baby to lick. The more he or she licks the mixture, the more the appetite will come back.

MONITOR YOUR DIET. One possible reason for a baby's apparent lack of appetite is that your milk may not taste good to the child. If you tend to have excess pitta in your constitution, and especially if your diet is hot and spicy or includes sour foods and fruits, your milk may become bitter, and the baby won't like it. This unpleasant taste could be the cause of the child's apparent lack of appetite. So it is important to determine the mother's *prakruti* (constitutional type) and to be sure the diet she is eating is appropriate.

EMPTY YOUR BREASTS. If your child has a diminished appetite and you are secreting more milk than gets used, it is important to empty your breasts. This will avoid congestion of the mastic and lymphatic tissue. Be sure the breasts are emptied of milk at least 2 or 3 times a day.

IF YOU DECIDE NOT TO BREASTFEED. A related situation occurs when a woman chooses not to breastfeed her child. Then the milk is stagnant, which may be one of the causes of fibrocystic changes in the breast. So it is important to empty the breasts whenever milk is present.

THERE IS INSUFFICIENT MILK

The child has a strong appetite, but lactation is scanty. This problem is the reverse of the first. Here are several suggestions to increase the quality and quantity of milk.

***SHATAVARI KALPA*.** To increase lactation, Ayurveda recommends a delicious concoction called *shatavari kalpa*: the herb *shatavari* roasted in a pan with ghee and natural brown sugar. Take one teaspoon of that sweet, roasted *shatavari* in warm milk 2 or 3 times a day.

PLAIN *SHATAVARI*. You can also use plain *shatavari* with ghee and sugar. Mix together equal amounts of *shatavari* and natural sugar, and take 1 teaspoon of the mixture with 1 teaspoon of ghee along with a cup of hot milk.

ALMOND MILK. Another formula to increase breast milk is almond milk. Soak 10 almonds overnight in water. In the morning, peel them and blend them in the blender with a cup of hot water or hot milk. Pour the mixture into a cup or glass, and add 1 teaspoon honey or date sugar, and a pinch each of ginger, cardamom, and saffron. Drink twice a day.

HERBAL FORMULA. To maintain healthy lactation, use this herbal formula:

kutki 2 *parts*
shilajit 2 *parts*
shatavari 3 *parts*

Take 1/4 teaspoon of this mixture 2 or 3 times a day with a spoonful of honey. If you wish, you may use this formula the entire time you are breastfeeding.

INFECTED NIPPLE

A third problem is that during the time you are nursing your child, the nipple is not properly cleaned and a fungal infection develops. So take care to wash carefully to prevent this from happening.

PREVENTION

To prevent breast abscess, mastitis, congestion, and stagnation of milk in the breast, gently massage your breasts with warm castor oil. Take 1 teaspoon of the oil, and gently massage the breast from inside outward—that is, from the sternum (breastbone) back toward the armpit, both underneath and around the nipple, and to the side.

Do not apply the castor oil to the areola and nipple. If you apply castor oil to the nipple and your baby sucks the oil, he or she may get diarrhea. So either avoid the nipple or wash off the oil before nursing the child.

Breasts, Sore

Sore breasts are generally symptomatic of hormonal imbalance, lymphatic congestion, or premenstrual syndrome. Or the physical discomfort may be associated with some emotional factor, such as grief or sadness. Here are several suggestions for effective self-treatment:

GENTLE MASSAGE. Take 1 teaspoon of warm castor oil, and gently massage the breast from inside outward, that is, from the sternum (breastbone) back toward the armpit, both underneath and around the nipple, and to the side. This kind of gentle massage before the morning bath, as well as at bedtime, will help to relieve the soreness.

HERBS FOR WATER RETENTION. Water retention may also be responsible for sore breasts. The breasts become tender, swollen, and enlarged, and the bra becomes tight. To reduce the swelling, make the following herbal mixture:

For a Constipated Baby

In India, if a nursing baby becomes constipated, the mother intentionally applies a few drops of castor oil to her nipple. Then, when the baby sucks the milk, those few drops of castor oil are taken in along with the milk, and the constipation is relieved in a gentle way.

punarnava 1 *part*
shatavari 1 *part*
musta 1 *part*

Use 1/2 teaspoon of this mix in 1 cup hot water to make a tea, and drink it. Then massage the breasts as above, and you will see remarkable improvement. You may drink the tea twice a day until the soreness goes away.

ANOTHER EFFECTIVE HERBAL REMEDY. Sore breasts can also be treated with another herbal combination:

jatamamsi 2 *parts*
shatavari 3 *parts*
tagar 3 *parts*

Mix the herbs together in the above proportions, and use 1/2 teaspoon in a cup of water to make a tea. Steep for 5 to 10 minutes, and drink. You can use this tea twice a day until the soreness is gone.

NOTE: Never use an overly tight bra for long periods of time. The pressure obstructs circulation, and the breast tissue stops breathing. It is better to use a cotton bra that allows proper breathing of the mastic tissue.

Brittle Nails

The nails of our fingers and toes are considered in Ayurveda to be a by-product of bone formation (*asthi dhatu*). Proper nutrition for building strong bones is thus essential if you want to have healthy nails. If there is insufficient intake of calcium and magnesium, or malabsorption of these minerals, the nails become rough, brittle, cracked, and split, and ridges and creases may appear. If you have these symptoms, you can be sure they are signs of malnutrition of the bone tissue.

To strengthen the bones and nails, take over-the-counter supplements of calcium, magnesium, and zinc. Your formula should include a daily dose of approximately

calcium	1,200 mg.
magnesium	600 mg.
zinc	60 mg.

Take the supplements at bedtime for best results. A general mineral supplement might also be helpful.

You may be getting enough minerals, but toxins in the colon may be preventing their complete absorption. If you are taking calcium, magnesium, and zinc as a dietary supplement and your nails are still brittle, that indicates that you are not absorbing these minerals. The culprit is overaccumulation of toxins (ama) in the colon.

A safe and simple way to cleanse the colon of the ama is to regularly take the herbal compound *triphala* (see appendix 2). Steep about 1/2 teaspoon in 1/2 to 1 full cup of warm water, strain, and drink. You can take this at night before going to bed, or steep it overnight in cold water and drink it first thing in the morning. It will gradually eliminate the ama.

Another way to promote the growth and strength of your nails is to eat a handful of white sesame seeds every day. A handful of sesame seeds contains about 1,200 mg. of calcium and magnesium.

Either one of the Ayurvedic herbs *ashwa-*

gandha or *shatavari* (1/2 teaspoon) taken in a cup of hot milk twice a day may also help to prevent brittle nails.

Aerobic exercise such as swimming, jogging, or aerobic dance, or the sequence of yoga postures known as the Sun Salutation (see illustration in appendix 4), should also be helpful. Exercise improves the circulation and helps carry the minerals to the tissue at the root of the nails.

Because the nails are connected with the *asthi dhatu* (bone tissue), strengthening *asthi* will be helpful. Taking *triphala guggulu* tablets (200 mg.) twice a day, after lunch and dinner, will help to strengthen your nails.

In some individuals, brittle nails and bone loss go together. Specifically, in women of menopausal age, brittle nails may suggest weakness in the *asthi dhatu*. So if you have brittle nails, it would be wise to investigate the possibility that osteoporosis may be developing.

Burns

Many people believe the best thing you can do for a burn is to put something fatty or greasy on it, such as butter. But this is not true. Any burn is pitta, the dosha of fire. The hot, sharp, burning quality of pitta immediately creates searing pain and inflammation. A fatty substance is in fact contraindicated, as it would serve to aggravate the pitta.

> **Time to See the Doctor**
>
> We are not discussing serious burns in this section but common household burns, such as from inadvertently touching an iron, a skillet, or a cigarette. For serious burns, particularly over a larger area of the body, a person needs hospitalization, plasma, and intensive care.

The most effective way to treat a burn is with cold. Immediate application of something cold, such as ice or cold water, is the best remedy. If you have no ice cubes, use a bag of frozen vegetables from the freezer.

After applying cold, make a paste of sandalwood and turmeric powders (equal amounts) mixed *not* in water but in aloe vera gel. Use about 1 tablespoon aloe vera and 1/4 teaspoon each of the sandalwood and turmeric. Mix them together, and apply the paste topically. This will be soothing and healing.

Or, after the ice, when the burning sensation stops, apply bitter ghee (*tikta ghrita*).

Cilantro is beneficial for burns. Make fresh cilantro juice by placing a handful of cilantro in the blender with about 1/3 cup of water. Strain. Take the juice internally (2 teaspoons 3 times a day), and put some of the pulp directly on the skin.

It is important not to apply a bandage to cover the burn. Keep it open to the air. If you apply a bandage, the body's heat may affect the burn adversely. So apply the herbal paste or bitter ghee, and leave it alone. If you have to cover it to keep the medication from rubbing off, use some light gauze.

Bursitis

See also "Arthritis"

Bursitis is an inflammation of the bursae, the little fluid sacs around the shoulder, knee, and other parts of the body. Bursitis is a pitta condition that is similar to arthritis. Effective treatment for it is similar to the treatment for pitta arthritis.

Taking *kaishore guggulu* (1 tablet 3 times a day) should help. This herbal remedy is available by mail from various sources of Ayurvedic herbs (see Resources).

Application of sandalwood paste will be soothing. Make the paste by taking 1 teaspoon of sandalwood powder and adding sufficient water to form a paste. Rub it gently onto the painful area.

Nasya, or the application of warm ghee nose drops to the nostrils (5 drops in each nostril), will help to relieve the pain. *Nasya* opens up the flow of *prana* and helps the *prana* to flow freely through the connective tissue of the joint, which will alleviate pain. (For instructions, see appendix 3.)

Topically, try gently rubbing some sesame oil, eucalyptus oil, tea tree oil, *mahanarayan* oil, or *neem* oil into the swollen joint or other painful area.

As with arthritis, the pathological process of bursitis begins with toxicity accumulated in the colon. These toxins get absorbed in the bloodstream, go into the general circulation, and lodge in the bursae, leading to the symptoms of bursitis. So it is important to keep the colon clean by using the following strategies:

- Before going to bed at night, take 1 cup of hot milk with 2 teaspoons of castor oil added. The laxative effect will eliminate pitta-type toxicity in the colon. If 2 teaspoons do not work, use 3 teaspoons the following night, adjusting your own dose. You should get a couple of good bowel movements in the morning, which will help to cleanse the impurities of the colon. You may continue using this remedy until your symptoms clear up.
- As a second choice, you can take *triphala* or *amalaki* (1 teaspoon) at night in 1 cup of warm water.

Your diet should be pitta-soothing but not vata-provoking. Strictly avoid hot, spicy foods and fermented foods such as pickles. Also avoid raw vegetables and salad. Strictly avoid ice water and other ice-cold drinks. Don't eat beans (pinto beans, adzuki beans, black beans, or garbanzos).

As long as you have bursitis, you should not do strenuous exercise. Gentle yoga stretching is beneficial. Try the Camel, Cobra, Cow, and Cat poses, the Spinal Twist, and Forward Bend—under the guidance of a yoga teacher.

Canker Sores

Canker sores are generally traumatic, that is, they are due to a cut or bruise in the mouth. When people eat some sharp, dried, or hard foods, such as popcorn, corn chips, crackers, or dried bread, or chew fennel seeds after a meal, the hard, sharp food can hurt the oral mucous membrane, and within a couple of days it will manifest as a canker sore.

People who use a rough, hard-bristled toothbrush, or who press unduly hard while brushing their teeth, may irritate the mucous membranes and create a canker sore. Some individuals inadvertently bite the delicate tissues in their cheeks or lips during sleep, or even while chewing or talking. This is more likely if they have TMJ and their bite is uneven, which can easily lead to lacerations and canker sores. If they have high pitta in their saliva, their teeth may be sharp because the crown of the tooth becomes eroded, a combination that may result in repeated sores.

TOPICAL REMEDIES

• The simplest Ayurvedic solution to canker sores is local application of turmeric and honey. Mix together 1 teaspoon honey with 1/4 teaspoon turmeric, and rub it on the sore. It will burn a little at first, but the sore area will heal quickly.

• Rinse your mouth several times a day with a little aloe vera juice.

• Aloe vera gel, 2 tablespoons 3 times a day, can also help heal canker sores.

• Mixing aloe vera gel with *neem* powder is also helpful. Use 1 teaspoon of gel with a pinch of *neem* powder, mix together, and apply directly to the canker sore.

• Put 10 drops of tea tree oil in 1/3 cup of water, and swish the liquid in your mouth. The mild solution will act as an antiseptic to help prevent secondary infection, and it will also help to heal the sore.

• Another topical Ayurvedic remedy is the herb *kama dudha*. Take 1/4 teaspoon and 1 teaspoon fresh cream. Mix together and rub it on the sore.

INTERNAL REMEDIES

• Generally, people with high pitta are more likely to get canker sores. So follow the pitta-soothing diet, avoiding hot, spicy foods and fermented food (chapter 8). Also keep away from strong alcoholic drinks, which will aggravate the sores.

• Between meals, drink 1/2 cup cranberry juice. That will help to heal the sore and relieve the burning sensation and irritation.

• Eating a mixture of rock candy powder (1/2 teaspoon) and cumin powder (1/2 teaspoon) will help stop the pain, as well as reduce inflammation and irritation.

• Sometimes canker sores are accompanied by either diarrhea or constipation. Taking 1/2 teaspoon arrowroot with 1 cup warm milk helps relieve constipation; taking 1/4 teaspoon arrowroot with 1 teaspoon ghee corrects diarrhea.

Cataracts

Cataracts are a kapha disorder. Molecules of kapha accumulate in the lens of the eye and affect its translucence and transparency, making it increasingly opaque. As the cataract grows, it creates increasingly smoky, blurred vision. Generally persons with diabetes are prone to cataracts, as are young people with juvenile diabetes, though cataracts are primarily associated with elderly people.

EFFECTIVE HERBAL EYEWASH. If your eye doctor has detected an early sign of cataracts developing, this *triphala* tea eyewash will be effective in dissolving the molecules of kapha that cause the cataract.

Boil 1 teaspoon *triphala* in a cup of water for 2 to 3 minutes. Let the tea cool, and strain it with a double or triple layer of cheesecloth so that not a single particle of *triphala* is left in the strained tea. Then, with an eye cup, wash your eyes with the *triphala* tea. You may wish to repeat the wash 2 or 3 times, depending on how it feels and how much tea actually got into the eye.

To keep the lens clear and prevent the further growth of cataracts, wash your eyes with *triphala* tea in the morning and at bedtime. Do it regularly for one month, and if it proves effective, you can continue indefinitely. It will help to arrest the process of cataract formation.

CASTOR OIL EYE DROPS. One drop of pure castor oil (without preservatives) placed in the eye at bedtime lubricates the cornea and the conjunctiva and helps to remove molecules of kapha from the lens. In this way one can prevent cataracts from developing.

HERBAL REMEDY. A third approach is to take this herbal mixture internally:

punarnava 5 *parts*
shatavari 3 *parts*
brahmi 3 *parts*

Take 1/2 teaspoon of this herbal mixture twice a day with warm water as a preventative measure against cataracts. As with the triphala eyewash, you may continue using this formula as long as you wish.

Cellulite

Cellulite is more a sociological problem than a health problem! Subcutaneous fat that accumulates under the skin and causes little dimples on the skin surface, cellulite is certainly not a disease. People with high cholesterol, who eat fried, fatty food and whose diet is excessively kapha-provoking, appear to be more likely to have it, as do individuals who use a lot of olive oil in their cooking. As cellulite may gradually lead to obesity, this condition can be seen as an early phase of being overweight.

In Ayurvedic terms, *meda* agni (the agni or fiery quality responsible for metabolizing fat) under the skin becomes low. Unprocessed fatty molecules lodge there and create cellulite. The Ayurvedic aim in treatment is to kindle or enliven the *meda* agni.

EXERCISE. Regular exercise is the first approach. Walking, swimming, or other aerobic exercise is important, and at least some of the exercise should be "local" to the area where the cellulite is forming. In other words, if cellulite is developing on the thighs, don't restrict your exercise to weight lifting and upper-body development!

WATCH OUT FOR KAPHA. Watch your diet and be sure it isn't kapha-increasing (see chapter 8). Minimize dairy products, sweets, cold food and drinks, and fatty fried food. Strictly avoid olive oil in cooking.

VITAMIN K. Rub vitamin K cream onto the skin. This cream will remove spider veins and minimize cellulite.

LOCALIZED MASSAGE. Massage the affected area with sesame oil and mustard oil, mixed half and half. After the massage, dust with a powder of the herb *vacha* (calamus), and rub the skin. This will help remove the cellulite.

Cholesterol

High cholesterol means increased lipids (fats) in the blood. It is essentially a metabolic disorder. People having low liver function or diminished thyroid activity, who have taken steroids in the past, or whose diet is very kaphagenic, seem most prone to develop high cholesterol.

Your cholesterol level should be below 200. About 160 to 190 is normal, but a cholesterol reading of 200 or above is worrisome, as a high cholesterol level in the blood tends to create plaque on the artery walls, resulting in atherosclerotic changes, cardiovascular disorders, hypertension, stroke, and heart problems.

There are two kinds of cholesterol, HDL (high-density lipoprotein), which is the "good" cholesterol, and LDL (low-density lipoprotein), which is the "bad" cholesterol. Researchers these days are saying that what is more important than the total level of cholesterol, as a predictive factor for cardiovascular and other health problems, is the ratio of total cholesterol to HDL.

To reduce high cholesterol levels, and to prevent cholesterol from building up any higher, follow these guidelines.

WATCH YOUR DIET. Stick to a kapha-pacifying diet (chapter 8). No fatty fried food. No cheese. No high-fat milk or yogurt. Minimize sweets and cold food and drinks. Use garlic and onion in cooking.

GET REGULAR EXERCISE. Each day from Monday to Friday, walk for at least half an hour. Go swimming or participate in some other aerobic exercise at least three times each week.

Just by regulating diet and exercise, you can control cholesterol. But there is much more that you can do.

HERBS TO COMBAT CHOLESTEROL. Garlic is effective against high cholesterol. Mix together 1 clove of fresh garlic chopped fine, 1/2 teaspoon grated ginger root, and 1/2 teaspoon lime juice; eat before each meal.

- Drink a tea made of 1 teaspoon cinnamon and 1/4 teaspoon of the herbal mixture *trikatu.* Steep it for 10 minutes in a cupful of water, add 1 teaspoon honey, and drink. Take it twice a day.
- Taking 1/2 teaspoon *trikatu* with 1 teaspoon honey 2 or 3 times a day is good for burning ama and excess kapha and helps to regulate cholesterol.
- This herbal mixture can help control high cholesterol levels:

kutki 3 *parts*
chitrak 3 *parts*
shilajit 1/4 *part*

Take 1/2 teaspoon twice a day, with honey and hot water.

- Take one 200-mg. tablet of *triphala guggulu* 3 times a day.
- Another herb that has been remarkably effective in bringing down cholesterol levels is *chitrak-adhivati.* Taking 1 200-mg. tablet twice a day, after lunch and dinner, will help bring cholesterol back to normal.

HOT WATER AND HONEY. Early in the morning, drink 1 cup of hot water into which you add 1 teaspoon of honey. This will help to "scrape" fat from your system and reduce cholesterol. Adding 1 teaspoon of lime juice or 10 drops of apple cider vinegar will make the drink more effective.

FOODS THAT REDUCE CHOLESTEROL. In addition to avoiding high-fat foods, you can eat certain foods that in themselves help to reduce cholesterol. These include blue corn, quinoa, millet, and oatmeal. Some research suggests that apples, grapefruit, and almonds can also help reduce cholesterol.

YOGA POSTURES. Yoga postures that are good for controlling cholesterol include the Sun Salutation, Shoulder Stand, Peacock, Cobra, Spinal Twist, Locust, and Lotus.

BREATHING EXERCISE. The breathing exercise known as Breath of Fire *(bhastrika)* is also helpful. (See chapter 6 for instructions.)

Chronic Fatigue

See "Fatigue and Chronic Fatigue"

Colds and Flu

Individuals often get colds and flu during the winter and spring seasons. The symptoms are all too familiar: runny nose, cough, congestion, headache, an achy body, and sometimes fever.

Ayurvedically speaking, colds are a kapha–vata disorder. The body builds up an excess of cool and moist kapha qualities, resulting in congestion and a runny nose, and at the same time it may suffer from excess vata, which reduces agni (gastric fire), leading to chills, loss of appetite, and/or poor digestion.

GINGER REMEDIES

The best remedy for colds is ginger. Here are several simple home remedies using ginger that will greatly relieve your cold symptoms and hasten full recovery.

• Combine the following herbs together:

ginger 1 part
cinnamon 1 part
lemongrass 2 parts

Steep 1 teaspoon of this formula for about 10 minutes in 1 cup of hot water; strain it, and add honey for sweetness if you like. If you drink this delicious tea several times a day, it will help to take care of cold, congestion, and flu.

• Another excellent remedy is ginger-cardamom-cinnamon tea. Here is the formula:

ginger 2 parts
cinnamon 3 parts
cardamom just a pinch

Steep 1 teaspoon in a cup of hot water for 10 to 15 minutes. When the tea has cooled down somewhat, you can add about 1/2 to 1 teaspoon of honey for taste.

• Boil 1 teaspoon ginger, or a few eucalyptus leaves, in a pint of water. Turn off the stove, put a towel over your head, and inhale the steam. This will relieve congestion and help you feel much better. Just steam alone, with no herbs added at all, will also be beneficial.

ADDITIONAL HERBAL REMEDIES

• Try 1/2 teaspoon fennel seed powder mixed with 1 teaspoon natural sugar, 2 or 3 times a day.

• For a cold with cough and congestion, mix 1/2 teaspoon cinnamon and 1 teaspoon honey. Eat this mixture 2 or 3 times a day. (For help with your cough, please see "Cough.")

• For flu, make a tea from 1 teaspoon *tulsi* (holy basil) in 1 cup water. Boil for just 1 minute and then drink.

• An ancient Ayurvedic herbal formula that is effective for colds is the following:

sitopaladi *1 part*
maha sudarshan churna *1 part*

Combine these herbs in equal proportions and take 1/4 teaspoon with 1 teaspoon honey 2 or 3 times a day after eating.

• Western herbology has some helpful herbs for colds. Try this mixture:

echinacea *1 part*
goldenseal *1 part*
cinnamon *2 parts*

Take 1/4 teaspoon of this mixture with honey twice a day.

CAUTION: Don't Combine Ginger and Aspirin. Ginger and aspirin are both blood thinners and should not be taken together. Therefore it is wise to drink ginger tea—or use any other ginger remedy—either two hours before or two hours after you take any aspirin.

OTHER REMEDIES AND RECOMMENDATIONS

VITAMIN C. Taking some Vitamin C will be beneficial.

NATURAL NOSE DROPS. Put some liquefied ghee (3 to 5 drops) in each nostril in the morning and evening. This will lubricate the nasal passages and relieve the irritation and sneezing of a cold.

HOT WATER. Drinking hot water several times a day is an effective way to remove toxins from the system and hasten recovery from a cold.

NO DAIRY PRODUCTS. Strictly avoid dairy products such as yogurt, cottage cheese, and milk, and all cold drinks.

BE SURE TO REST. Rest is very important for healing. As much as possible, rest, read, and relax.

ONLY MILD EXERCISE. Ayurveda says that when you have a cold, it is best not to do vigorous exercise, which can set up the conditions for the cold to move into the chest. Just do some gentle yoga *asanas*. *Surya namaskar* (Sun Salutation) is beneficial. The inverted postures, including Shoulder Stand and Headstand (hold for only about 1 minute), as well as Forward Bend, help to prevent postnasal drip and help to drain the mucus through the nose.

BREATHING EXERCISE. Use the Breath of Fire breathing exercise to help burn up your cold. Inhale normally and passively, but exhale forcefully, and repeat rapidly several times. This exercise will help to eliminate mucus from the respiratory tract. For more detailed instructions, see chapter 6.

• Another effective breathing exercise is deep Alternate Nostril breathing, without retention of breath. This will also help to relieve congestion (see chapter 6).

PREVENTION. As a preventive measure, take the herb *amalaki*. It is a *rasayana* (rejuvenative tonic) and a good source of vitamin C and iron. Taking 1 teaspoon of *amalaki* daily, with warm water at night, will help to prevent the common cold.

If you are taking triphala at night, you are already taking *amalaki*; it is one of the three herbs that constitute *triphala* (along with *haritaki* and *bibhitaki*). Taking extra *amalaki* is not recommended, as it would create diarrhea.

Colitis

Colitis is caused when vata pushes pitta into the colon and inflammation occurs. The basic line of treatment is to pacify pitta.

HERBAL REMEDIES

• An excellent herbal remedy for colitis is:

shatavari 4 *parts*
shanka bhasma 1/8 *part*
kama dudha 1/8 *part*
sanjivani 2 *parts*

Take 1/4 teaspoon of this mixture with warm water 2 or 3 times a day for 1 or 2 months.

• You can also take aloe vera gel, 1 tablespoon twice a day. Aloe vera is cooling and good for reducing pitta.

ENEMAS

HEALING ENEMA FOR ULCERATIVE COLITIS. Ulcerative colitis is characterized by diarrhea, mucus, and blood from the rectum. For that condition, Ayurveda suggests a *basti* (enema) using (instead of plain water) a tea made from an astringent herb such as *bilva*, *ashoka*, sandalwood, or licorice root. This is how to prepare the enema:

Boil 1 tablespoon of the herb (such as licorice powder) in 1 pint of water for 5 minutes. Strain, and add about 2 tablespoons of ghee while the tea is still warm. Let the liquid cool to room temperature, and use it for an enema. Retain the liquid inside for 5 minutes if you can. Do this procedure once or twice a week. (More complete instructions for *basti* are found in appendix 3.)

Licorice contains food precursors of natural steroids, which will help heal the ulcer. This is a safe, simple way to correct colitis or ulcerative colitis.

SOOTHING OIL ENEMA. The colon is the seat of vata. This vata dosha is pulling or pushing pitta into the colon, which then causes the colitis. To combat the excess pitta and at the same time pacify vata, Ayurveda suggests injecting a cooling oil such as coconut oil into the rectum. Use about 1 cup of slightly warmed oil as a *basti,* and try to retain it for 5 minutes, but don't worry if it comes out more quickly.

DIETARY REMEDIES

TWO APPLE REMEDIES.

- A simple and beneficial remedy for colitis is to eat cooked apples with a pinch of nutmeg. Peel a couple of apples, remove the seeds, and cook. Make them into a pulp (you can use a potato masher), and add 1 teaspoon ghee and a pinch of nutmeg. This will help to pacify the irritation of colitis and ulcerative colitis.
- Apple juice will also help relieve the burning sensation.

DIETARY PRECAUTIONS. A person with ulcerative colitis should never eat hot spicy food, drink alcohol, or use tobacco, all of which provoke pitta and will significantly irritate the colon.

EXERCISES TO STRENGTHEN THE COLON

LEG LIFT. When a person has ulcerative colitis, the colon is very weak. To strengthen the wall of the colon, lie flat on your back and gradually lift both your legs, keeping the knees as straight as you can, until the legs are at a 45-degree angle to the floor. This exercise is called a Leg Lift. If you find it difficult to lift both legs together, you can lift one leg and then the other. Hold your legs in the raised position for just a few seconds at first, up to 1 minute after several weeks of practice.

YOGA POSTURES. Slowly move into the Chest-Knee pose, then the Plow pose, Locust pose, and if you can, the Elevated Lotus. Also, exercise your abdomen by drawing it gradually in and out. This will strengthen the wall of the colon. Illustrations of yoga postures are in appendix 4.

Conjunctivitis

This is a pitta condition involving inflammation of the conjunctiva of the eyes, which makes the eyes red and photophobic (highly sensitive to light), with discharge and a burning sensation. Here are some effective remedies:

CILANTRO LEAVES. Apply the pulp of fresh cilantro leaves on closed eyelids. Blend a handful of cilantro leaves with 1/4 to 1/3 cup water; strain out the juice, and apply the pulp to your closed eyelids. Drinking the liquid will also be beneficial.

CORIANDER EYEWASH. Make an eyewash by steeping 1 teaspoon of coriander seeds in 1 cup boiling water for at least 15 minutes. Strain thoroughly, and cool before using the water on your closed eyes. (Don't worry if a little goes into the eyes.) Careful: Don't use it either too hot or too cold.

GOAT'S MILK COMPRESS. Dip a sterilized cotton ball in goat's milk, and put it over your eyes. This will cool down pitta and allow conjunctivitis to be healed.

HERBAL REMEDY. Internally, you can take a mixture of equal parts of *kama dudha* and *gulwel sattva.* Take 1/4 teaspoon of this mixture with warm water twice a day for 1 week.

HOW TO HEAL CONJUNCTIVITIS IN CHILDREN

The best way to heal conjunctivitis in young children is to place a drop of mother's milk in the eye. Mother's milk is healing for her child. If the mother is still lactating, and her child gets conjunctivitis, with irritation and discharge in the eye, just one drop of her milk may heal it.

NATURAL HERBAL ANTIBIOTICS

• Make a turmeric solution by stirring some turmeric into a few ounces of pure water. Immerse a clean handkerchief into the solution, and let it dry. (It will be quite yellow.) Then use it to mop the affected eyes.

TIME TO SEE THE DOCTOR

If your conjunctivitis is not cleared up within 3 to 4 days, immediately see your doctor.

The natural antiseptic, antibiotic properties of the turmeric will help take care of the bacteria and facilitate healing.

• Herbal antibiotics are also helpful taken internally. You can make a mixture of these three:

turmeric 1 part
neem 1 part
manjistha 1 part

Take 1/2 teaspoon twice a day with warm water, after meals.

Constipation

Constipation is a vata condition expressing such vata qualities as dryness and hardness. It is caused by insufficient fiber in the diet, insufficient water intake, lack of exercise, heavy meat eating, and numerous other factors. Constipation may create distension and discomfort, flatulence and pain, headache and bad breath, and may lead to absorption of toxins from the colon. Thus it is best to prevent constipation by keeping vata in balance.

FOLLOW THE VATA-PACIFYING DIET. One of the best ways to prevent constipation, especially if you have a predominantly vata constitution, is to follow the vata-balancing diet (see chapter 8). Stay away from cold foods and drinks, dried fruit, salads, and most beans; favor warm foods, warm drinks, and well-cooked vegetables. Some oil in the diet is helpful.

TRIPHALA. Probably the best Ayurvedic remedy for constipation is *triphala,* a combination of three herbs beneficial for all doshic types (see appendix 2). Most problems with constipation can be corrected by taking $^1/_2$ to 1 teaspoon of *triphala* at night. Steep the herbs in a cup of hot water for 5 to 10 minutes, and drink.

Some people find that taking *triphala* at night creates a diuretic action and they have to get up several times to urinate. If that happens to you, you can steep the *triphala* in a cup of warm water overnight and drink it first thing in the morning. Actually, the best time to take *triphala* is in the very early morning, around 4 or 5 A.M., but do your best within your daily schedule.

Here are some further recommendations to help relieve constipation:

SNACK ON FRUIT. Many varieties of fruit can help remedy constipation. So in between meals, eat some fruit. A banana, for example, is a mild laxative. Two ripe yellow bananas, taken between meals, will help relieve constipation. (But don't eat the bananas with meals. They don't combine well with other foods. See chapter 8 for tips on healthy food combining.)

> NOTE: Bananas should be eaten when ripe. You can tell a ripe banana by its bright yellow skin. The inside will be studded with tiny black dots. Green bananas are constipating and should be avoided. Also avoid eating bananas once the skin turns black. They are overripe.

AN APPLE A DAY KEEPS THE DOCTOR AWAY. There is a lot of truth in this old folk saying. Apples are effective both to help regularize the bowels and to clean the tongue and teeth. To combat constipation, peel and thoroughly chew a raw apple about an hour after a meal.

Also effective:

- Pineapple juice
- Raisins—a handful every day, at least an hour after meals
- Prunes
- Peaches—one or two about an hour after meals

EAT MORE FIBER. Fiber in the diet, such as wheat bran, oatmeal, or oat bran, will help keep the bowels regular. Don't forget that fresh fruit and vegetables as well as whole grains are high in fiber, too.

MILK AND GHEE—MILD AND EFFECTIVE. Taking 1 or 2 teaspoonfuls of ghee in a cup of hot milk at bedtime is an effective but gentle means of relieving constipation. This is especially good for vata and pitta constitutions, but it may be too kapha-increasing for kapha types to use regularly.

CASTOR OIL. Castor oil can also be used, but only when the constipation is more obstinate. At bedtime, make yourself a cup of ginger tea (either by boiling some fresh, sliced ginger in water, or adding some powdered ginger to a cup of hot water), and then add 2 teaspoons of castor oil to the tea and drink it.

If 2 teaspoons don't bring the desired result, try the procedure again the next night, increasing the dose to 3 teaspoons, and then go to 4 teaspoons if necessary. Adjust your dose according to what works.

SUGGESTION: Use this castor oil laxative treatment on weekends, when you can stay home!

Castor oil tends to create dependency, in the sense that once you use it, other purgatives rarely work. That is why it is recommended to use castor oil for constipation only in severe cases or in emergencies, as a last resort, but not on a regular basis.

However, there is one way to avoid this dependency. Take 2 teaspoons of castor oil with 1 cup warm milk. This will give a good bowel movement without creating dependency.

FLAXSEED. At night, boil 1 tablespoon of flaxseed in a cup of water for at least 2 to 3 minutes. Then drink the whole cupful, including the tea and the seeds.

FOR CONSTIPATION IN CHILDREN. Give the child 3 figs soaked in warm water.

FOR SEVERE CONSTIPATION. If there is absolute constipation for three days, don't use purgatives. The use of drastic purgatives when constipation is severe can create an intestinal obstruction or even perforation, which can be dangerous. A better approach is to do an enema and then take steps to regulate the system.

Do the enema with plain warm water, or you can use *triphala* tea or *dashamoola* tea instead of plain water. That will relieve the immediate problem. Then, to regulate bowel movements, follow the suggestions in the following section.

PREVENTION. Here are several suggestions for avoiding constipation in the future.

- Follow the vata-pacifying diet (chapter 8).
- Use a lot of fiber in your diet.
- Drink 4 to 5 glasses of water a day, in addition to whatever juices or teas you may drink.
- Get regular exercise. Half an hour of walking, light jogging, swimming, or other aerobic exercise (suitable to your constitution, age, and level of fitness) from Monday to Friday will be very beneficial.
- Yoga *asanas* will also help prevent constipation. In particular, practice the Sun Salutation (12 cycles a day), Chest-Knee pose, and Leg Lift (see appendix 4).
- The yoga exercise known as *nauli* will also be beneficial (see appendix 3).

Constipation During Pregnancy

See also "Constipation"

The best remedy for constipation during pregnancy is the herb *sat isabgol* (psyllium husks). Take 1 teaspoon with a glass of warm milk.

A cup of hot milk with 1 teaspoon of ghee added is also effective. Ghee and milk mixed together is a wonderful combination for gentle, mild laxative action during pregnancy.

One of the most effective herbal remedies for constipation, *triphala,* should *not* be used during pregnancy. It will irritate the child, and the baby will become hyperactive.

Also, do not take castor oil or any other

drastic purgative during pregnancy; like *triphala,* it will make the baby hyperactive.

Cough

A tickling sensation in the throat, dryness, irritation, or inflammation of the trachea or bronchus can all cause a cough.

From an Ayurvedic perspective, most coughs are caused by excess pitta or kapha in the bronchial tree, causing congestion and irritation of the bronchial mucous membrane. The basic strategy for managing this condition is to reduce the unwanted pitta or kapha that is creating the congestion.

To treat a cough most effectively, you need to determine whether it is a dry cough (vata) or a productive cough with mucus coming up (kapha), or whether pitta has also become involved.

DRY COUGH

For a dry cough or a cough without much mucus, eat a ripe banana with 1 teaspoon of honey and 2 pinches of ground black pepper. You can eat this 2 or 3 times a day.

Rx for a Stubborn Cough

Chop a clove of garlic, and boil it in a cup of milk. Then add 1/4 teaspoon turmeric. This creates a golden yellow milk that tastes like garlic soup. This garlic-turmeric milk is effective for soothing and healing most types of cough.

- Try chewing 1/4 teaspoon of *ajwan* mixed with 1 teaspoon natural organic sugar.
- Make *talisadi* tea, made of

talisadi powder	*1/2 teaspoon*
licorice powder	*1/2 teaspoon*

with a little honey added. This tea is quite effective.

- Dry cough or irritation in the throat may be due to slight congestion in the tonsils, or a congestive condition in the throat such as pharyngitis or laryngitis. To relieve this condition, boil 1 cup milk with 1/2 teaspoon turmeric and 1/4 teaspoon ginger, making a golden yellow milk. If you drink this at night, it will relieve the irritation in the throat and take care of a dry cough.

PRODUCTIVE COUGH

For a productive or kapha cough, the simplest home remedy is black pepper. Mix 1/4 teaspoon of the powder with 1 teaspoon of honey, and eat it on a full stomach. (If your voice is hoarse, use 1 teaspoon of ghee instead of the honey.) The heating quality of black pepper helps relieve congestion and drives out the cough. Take 2 or 3 times a day for 3 to 5 days.

- A tea made from 1/2 teaspoon ginger powder, plus a pinch of clove and a pinch of cinnamon powder in a cupful of boiled water, can offer relief from your cough.
- If your cough persists, try this formula:

ground mustard 1/2 *teaspoon*
ginger powder 1/2 *teaspoon*

Mix together into 1 teaspoon of honey, and eat slowly. (Ginger relieves congestion, and mustard has a heating action.) You can use this mixture 2 to 3 times a day for as long as the cough persists.

• Another helpful natural remedy for a productive cough is the following:

bay leaf 1/2 *teaspoon*
pippali 1/4 *teaspoon*

Take this mixture in 1 teaspoon honey 2 or 3 times a day.

• You can also try 1 teaspoon honey mixed with a pinch of clove powder, 2 or 3 times a day.

OTHER COUGHS

PRODUCTIVE COUGH WITH GREENISH-YELLOWISH MUCUS. In such a cough there is some secondary infection due to the involvement of pitta dosha. For this condition, you can use a tea made of equal proportions of

sitopaladi
maha sudarshan

Use 1/4 teaspoon of the mixture to make a tea, and drink it 3 times a day with honey.

> **TIME TO SEE THE DOCTOR**
>
> If your cough persists for more than a week, you should see a doctor.

It will encourage elimination of the mucus and help heal the cough quickly.

FOR A CHILD'S COUGH. Try giving the child a drink of 1/2 cup pomegranate juice with a pinch of ginger powder and a pinch of *pippali* powder.

• Mix 1/4 teaspoon of *sitopaladi* with 1 teaspoon of honey as an effective cough remedy for children. However, if the mother is sensitive or allergic to pollen, the child may be allergic to honey. In that case, instead of honey, use maple syrup.

FOR A CHRONIC COUGH. Make a mixture of 4 parts garlic powder to 1 part *trikatu*. Add a little honey. Take this twice a day.

Cramps, Abdominal

See "Muscle Cramps and Spasms"

Cramps, Menstrual

See "Menstrual Difficulties"

Dandruff

Although dandruff can sometimes be caused by a fungal infection or other skin disease, in most cases it is produced when the scalp doesn't receive a sufficient supply of blood. Consequently there is a lack of protein in the skin, which becomes dry and flaky.

Dandruff may also be due to a deficiency of vitamin B-6, or to an excess of vata dosha, which also makes the skin dry.

The treatment is simple. To improve circulation to the scalp, massage for a few minutes daily with *neem* oil (in a sesame oil base). If a fungal infection of the skin is causing the dandruff, the *neem* oil, which has disinfectant properties, will help heal this also.

A second option is to use some eggwhite mixed with lime juice. Put two eggwhites in a small jar or container with the fresh juice of one lime, mix together, and apply to your hair. Let it stay in your hair for a half hour, then wash the hair with *neem* soap. The eggwhite will provide the scalp with the lacking protein, and the dandruff will soon disappear.

Depression

PLEASE NOTE: Depression is a serious medical condition that requires the supervision of a medical doctor. Mild or preclinical cases may sometimes be completely healed using these Ayurvedic recommendations, but they are not a substitute for consulting with a physician.

If you are already under a doctor's care for depression, the Ayurvedic remedies suggested here can be used in conjunction with the regimen outlined by your physician. But it is only fair and proper to do so with his or her approval and supervision.

Ask your doctor to carefully monitor your progress. As time goes by, you may be able to minimize or eliminate your dependence on strong medications if your body's balance can be brought to a point where diet, exercise, and other Ayurvedic programs are sufficient to control or eliminate the depression.

Clinical depression is more than just a low or heavy mood. The symptoms of depression include a loss of interest in friends and usual activities; sleep disturbances, such as insomnia, early morning awakening, or oversleeping; anxiety, irritability, or restlessness; low energy and fatigue; poor appetite and weight loss, or sometimes the reverse, overeating and weight gain; difficulty concentrating and making decisions; decreased sex drive; feelings of worthlessness and guilt; feelings of hopelessness and helplessness; frequent crying spells; and suicidal thoughts.

The genesis of depression, from an Ayurvedic perspective, is too complex to lay out here. In brief we can say that because of specific etiological factors, vata from the colon, pitta from the intestine, or kapha from the stomach enters the general circulation and lodges in the nervous system, interferes with normal functioning of the mind and nervous system, and causes depression.

The resulting depression may be vata, pitta, or kapha. Each of these three types of depression is treated in different ways, though the first step for each is to bring the diet in line with the guidelines for vata-, pitta-, and kapha-pacifying diets (see chapter 8). This is important—please don't overlook it!

VATA DEPRESSION

Vata-type depression is generally associated with fear, anxiety, nervousness, and insomnia. The following home remedies will help dissolve a mild vata depression:

• Drink *dashamoola* tea. Steep 1 teaspoon of the herb *dashamoola* in 1 cup of hot water, and drink. Take twice a day.

• Make a tea from equal proportions of *ashwagandha* and *brahmi* (about $^1/_3$ to $^1/_2$ teaspoon each), steep in a cup of water for about 10 minutes, and drink 2 or 3 times a day.

• Another domestic remedy for depression is a tea made of holy basil (*tulsi*) and sage. Use $^1/_4$ teaspoon *tulsi* and $^1/_2$ teaspoon of sage per cup of hot water; drink twice a day.

• Nose drops of warm sesame oil (3 to 5 drops in each nostril) are effective for relieving depression (see appendix 3). Do this *nasya* procedure morning and evening on an empty stomach.

• Rubbing the top of the head and the soles of the feet with sesame oil is quite soothing to vata and healing for vata depression.

• Psychologically, one factor that sustains vata depression is loneliness. Try to spend more time relating to people; it will help lift the depression.

PITTA DEPRESSION

Pitta-type depression is generally associated with anger, or with fear of failure, of losing control, or of making mistakes; it often involves thoughts of committing suicide. It is serious; you should consult your doctor.

Of course it *is* possible to have a mild pitta depression, caused by failing an examination, not getting a promotion at work, or some such thing. A pitta person can be quite addicted to success and, when he or she doesn't succeed, can easily become upset and depressed. This type of depression may not last long or be too severe.

Pittas are most vulnerable to SAD, seasonal affective disorder, a fairly mild form of depression that usually occurs in the winter.

For all types of pitta depression, use the following simple but effective remedies:

• Rub some coconut oil or sunflower oil onto your scalp and the soles of your feet at bedtime.

• Drink gotu kola or *brahmi* tea or ginkgo tea 2 or 3 times a day. Use $^1/_2$ teaspoon of herbs in a cup of hot water.

• Mix equal amounts of these three herbs:

brahmi
jatamamsi
shatavari

Take $^1/_2$ to 1 teaspoon of this mixture 2 or 3 times a day with warm water, as a tea.

• Use *brahmi* ghee nose drops, 3 to 5 drops in each nostril, twice a day on an empty stomach.

• Meditate. A few minutes of meditation will be helpful in healing pitta depression. See chapter 7 for some hints on meditation.

KAPHA DEPRESSION

Kapha depression creates a sense of mental heaviness and is associated with excess sleep, weight gain, drowsiness, and lousiness! The following natural remedies may bring great relief from kapha depression:

• Fast for 3 to 4 days on apple juice. This will work wonders to lighten the heaviness of a kapha depression.

• Increase the amount of exercise you do.

• Drink ginger tea ($^1/_2$ to 1 teaspoon of

Time to See the Doctor

If your depression doesn't soon begin to lift as a result of using these Ayurvedic home remedies, please consult a doctor.

ginger powder steeped in hot water) twice a day.

• Make the following herbal compound:

sarasvati 2 *parts*
punarnava 3 *parts*
chitrak 3 *parts*

Take this mixture 3 times a day. Put 1/2 teaspoon of the powder on your tongue, and wash it down with warm water.

• Put 5 drops of *punarnava* ghee in each nostril twice a day. (See appendix 2 for instructions on how to prepare your own medicated ghees and oils.)

• The Sun Salutation (12 repetitions a day), Shoulder Stand, and Plow pose are recommended yoga *asanas* for depression. Also do the Maha Mudra. Other recommended postures are the Bow pose and the Vajrasana (Sitting on the Heels). (Illustrations of yoga *asanas* appear in appendix 4.)

• The breathing exercise known as *ujjayi pranayama* is also beneficial for healing kapha depression. (See instructions in chapter 6.)

Diabetes

Diabetes is a metabolic kapha type of disorder in which diminished functioning of agni (digestive fire) leads to a tendency toward high blood sugar. To control high blood sugar, Ayurveda uses the following herbal mixture:

guduchi 1 *part*
shardunika 1 *part*
kutki 1 *part*
punarnava 2 *parts*

Take 1/2 teaspoon 2 or 3 times a day with warm water.

• Another simple and effective herbal way to control blood sugar is to use turmeric. Fill some 00-size capsules (available at a pharmacy or natural food store) with turmeric, and take 2 capsules 3 times a day, a few minutes before meals. You can continue this program for up to a month, and then reevalulate your condition. Clinical observation suggests that a person who is insulin dependent will experience a markedly diminished requirement for insulin; the diabetes can often be brought under control.

• To help regulate your blood sugar level, you can try taking 1/2 teaspoon of ground bay leaf and 1/2 teaspoon turmeric, mixed in 1 tablespoon aloe vera gel. Take the mixture twice a day before lunch and dinner.

DIET. To reduce kapha, you should follow the kapha-pacifying diet (see chapter 8), especially avoiding excess intake of sweets, carbohydrates, and dairy products. Take more fresh vegetables and bitter herbs.

COPPER WATER. Put one cup of water into a copper vessel at night, and drink the water in the morning.

YOGA POSTURES. Beneficial yoga postures for diabetic conditions include the Sun Salutation and the Peacock pose, Locust pose, Leg Lift, and Chest-Knee pose. Alternate Nostril breathing is also helpful. (Please see illustrations for yoga postures in appendix 4, and the *pranayama* instructions in chapter 6.)

Diarrhea

See also "Diarrhea—Babies"

Generally, diarrhea occurs when agni (the digestive fire) becomes weak. As a result, absorption and assimilation become minimal, and the undigested foodstuff gets eliminated as a liquid, watery stool. To relieve diarrhea, Ayurveda aims to strengthen agni and to pacify whatever dosha—generally pitta—is aggravated.

Indigestion, nervousness, or eating some wrong food or food combination can also create diarrhea.

PACIFY PITTA

The first line of defense against diarrhea is to immediately reduce pitta in your diet. Follow the guidelines for the pitta-pacifying diet (see chapter 8), especially keeping away from spicy and fermented foods.

> **TIME TO SEE THE DOCTOR**
>
> If there is no serious illness, diarrhea is usually quite easy to control. However, this condition can also be a symptom of a more serious illness, so if these home remedies don't work in 2 or 3 days, consult a doctor.

FOUR FOOD CURES

- Cook one or two apples until they are mushy, then add 1 teaspoon ghee, a pinch of cardamom, and a pinch of nutmeg. Eat slowly. This mixture is not only delicious, it will also help stop diarrhea right away.
- If you don't have apples, you can use bananas, only you don't have to cook them. Chop 1 or 2 ripe bananas into pieces, and as with the apples, add 1 teaspoon of warm ghee and a pinch each of cardamom and nutmeg. Bananas are high in potassium, which helps to bind the stool.
- Another effective remedy for diarrhea is cooked rice with yogurt. Take about a cupful of cooked basmati rice, add 1 tablespoon of ghee and 3 or 4 tablespoons of plain fresh yogurt, stir together, and eat.
- Another remedy using yogurt is to blend together equal parts of yogurt and water (about 1/2 cup each), add about 1/8 teaspoon of fresh grated ginger, and drink.

HERBAL REMEDIES

- Try ginger powder (about 1/2 teaspoon) with 1 teaspoon raw natural sugar. Mix together, and chew the mixture with some warm water. Take 2 or 3 times a day for 2 to 3 days.
- Another simple remedy is the following:

ghee 1 *teaspoon*
nutmeg 1/4 *teaspoon*
ginger powder 1/4 *teaspoon*
natural sugar 1 *teaspoon*

Mix together and eat. Like the ginger-sugar mixture above, take this formula 2 or 3 times a day for 2 to 3 days.

• For acute diarrhea, mix ½ teaspoon fennel powder with ½ teaspoon ginger powder, and chew this mixture 2 or 3 times a day.

• Try drinking a cup of hot black coffee with a little lime juice (about 10 drops) and a pinch of cardamom or nutmeg.

• If your diarrhea appears to be the result of high pitta, use this herbal formula:

shatavari ½ *teaspoon*
arrowroot ½ *teaspoon*

Mix together, and take with ½ cup warm water 2 or 3 times a day.

• You can also use *sat isabgol* (psyllium husks) to combat pitta diarrhea. This may sound strange, as psyllium is often used as a laxative. However, in pitta diarrhea, an excess of pitta accumulates in the gastrointestinal tract and irritates the wall of the colon, creating the diarrhea. So at bedtime, take 1 teaspoon *sat isabgol* mixed into a cup of fresh yogurt. That will absorb pitta and bind the stool, helping to correct the diarrhea. Be sure the yogurt is freshly made, not old.

AVOID DEHYDRATION

Diarrhea can sometimes cause dehydration. To prevent this from happening, add 1 teaspoon of natural sugar, 1 teaspoon of lime juice, and a pinch of salt to a pint of room-temperature water, and sip throughout the day.

NOTE: If the diarrhea continues beyond three days, it would be wise to consult a doctor.

Diarrhea-Babies

Diarrhea in the babies of nursing mothers may be due to the mother's diet. For example, if the mother eats stale and leftover food, or food that is heavy to digest, then her milk will become harder for the child to digest. As a general rule, Ayurveda suggests that when babies six months old or younger get diarrhea, the mother should follow a pitta-pacifying diet.

AN APPLE A DAY... A baby's diarrhea can usually be corrected simply by feeding the child some cooked apple. Remove the skin and seeds, cook the apple, and add ½ teaspoon ghee, a pinch of cardamom, and a small pinch of ginger. Stir it up well, and cool to room temperature.

SUGGESTION: To feed this applesauce to your child, use a standard baby bottle. With a clean scissors, cut off the tip of the nipple, making an opening large enough for the applesauce to flow through.

MAKE WHEY. Whey is a natural source of lactobacillus. Since a baby's diarrhea is often due to altered flora in the gastrointestinal tract, the whey should help restore the normal flora. It is also a good source of potassium and of calcium, which binds the stool.

Bring 1 cup of milk to a boil; when it just begins to boil, squeeze a little lime juice (about ½ teaspoon) into the pot. The milk will curdle. Then strain the thick part out by pouring the mixture through cheesecloth or a sieve.

The remaining watery part is the whey. Giving 4 to 5 teaspoons of the whey to the child every 10 to 15 minutes should stop the diarrhea.

(The thick, solid part is a delicious fresh cheese called *paneer,* much used in Indian cooking. Try it!)

A SIMPLE HERBAL REMEDY. Another simple domestic remedy is to mix 1 teaspoon honey, 1/2 teaspoon ghee, a pinch of nutmeg, and a pinch of saffron.

POPPYSEED PORRIDGE. You can also make your child a porridge of poppy seeds. Bring 1/2 cup milk and 1/2 cup water to a boil, then add about 1 teaspoon poppy seeds. The seeds will swell and become soft; they will make a nice, easily digested porridge. It is a good food that helps to stop diarrhea. As a bonus, your child will also sleep soundly.

> **TIME TO SEE THE DOCTOR**
>
> If your infant has diarrhea, watch him or her carefully. If bowel movements are becoming less frequent and are firmer and denser, your child is getting better. But if the stools continue to be watery and occur several times in a day, and if your baby's eyes appear sunken, the lips are dry, and she or he looks drowsy, these are all warning signs of dehydration. This is a serious condition, and you need to consult a doctor.

CALCIUM SUPPLEMENT. Babies may also get diarrhea when they are teething. Teeth are a by-product of *asthi dhatu,* or bone formation. When babies start growing teeth, especially the incisors or canine teeth, vata in the *asthi dhatu* gets provoked, their digestive fire becomes weak, and they may get diarrhea. At that time, they need more calcium. You can give the child a simple calcium supplement in the correct dose for children.

Dizziness

See "Fainting and Dizziness"

Dry Skin

See also "Skin—Ayurvedic Care"

Dry skin can have several causes. It may be due to a lack of sebaceous (oily) secretions; insufficient sweating; an excess of hot, sharp pitta; or too much vata. External causes of dry skin include sun, wind, hot dry air, excess washing, and excess use of soap or dishwashing soap.

MOISTURIZING CREAM MAY NOT BE THE ANSWER. Many people use moisturizing creams to counteract dry skin. But dryness of the skin usually comes from within rather than from external causes. For this reason, mere application of a moisturizer doesn't truly solve the problem.

In general, moisturizing creams work only temporarily. They stimulate secretions of the sebaceous glands, and for a while the skin looks soft and oily. But then the glands become tired and exhausted, resulting in more dryness. You will have much greater success if you treat the dryness both externally, with natural oils, and internally, by lubrication of the colon with oil enemas.

Here are several effective Ayurvedic home remedies to keep your skin smooth and lustrous.

APPLY SOME OIL. In some cases, applying some oil to your skin may be all you need to eliminate dry skin. If your constitution is predominantly vata, apply sesame oil; if you are pitta, apply sunflower or coconut oil. If you are kapha, apply corn oil.

However, application of oil to the skin will probably not be sufficient. To treat the internal cause of the dryness, you'll have to lubricate the colon with a gentle oil enema.

OIL ENEMA. Here is the procedure:

- *Step 1:* Begin with a cleansing enema. Either in the morning or evening, give yourself a regular water enema. After a good bowel movement, wait one hour before proceeding to step 2.
- *Step 2:* For the oil enema, use 1 cup of sesame, sunflower, or corn oil, according to the above vata–pitta–kapha recommendations. Inject the oil into the rectum (using a hot water bottle or a syringe), and try to retain it for 5 to 10 minutes. If it goes out, don't worry, let it out. (More complete guidelines on how to do an enema are in appendix 3.)

This simple oil enema will make your skin soft, delicate, and gorgeous. The colon is an important part of the absorption process for food nutrients. Similarly, the oil in the colon from the enema easily gets absorbed into the system and helps to lubricate the skin from within.

For best results, perform the oil enema according to this schedule:

Week 1	Every day
Week 2	Every 2 days
Week 3	Every 3 days
Week 4	Once

CHERRY MASK. You may also find relief from dry skin by applying a pulp of fresh cherries to your face at night, before going to bed. Leave it on for 15 minutes, and then rinse off. This will give you a beautiful complexion.

Earache

If the ear passage gets dried and crusty due to excess vata, it may start aching. The eardrum may even become tight and painful.

However, before treating earache, it is important to first rule out several possibilities, such as infection (*otitis externa* or *otitis interna*), perforated eardrum, or excess wax causing pressure on the ear (see "Earwax"). Having ruled these out, one can then treat the vata problem.

TEA TREE OIL. Begin by pulling down on the lobe of your painful ear. If this hurts, it means there is *otitis externa*, external ear infection. To heal the infection, take a cotton swab and dip it into tea tree oil, a wonderful natural disinfectant widely available at natural food stores and some pharmacies. Then apply the oil to the ear with the swab.

NOTE: Using plain tea tree oil may create a burning sensation on sensitive skin, so it is usually best to dilute it, using 10 to 20 drops of tea tree oil mixed in 1 ounce of sesame oil.

TEA TREE OIL WITH *NEEM*. For an even more effective treatment, combine the tea tree oil with *neem* oil. Here again, don't use pure *neem* extract. Mix 10 to 20 drops of *neem* in sesame oil, then add it to the tea tree oil. Gently apply a few drops of the oil mixture to the ear passage.

ANTIBIOTIC HERBS. At the same time you are treating the infection on the outside with tea tree oil, internally you can take turmeric-echinacea-goldenseal tea:

turmeric 1 part
goldenseal 1 part
echinacea 1 part

Stir $^1/_2$ teaspoon of this mixture into hot water, steep for a few minutes, and drink. Alternatively, simply swallow $^1/_2$ teaspoon of the powder mixed in 1 teaspoon of honey. Take 3 times a day after food, for 1 week. This powerful antiseptic, antibiotic formula will help control the ear infection.

ASAFETIDA. You can also take a small amount of cotton, put a pinch of asafetida into it, and roll it into a capsulelike shape. Place that ball of cotton into the outer ear. The fumes of the asafetida will quickly relieve ear pain.

ONION JUICE. Combine 1 teaspoon fresh onion juice with $^1/_2$ teaspoon honey. Mix well; introduce 5 to 10 drops into the affected ear. The mixture should be room temperature or a little warmer before you put it in your ear.

HEAT. Earache can also be moderated by heat. Take a handkerchief and put it on a warm (not hot) pan, fold it, and place it on the ear to give a little soothing external heat.

Ears, Ringing

See "Tinnitus"

Earwax

Earwax is one of the natural secretions of the body. It has the function of protecting the eardrum from dust, and it also keeps the ear canal lubricated. But because it is constantly exposed to the air, the wax may accumulate dust and dirt and become tarry black or brown-black and thick, packed tightly into the ear canal. It may obstruct hearing or create uncomfortable pressure, and so it has to be periodically removed.

WASH IT OUT. Gentle irrigation of the ear canal with warm water will usually take care of it. You can pick up an ear syringe in a pharmacy quite inexpensively. Prepare a pint of warm water (body temperature), add about $^1/_2$ teaspoon of baking soda, and use that water to clean the ear. Follow the directions that come with the syringe, which essentially are to hold the syringe at the edge of the ear canal (do not insert it; the water has to be free to come out again), and squirt the water *gently* into the ear. You will want to tilt your head toward the shoulder of the ear you are cleaning and hold your head over a basin or over the sink. Do a final rinse with plain warm water.

After irrigating the ear, it is important to dry the ear thoroughly. A good way is to dip a cotton swab into some rubbing alcohol, and wipe the ear with the swab.

SOFTEN IT WITH OIL. Sometimes the wax is stubborn and doesn't come out easily. In that case, for a day or two before doing the irrigation, soften the wax in the ear canal by lubricating it with warm garlic oil. Take about 1 tablespoon of sesame oil, add 1/2 clove of freshly chopped garlic, and boil it until the garlic pieces turn brown. It will have a pleasant smell. Then press the oil from the garlic, and strain it into a jar or other container. (Plain sesame oil will also work, but the garlic oil will be more effective.)

Then, 2 or 3 times a day, put a few drops of that oil—when it is warm, not hot—into the ear. That will lubricate the ear passage and soften the wax for easy removal.

DISSOLVE IT WITH HYDROGEN PEROXIDE. You can also use a mild hydrogen peroxide solution (about a 3 percent solution) to dissolve the wax. You can buy this solution in most pharmacies. Put a few drops in the ear. It will oxygenate the ear, and the wax will simply dissolve. When you're finished, clean the ear with some warm sesame oil.

MASSAGE TO LOOSEN STUBBORN WAX. For stubborn earwax, massage the outside of the ear. Put a little sesame oil or castor oil on the mastoid bone (the bone behind the ear), and gently massage. Pull the ear lobe, and at the same time open your mouth. This will help to loosen the ear wax, and it will come out quite easily when you irrigate with water.

HERBAL REMEDY. The root cause of excessive earwax production is increased vata in the *mamsa dhatu* (muscle tissue). To deal with this, take *triphala guggulu* tablets, 200 mg. twice a day, for one month. That will definitely break down the body's habit of forming excess earwax.

PREVENTION. Here is another excellent way to prevent the buildup of earwax. Once a month, sleep on your left side. Fill your right ear with warm sesame oil, and go to bed. (Put an old towel on the pillow to catch the excess oil.) The whole night, the ear passage will be soaked in the sesame oil. The wax will rise up toward the surface of the ear canal, and you can clean it out in the morning with a dry cotton swab. (Don't stay awake all night trying not to turn over; just sleep comfortably. Even a couple of hours with the oil filling the canal will do the trick.)

The next night, sleep on the other side and treat the other ear in the same way. This way you can avoid the tendency for excess earwax to form.

Eating Disorders

See also "Overeating" and "Obesity"

NOTE: The Ayurvedic recommendations in this and related sections can help you deal with eating disorders, but to fully heal them you may also require psychiatric counseling.

KINDS OF EATING DISORDERS

BULIMIA AND BINGE EATING. Almost everyone does some extra munching now and then. But if you often continue eating even though you are full, you might be a victim of binge eating disorder or bulimia.

Individuals with bulimia eat to excess and then induce vomiting to avoid gaining weight, while those with binge eating disorder overeat but don't induce vomiting. Binge eating may lead to obesity, and bulimia may lead to metabolic disorders.

OVEREATING. Overeating of all kinds is most often the result of psychological and emotional factors, such as low self-esteem, anxiety, grief, and sadness. To compensate for those emotions, people go on eating.

ANOREXIA. Anorexia nervosa is a serious problem, usually among young women who have a fear of being fat and purposefully starve themselves. The root cause of anorexia is often depression.

SUGGESTED REMEDIES

Here are some brief suggestions to help you deal effectively with these eating disorders. For more complete treatments, please see "Overeating" and "Obesity."

FOLLOW A LOW-FAT DIET. Avoid fatty fried food, cheese, yogurt, excess carbohydrates, ice cream. These kapha-inducing substances lead to weight gain and possibly to obesity.

EAT HOT SPICY FOOD. When cooking, add garam masala, chili pepper, cayenne pepper, curry pepper, turmeric, cumin, and the like to your food. These spices will burn the ama that causes overeating.

EAT TWO OR THREE MEALS A DAY. That's all. Eat breakfast, lunch, and dinner, but skip between-meal snacking. While eating, play some soft, gentle music such as classical Indian music; choose a gentle, loving raga. Don't listen to jazz or rock; that loud music will overstimulate the system and cause you to eat more.

LICORICE. Whenever you desire to munch, eat licorice candy, which is a mild diuretic that acts to reduce kapha. Or eat a handful of raisins.

HERBAL TEA. To help heal the emotional factor in all eating disorders, drink herbal tea. Excellent choices are chamomile, comfrey, *brahmi*, or *jatamamsi*. These are good individually, but a tea made from all of these mixed together in equal amounts is especially effective to reduce stress and balance the emotions. Use 1/2 to 1 teaspoon of herbs steeped in boiling water for 10 minutes.

> NOTE: If there is depression, *jatamamsi* or *brahmi* tea will help, but it may also be necessary to see a psychiatrist or other mental health professional.

OIL MASSAGE. Rub some *bhringaraj* oil on the soles of the feet and on the scalp at night. That will help you relax and sleep. Lightly massaging with a little of the oil in the morning will also help you deal with the stress.

YOGA POSTURES. Good yoga *asanas* for eating disorders include the Bow, Boat, Peacock, and Rooster poses. The Lion pose is also quite effective for reducing stress (see appendix 4).

BREATHING AND MEDITATION. *Ujjayi pranayama* and *So-Hum* meditation will also be helpful (see chapters 6 and 7).

Edema

See also "Swelling During Pregnancy"

Suddenly one morning a person may wake up with swollen eyes, a swollen foot, a swollen nose, or a swollen toe—any part of the body can swell. There may be associated symptoms such as pain or itching. Sometimes the edema may be related to an injury, such as a bump, or it may be due to torn ligaments. Or fluid may seep from the blood vessels due to prolonged standing or walking. Because of poor circulation, a person's feet or ankles may swell. Edema may also be an allergic reaction, or the result of an insect bite.

Because there are so many possible reasons for the swelling, finding out the cause is essential for maximally effective treatment. Nevertheless, the following recommendations should prove helpful.

APPLY A HEALING PASTE. At the site of the swelling, apply a paste made of turmeric and red sandalwood. Mix an equal amount of the herbal powders together, add sufficient water to make a paste, and apply.

NOTE: Don't get this mixture of turmeric and sandalwood in your eyes; it may irritate the eye and create conjunctivitis.

GIVE YOUR FEET A RAISE. If the edema is in your feet, raise the feet. Sit in a comfortable chair with your legs resting on a footstool, or use a small table and place a couple of pillows under your feet. When you go to bed, place pillows under your feet. This will gradually drain the excess water and relieve the swelling.

FOR INSECT BITES. For swelling due to insect bites, use *neem* and tea tree oil topically. The venom of the insect irritates the skin, and *neem* and tea tree oil mixed together in equal proportion will neutralize the venom toxicity and minimize the edema. *Neem* oil is also effective by itself. (See "Bites and Stings" for further suggestions.)

NATURAL ANTIHISTAMINE FOR ALLERGIES. If the swelling is due to allergy, take antihistamine in the form of fresh cilantro juice. Chop some fresh cilantro and place in the blender with $1/3$ cup of water. Blend, strain, and drink immediately. Also apply the pulp locally to the swollen area. (See "Allergies" for many more suggestions.)

FINGER RING SWELLING. Swelling on a finger may be due to a too-tight ring. Simply remove the ring. If it will not easily slip off, raise your hand high above your head or soak your hand in ice water for a few minutes, then use some soap or oil to make your finger slippery. If this does not work, the ring may have to be cut. That will release the blood flow and relieve the edema.

HERBS TO IMPROVE CIRCULATION. Poor circulation can lead to edema. To increase circulation, mix:

punarnava 5 *parts*
manjistha 3 *parts*
gokshura 3 *parts*

Take 1/2 teaspoon twice a day with warm water, after meals.

LOCAL EXERCISE TO IMPROVE CIRCULATION. In addition to the above herbal formula, giving some exercise to the part of the body that is swollen should improve circulation and reduce the swelling. Fill a pan or bucket with hot water, and steep a "teabag" of mustard seeds in it. Make the bag by wrapping 2 tablespoons of mustard seeds in a handkerchief or some cheesecloth. Put it into the bucket you're using to soak your ankle, finger, or whatever part is swollen. While you soak, flex the swollen part and do some underwater exercises to increase circulation.

REMEDIES FOR LOCALIZED SWELLING

• *For swelling of the nose,* do *nasya* using *brahmi* oil or plain ghee (see appendix 3).

• *For swelling of the eyes,* apply a few drops of pure rose water. You can generally buy a 3 percent solution of rose water; to make it at home, use organic roses and soak both petals and the hip in distilled water for several hours, then strain and use the water.

• *For swollen toes,* apply a paste of turmeric and red sandalwood.

• *For a torn ligament,* apply some *mahanarayan* oil topically. Internally, take *kaishore guggulu,* 200 mg. twice a day.

• *For facial swelling.* Some parasites, such as amoebas, giardia, and pinworms, can create swelling of the face. If you have determined that this is the cause of your facial swelling, the following formula will be effective:

vidanga 3 *parts*
neem 3 *parts*
shardunika 3 *parts*

Take 1/2 teaspoon twice a day after lunch and dinner.

Eye Irritation

See also "Eyes—Ayurvedic Care"

Around the age of 40, *alochaka* pitta (a subtype of pitta associated with vision) tends to become low, and people frequently find that their eyes become irritated. Individuals who work in front of a computer for a long time, watch a lot of TV or movies, or do a lot of driving or close-up work, or who live in a city with high air pollution, may find that their eyes become irritated and build up quite a lot of strain.

The irritation may be due to dryness of the conjunctiva (which results from excess vata), or it may be related to excess hyperacidity or pitta in the stomach. Or, because the liver and eyes are closely related, high or stagnant pitta in the liver may be a causal factor. It is important to pin down the cause in order to treat it with maximum effectiveness. But most of the following remedies will be helpful in all situations.

TAKE A BREAK. If you are using your eyes a lot, perhaps in front of a computer or driving, stop every hour or two for a few minutes to give your eyes a rest.

USE A PROTECTIVE SCREEN. Use a protective screen on your video terminal, to cut radiation and glare.

CHANGE YOUR FOCUS. If you are doing a lot of reading, stop for a minute or two and refocus on a distant object. Every half hour, close the book and look at something across the room or out the window. Doing something different with the eyes is restful and will help prevent eye irritation.

TAKE A TEA BREAK. In the midst of a lot of close-up work or sitting at the computer, stop for a few minutes and have a cup of tea: chamomile, comfrey, mint, or even *chai* (which has some caffeine and will not be as soothing as the other three). This will be relaxing and will help to relieve the irritation and strain.

ROSE WATER EYE DROPS. You can also prepare a solution of rose water. Take 1 ounce of distilled or purified water, add 5 drops of pure rose water, and use the solution to rinse your eyes. Use a dropper or an eye cup, and be sure the water is neither too cold nor too hot. This solution will immediately soothe any eye irritation.

SPLASH YOUR EYES WITH WATER. Simply washing the eyes with clean water will also help. As if rinsing your face after washing, splash some water onto your eyes, opening the eyes for a moment to allow some water to go in. Or you can use an eye cup and rinse the eyes.

THE SIMPLEST AND BEST REMEDY FOR IRRITATED EYES. Put a single drop of pure, genuine castor oil (without preservatives) into your eyes at bedtime. Rubbing a little castor oil on the soles of your feet at bedtime also helps; remember to wear some old socks to prevent the oil from staining your sheets.

FOR BLOODSHOT EYES. If your eyes are irritated and bloodshot, drink a cup of fresh orange juice with 1/2 teaspoon of natural sugar and a pinch of cumin.

TO PACIFY ACIDITY. If excess acid and high pitta in your system seems to be the cause of the eye irritation, take some *shatavari* (1/2 teaspoon), add just a pinch of *shanka bhasma,* and take it twice a day for 2 weeks, with a little warm water.

• Aloe vera gel (2 tablespoons 3 times a day) also pacifies acidity.

• If you determine that high pitta might be the cause of the eye irritation, make a mixture of the herbs *shanka pushpi* and *jatamamsi* in equal proportions. Take 1/2 teaspoon twice a day for 2 weeks.

Eyes—Ayurvedic Care

Ayurveda has a number of excellent suggestions for maintaining your eyes in strength and health.

COOL WATER WASH. Early in the morning, when you wash your face, fill your mouth with cool water and hold it there; then splash cool water over your open eyes. Traditionally, you're not supposed to swallow or spit out the water, but keep it in your mouth as you sprinkle the cool water on your eyes. This has a double cooling effect, both from outside and from the oral cavity, that will make your eyes feel fresh, happy, and cheerful. (If you prefer, you can use an eye cup instead.)

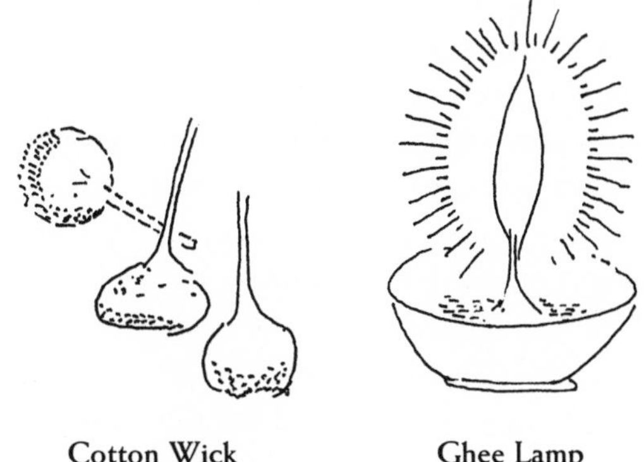

Cotton Wick Ghee Lamp

GHEE LAMP. A traditional Ayurvedic way to strengthen and soothe the eyes is to gaze at

Ayurvedic Eye Exercises

The following exercises will strengthen your eyes.

• First, blink the eyes rapidly several times. Then, with eyes open, move your eyes in this pattern:

up and down
side to side
diagonally from top left to bottom right
diagonally from top right to bottom left
clockwise in a circle
counterclockwise in a circle

• Hold your arm outstretched in front of you. Look at the tip of your index finger, and gradually bring the finger close to you, following it with your eyes, until it touches your "third eye," between the eyebrows.

• Look at the tip of your nose, and then up toward your "third eye."

• Finally, close your eyes tightly, then release. These exercises are beneficial for improving the circulation of the eccentric muscles of the eyeball.

After finishing the exercises, or anytime your eyes feel tired or strained, rub your palms vigorously together for a few seconds to generate some warmth, then place them *lightly* over your eyes. Feel how soothing the warmth is! Keep them there for a minute or two to strengthen and nourish your eyes.

the flame of a ghee lamp. Prepare a ghee lamp by taking a small bowl, placing a cotton wick in it, and adding ghee. Be sure the wick is made of genuine cotton; synthetic cotton will burn up in an instant. Also be sure the wick is not too thick. Apply a little ghee to the tip of the wick and then light it.

Set the ghee lamp at a distance of 2 or 3 feet from you, remove your glasses, and gaze at the flame for 2 or 3 minutes *without blinking*. This procedure will improve the *tejas* or lustrous quality of the eyes.

SALUTE THE SUN. Another effective way to keep eyes strong is to do the Sun Salutation exercise. Performing 12 sets of Sun Salutations is one of the best exercises for the entire body, including the eyes (see appendix 4).

FOR PITTA TYPES

The following six remedies are especially helpful for pitta types, who are more likely to find their eyes burning.

***TRIPHALA* EYEWASH.** Boil 1 teaspoon of *triphala* in a cup of water for 3 minutes. Cool the tea, and strain it with double- or triple-folded cheesecloth or a paper coffee filter so that no particle of *triphala* is left in the tea. Then wash your eyes with the tea.

CASTOR OIL REMEDY. At bedtime, put 1 drop of pure castor oil, with no preservatives, into each eye. Also rub 1 teaspoon of the oil into the soles of your feet. Next morning your eyes will feel really happy and fresh!

TO SOOTHE BURNING EYES. For a burning sensation in the eyes, put 1 drop of lukewarm liquid ghee in each eye at bedtime. That will lubricate the eyelid and eyelashes and will also soothe and strengthen your eyes.

ROSE WATER. You can also put 3 drops of pure rose water into each affected eye. Rose water is cooling.

A HEALING SALVE. Collyrium is effective for soothing your eyes. (It is available in most Indian grocery stores. Ask for *kajal*.) It is made of castor oil and natural camphor. It is black and people use it cosmetically as an eye liner, but it is actually medicinal and good for the eyes. Scoop out a small amount of salve with your little finger. Make sure the nail is well trimmed. With the other hand, pull the lower eyelid down while looking in the mirror and with your little finger apply the salve sparingly to the inner edge of the eyelid.

STRESS REDUCER. For eyestrain, Ayurveda also suggests taking a sterilized cotton ball or a piece of gauze, dipping it into cool goat's milk, and putting it over your closed eyes. This will ease stress and make your eyes feel better. (If goat's milk is not available, you may use cow's milk, but goat's milk is preferable.)

ADDITIONAL SUGGESTIONS

READ SITTING UP. While reading, keep your vertebral column straight. Avoid reading while lying down.

USE A NONGLARE COMPUTER SCREEN. If you are using a computer, be sure it has a nonglare screen, or use a protecting filter to reduce glare so it won't hurt your eyes.

Eyestrain

See "Eyes—Ayurvedic Care" and "Eye Irritation"

Fainting and Dizziness

Increased vata dosha, along with excess pitta moving in the nervous system, cause fainting and dizziness. There are two types of dizziness:

In the first kind, one feels that external objects in the environment are moving: "I am still, but the room is moving around me." That is called *objective dizziness,* and it is primarily due to aggravated vata.

The second type is called *subjective dizziness.* Here, one has the feeling of swinging or disequilibrium, of being subjectively in motion. This type of dizziness is caused primarily by excess pitta. The difference between the two is subtle and not easy to pinpoint, especially since vata and pitta are both always involved. But it is helpful to distinguish between the two, as some aspects of treatment will be different.

> **Time to See the Doctor**
>
> The remedies in this section are simple, effective means of relieving dizziness. But if dizziness or fainting persists after using them, it would be wise to see a neurologist or another medical expert, because the dizziness might be due to some serious pathology.

Vertigo, a spinning, merry-go-round kind of feeling, may be related to infection in the inner ear, head injury, or viral infection. It may be due to Ménière's disease, a condition in which increased pressure in the middle ear generates a feeling of vertigo. Ménière's disease will result in progressive hearing loss if it's not treated. All these conditions have to be suspected and ruled out before undertaking home treatment for dizziness. However, the domestic remedies below will help most cases of dizziness.

Dizziness or feeling faint may also occur when there is insufficient oxygen in the room.

If you feel dizzy and you're not sure whether you're spinning or the room is moving, focus on a fixed point, such as a window frame. When the eyeball becomes steady by focusing on a stable point, it sends a message to the brain that calms down the *rajasic* quality of vata dosha. This works well for objective dizziness.

The kind of dizziness known as *motion sickness* is often associated with nausea and vomiting. To help with motion sickness, before starting the trip, take one 00-size capsule filled with ginger powder. Bring some more along on the trip. You might also bring some candied ginger and chew on a piece of it from time to time. If you are in a car and you feel that everything seems to be in motion, try to look at a fixed point, such as the horizon or a distant unmoving object. This should help to stop the dizziness.

Sometimes people feel dizzy when they stand up quickly. There are many possible causes for this, including low adrenal energy, low blood pressure, or the use of some anti-hypertensive drugs, especially beta blockers, which may weaken the adrenals. If you find yourself getting dizzy upon standing up, simply get up *slowly.* This will help.

Pitta individuals with hypoglycemia may experience sweating and dizziness and may even verge on fainting if they go too long without eating. This is a form of subjective dizziness. Hypoglycemics have to eat on time, or they may even become unconscious. Drinking some apple juice or any sweet fruit juice will be effective.

QUICK REMEDY FOR FAINTING. If a person faints, collapses, and becomes unconscious, sprinkle some cold water on the face.

DIZZINESS FROM EXERCISING. Individuals who exercise vigorously may become dehydrated from sweating a lot, which may bring on dizziness. The cure for this is about as simple as it gets: Drink some water. Even just one glass of cool water will help to reduce pitta as well as correct the dehydration, and the dizziness will subside.

DEEP BREATHING. Another simple remedy for dizziness is breathing deeply, as in *ujjayi pranayama* (see chapter 6) and holding the breath behind the belly button.

EAR PULL. Here's another simple remedy: Insert your index finger into your ear and gently pull the ear upward, forward, and downward. This will regulate intracranial pressure, which will greatly if not entirely relieve the feeling of faintness or dizziness.

NATURAL SMELLING SALTS. For dizziness or when feeling faint, slice or chop up an onion and inhale the smell forcibly until tears come to your eyes. Onions contain a lot of ammonia; inhaling them produces vasodilation, which brings more blood supply to the brain, and dizziness is automatically corrected.

HERBAL FORMULAS. If you determine that the dizziness is primarily due to pitta, a wonderful Ayurvedic herbal formula may prove helpful. Mix these herbs:

brahmi 1 part
jatamamsi 1 part
saraswati 1/4 part

Take 1/2 teaspoon of the mixture 2 or 3 times a day with water after meals.

The following formula is also helpful when dizziness is due to excess pitta:

shatavari 1 part
jatamamsi 1 part
kama dudha 2 pinches

If you take 1/2 teaspoon of this mixture a couple of times a day with warm water, it will help take care of your dizziness.

SANDALWOOD. Pitta-type dizziness can also be helped by the smell of sandalwood oil or incense.

GHEE NOSE DROPS. Using ghee nose drops will also help. Warm up a little bit of ghee until it is liquefied. When cool enough not to injure delicate tissue, put 3 to 5 drops in each nostril, and inhale. This will improve blood supply to the brain and will relieve the dizziness.

COLON CLEANSING. Sometimes dizzy spells are due to chronic constipation and gases. So keep the colon clean with *triphala,* 1/2 teaspoon taken at bedtime in a cupful of warm water.

Fatigue and Chronic Fatigue

Fatigue is physical and mental stress. However, it is not always due to overwork. In fact, sometimes people feel tired because they're not doing enough, not working hard enough. For such people, fatigue can be due to boredom or lack of motivation.

In such cases, I've had to ask patients to walk or to do some physical work in order to get rid of fatigue and increase their energy level. So the first thing to determine is whether the tiredness is due to too much physical work or too much idleness!

Fatigue may be due to low gastric fire, weakness of the liver, low adrenal energy, or anemia. It may be caused by Epstein-Barr virus, a form of chronic fatigue syndrome related to high stagnant pitta in the liver. People having a history of infectious mononucleosis can feel very tired.

Here are some treatment recommendations for fatigue of various causes:

FOR FATIGUE AFTER EXERCISE OR HARD PHYSICAL WORK. Drink a cup of fresh orange juice with a pinch of rock salt. Adding 10 drops of fresh lime juice will help pacify pitta.

• Drinking 1 cup of ginseng or *ashwagandha* tea once or twice a day will help.

FOR ANEMIA. If the fatigue is due to anemia, treat the anemia with blood builders such as pomegranate juice, grapes and/or grape juice, beets or beet/carrot juice, or the herbs *abrak bhasma* and *loha bhasma.* (See "Anemia" for many more recommendations.)

FOR EPSTEIN-BARR VIRUS. If the fatigue is due to Epstein-Barr virus, treat it as a pitta disorder.

• Follow the pitta-pacifying diet (see chapter 8).

• Use the following herbal formula:

shatavari 5 parts
bala 4 parts
vidari 3 parts
kama dudha 1/4 part

Take 1/2 teaspoon of this mixture 2 or 3 times a day with 1 teaspoon of *shatavari* ghee. This will strengthen the liver and help to remedy chronic fatigue syndrome (see the *shatavari* ghee recipe in appendix 2).

TO STRENGTHEN GASTRIC FIRE

When your agni (gastric fire) is low and your digestion slow, nourishment from the food you eat will be poorly absorbed and assimilated. If the nourishment you derive from eating is insufficient, naturally your energy will be low.

• One of the best ways to kindle agni is to use some ginger. Before each meal, chop or grate a little fresh ginger, add a few drops of lime juice and a pinch of salt, and chew it up. Or just cut a thin slice of fresh ginger, put on a pinch of salt, and chew that.

• Avoid cold and iced drinks, especially during or after meals. They counteract agni and impede effective digestion. Take small sips of warm water during the meal.

• Taking *chitrak-adivati,* one 200-mg. tablet twice a day, after lunch and dinner, will help kindle the fire and the fatigue will go.

Time to See the Doctor

Unusual exertion, stress, lack of sleep, and a number of other factors can make you understandably tired. But if you use the Ayurvedic remedies recommended for fatigue for a few weeks and you still have unexplainable feelings of exhaustion or continue to feel unusually listless, lethargic, and drained of energy, your tiredness may be due to a more serious illness. Fatigue is a symptom of many illnesses, including anemia, lung disease, diabetes, hepatitis, mononucleosis, thyroid disease, and cancer. You may also have developed chronic fatigue syndrome. So please be wise and consult a physician.

• You will find many additional tips for strengthening the digestive fire in "Indigestion."

YOGA POSTURES AND *PRANAYAMA*. Alternate Nostril Breathing and some gentle yoga stretching can be beneficial to kindle the gastric fire. See appendix 4 and chapter 6 for help with yoga postures and *pranayama*. In general, unless fatigue is due to idleness, Ayurveda does not recommend much exercise for cases of fatigue. Exercise will burn *ojas* and may increase rather than decrease the feelings of fatigue.

TO BUILD STRENGTH AND ENERGY

Use the following food remedies for added nourishment and strength.

DATES. Soak 10 fresh dates in a quart jar of ghee. Add 1 teaspoon ginger, $1/8$ teaspoon cardamom, and a pinch of saffron. Cover and keep in a warm place for at least 2 weeks. Then eat 1 date daily, in the early morning. Believe it or not, it tastes delicious, and it works to remedy anemia, sexual debility, and chronic fatigue.

A simpler tonic using dates is this date drink: Soak 5 fresh dates in a glass of water overnight. Next morning, liquefy in a blender and drink. It will give you energy and vitality. (Be sure to remove the pits before blending!)

MANGOES. Eating one ripe mango daily, and an hour or so later drinking 1 cup of warm milk with 1 teaspoon ghee added, is also good for increasing vitality.

A variation is to drink 1 cup of fresh mango juice, followed an hour or so later by ½ cup of warm milk with a pinch of cardamom, a pinch of nutmeg, and 1 teaspoon of ghee.

Fever

Fever is a sign of ama (toxins) moving in the circulatory system. Contrary to what some people believe, fever is not often a sign of infection. In some cases there *is* infection, but most of the time the fever is due to toxicity in the *rasa dhatu*, the body's basic vital tissue (see page 31). When the ama has been eliminated, the fever will subside.

DON'T EAT. There is an old saying, "Feed a cold and starve a fever," and truly the first treatment recommended by Ayurveda for a fever is to observe a fast. For acute fever, a total fast is recommended if the person is strong enough. If the person is debilitated or weak, it is better to drink water, some kind of fruit juice, or one of the herbal teas suggested below, such as holy basil *(tulsi)* or lemongrass. *Don't drink milk;* it will worsen the fever and create diarrhea.

In addition to fasting, the following recommendations will be helpful.

HERBAL REMEDIES

The simplest herbal remedy for fever is cilantro juice. Put a handful of cilantro leaves in a blender with about ⅓ cup water, and blend thoroughly. Strain out the pulp. Take 2 teaspoons of the remaining liquid 3 times a day to help lower the fever.

• You can make an effective herbal tea for fever consisting of

lemongrass
tulsi (holy basil)
fennel

in equal proportions. For each cup, use 1 teaspoon of the mixture and steep in boiling water for 10 minutes; strain and drink. This is an excellent diaphoretic; that is, it

Time to See the Doctor

Fever is a sign that your body is fighting toxins and/or infection and is healing and purifying itself. It is usually self-limiting—that is, it will disappear when the needed healing is done. But there are definitely times when fever requires the attention of a medical professional:

- any fever in a baby under 4 months old
- fever above 104 degrees Fahrenheit in an adult
- fever above 101 degrees in a person over age 60
- fever that lasts longer than 3 days
- fever accompanied by a severe headache and a stiff neck
- any fever in a person who has a chronic illness such as heart disease, diabetes, or respiratory disease

If any of these conditions are present, call a doctor or seek immediate attention.

makes you sweat, which brings down the temperature.

• Another excellent herbal remedy for reducing fever is a tea made of

coriander 2 *parts*
cinnamon 2 *parts*
ginger 1 *part*

Steep 1 teaspoon of this mixture in a cup of hot water for 10 minutes before drinking. You can drink this every few hours until the fever breaks.

• Another simple three-ingredient tea made of household herbs is this one:

cumin seeds
coriander seeds
fennel seeds

Mix seeds in equal proportions. Use 1 teaspoon of your mixture in a cup of boiling water; steep for 10 minutes, strain, and drink.

OTHER REMEDIES AND RECOMMENDATIONS

GRAPE JUICE WITH HERBS. Grapes are cooling. Into a cup of grape juice add 1/2 teaspoon cumin, 1/2 teaspoon fennel, and 1/2 teaspoon sandalwood powder, and drink. This will help to relieve fever.

AVOID COLD DRINKS. When you have a fever, it's best not to drink anything cold. Use the lemongrass-tulsi-fennel tea mentioned above, or any of the other herbal suggestions. Any hot tea will help to kindle the body's digestive fire (agni) and burn the ama

If the Fever Is High

If the temperature is high, prepare a bowl of cool water into which you have added 1 teaspoon of salt. Fold two pieces of clean cloth (such as handkerchiefs), dip them into the water, and put one on the forehead and one over the belly button. Repeat as needed. This will bring down the temperature quickly.

If you can get *maha sudarshan churna* from an Ayurvedic pharmacy, take 1/2 teaspoon twice a day with warm water. This formula will bring down any kind of fever.

If the person with high fever has a pitta constitution, there may be a danger of febrile convulsions. To help relieve this condition, make a slight modification of the procedure described above. Grate an onion and wrap half in one of the damp handkerchiefs, the other half in the second handkerchief. Place on the forehead and belly button, as above.

The belly is the seat of pitta, and the onion will help absorb the pitta. Tears will come to the eyes, the convulsions will stop, and the temperature will come down. If this procedure doesn't bring the fever down, see a doctor.

(toxins). Again, fever is a sign of ama in the system; once the ama is burned out, the body's temperature will come back to normal.

STAY PUT. It is not a good idea to exercise or to travel when you have a fever. If you do get a fever when on a journey, follow any of the above recommendations that you can; if possible, take *maha sudarshan churna* ($^1/_2$ teaspoon with a little warm water).

FOR CHRONIC FEVER. Make a tea of 1 teaspoon holy basil *(tulsi)* steeped in 1 cup hot water. Add $^1/_4$ teaspoon black pepper and 1 teaspoon honey. Take this 2 or 3 times a day.

• Another excellent formula to bring down chronic fever is $^1/_2$ teaspoon *maha sudarshan churna* mixed with 1 teaspoon *tikta ghrita* (bitter ghee). Take this 3 times a day on an empty stomach.

Fibrocystic Breast Disease

According to Ayurvedic principles, fibrocystic breast disease is a kapha disorder. Excess kapha builds up, leading to congestion, enlargement of the breasts, tenderness, and development of fibrocystic tissue.

GENTLE MASSAGE. To help reduce the accumulation of kapha, apply 1 teaspoon of warm castor oil to the breasts, and gently massage from inside to outside, that is, from the breastbone toward the armpits. Do this gentle massage before taking a warm shower. Or you can do a soap massage of the breasts during your shower, again massaging from the center of your chest outward.

Massaging the breasts in this way will improve the circulation of the mastic tissue and encourage lymphatic drainage into the armpits; in this way, fibrocystic changes can be minimized.

This massage will also take care of tenderness in the breasts. (See "Breasts, Sore" for more suggestions.)

EFFECTIVE HERBAL REMEDY. To help prevent fibrocystic breasts, use the following herbal formula:

kutki 2 parts
chitrak 2 parts
punarnava 5 parts

This herbal combination ($^1/_2$ teaspoon twice a day) will help to prevent the accumulation of kapha in the breast that leads to the development of fibrocystic tissue.

KAPHA-REDUCING DIET. As fibrocystic breasts are due to excess kapha, you will find it helpful to follow the kapha-reducing diet. Avoid dairy products, cold food and drink, heavy meats, wheat, and all sweets except honey. (See dietary guidelines in chapter 8.)

YOGA POSTURES. Doing some yoga postures daily will be helpful. Include the Locust, Bow, Boat, Spinal Twist, and Shoulder Stand in your "routine" of postures. (See appendix 4 for illustrations.)

Food Allergies

See also "Allergies"

To deal effectively with food allergies and minimize their negative impact on your life, begin by making a list of foods you appear to be allergic to. You will usually find, according to Ayurvedic dietetics, that you have reactions to foods with the same doshic quality as your constitution, particularly if you have an excess of that quality at the present time.

DETERMINING YOUR FOOD ALLERGY TYPE

The following descriptions should help you determine the type of food allergy you have.

- Kapha-type individuals, with excess kapha in their system, will be allergic to kapha foods, including dairy products such as milk, yogurt, and cheese; wheat; cucumber; and watermelon. Their food allergies may manifest as heaviness in the stomach, slow digestion, sleeping disorders, colds, congestion, cough, or water retention. In more serious conditions kapha food allergies may lead to bronchial congestion and kapha-type asthma.
- Pitta individuals, whose systemic pitta is unduly high, will show allergic reactions to such high-pitta foods as hot, spicy dishes; citrus fruits; sour fruits; tomatoes; potatoes; eggplant; and fermented foods. Their symptoms are likely to include heartburn, acid indigestion, stomach upset, nausea, and even vomiting. The person may suddenly get hot flashes, and may have bloodshot eyes.
- Vata individuals, especially when vata is in excess, are prone to get allergies to raw foods; beans (black beans, adzuki beans, pinto beans, and so on) and certain animal proteins. Vata food allergies are likely to manifest as bloating of the stomach, burping, gas, gurgling of the stomach, and vague abdominal discomfort and pain. It may also lead to insomnia and nightmares, pain in the joint, sciatica, muscle twitching, and muscle spasms.

So food allergies need to be studied according to an individual's *prakruti* (constitution) and *vikruti* (current status of the doshas).

TREATMENT

The best approach is simply to avoid the problematic food items and to follow the diet appropriate for your body type. For example, a vata person having vata-type food allergies should avoid a vata-provoking diet and should eat vata-pacifying foods. The same is true for pitta and kapha. (See the diet recommendations in chapter 8.)

Here are some additional suggestions for each of the three main types of food allergy.

FOR VATA-TYPE FOOD ALLERGIES. An effective way to help bring vata food allergies under control is to take a *dashamoola basti* (enema) twice a week, such as on Sunday and Thursday. Boil up 1 pint of water with 1 tablespoon of *dashamoola,* and use the resulting tea (after it cools down) for the enema. Try to retain the liquid at least 10 minutes. (For more on enemas, see appendix 3.) This herbal enema will help to pacify vata and remove toxicity from the colon, and vata-type food allergies can be minimized. Continue taking the *dashamoola* enema twice a week for one month.

Drinking licorice tea made from 1/2 teaspoon licorice root powder, 1/2 teaspoon honey, and 1 teaspoon ghee can also be helpful. Sip a little of the tea every half hour to an hour throughout the day until symptoms are relieved. Don't forget to add the honey only after the tea starts to cool; honey should never be cooked. *Note:* People with high blood pressure should not drink licorice tea. Substitute 1/2 teaspoon cinnamon and 2 to 3 cloves for the licorice, and make the tea as above.

FOR PITTA FOOD ALLERGIES. To control pitta food allergies, it is helpful to do *virechana chikitsa* (purgation). Take 1 teaspoon of *amalaki* or *sat isabgol* (psyllium husks) at night. Add the herbs to 1 cup of hot water, let it stand for 10 to 15 minutes, and drink. Stagnation of pitta in the small intestine is the root cause of a pitta-type food allergy. Purgation therapy clears away the pitta so that the allergy can be brought under control. Continue with *virechana* daily for a month, or until the allergy subsides.

You will also find it helpful to eat cooked apples. Peel and core a couple of apples, cook them a few minutes to soften them, and mash them up with a pinch of cumin and 1 teaspoon ghee. Eat about 1/2 cup once or twice daily, at least an hour before or after meals.

FOR KAPHA FOOD ALLERGIES. The Ayurvedic purification known as *vamana* (vomiting) will be helpful. Every Sunday (or at least for a couple of weeks) in the early morning, drink 2 pints of salt water. Add 2 teaspoons of salt to 2 pints of water, drink it down, and then try to vomit it out. (Rubbing the back part of your tongue until you get a "gag" reflex will help.) This purification process will remove a lot of excess mucus from the stomach and help to clear up food allergies.

If vomiting doesn't take place, don't worry about it; the remaining salty water won't hurt you. It will simply go through your system and will actually have some beneficial cleansing effect.

NOTE: Many people feel a lot of fear or discomfort with the idea or the actuality of vomiting. If you feel this way, do not force yourself to do this purification. Do *vamana* only if it is comfortable for you to do so.

Kaphas should also fast on Sunday. The fasting is important; it will help cleanse the system.

Make a tea out of 1/2 teaspoon licorice root powder, 1/4 teaspoon cinnamon, and 1/2 teaspoon coriander. Steep in 1 cup of water for 10 minutes, strain, and sip a little of the tea throughout the day, about an ounce every half hour to an hour. Again, people with high blood pressure should not drink licorice tea. Substitute 1/2 teaspoon cinnamon and 2 to 3 cloves for the licorice.

FOR ALL FOOD ALLERGIES. If you don't know whether the allergy is vata, pitta, or kapha, then try this simple remedy that is effective for all types: Roast some cumin, fennel, and white sesame seeds, and eat a handful after meals.

To prepare the mixture, take one ounce of each kind of seed, and dry-roast it *separately* (one type at a time) on a heavy cast-iron pan. You will have to stir the seeds constantly to keep them from burning. The fennel takes a few minutes, the others only about a minute or two before they become fragrant and slightly brown. Put the seeds together, add about 1/2 teaspoon rock salt (don't use sea salt), and mix it all up. Store in a glass jar.

Chewing a little of this mixture after eating any food will aid digestion and help prevent any kind of food allergy.

Frequent Urination

See "Bladder Problems," "Prostate Problems," and "Urinary Incontinence"

Frequent Urination During Pregnancy

Frequent urination during pregnancy is an entirely natural phenomenon. When the uterus becomes enlarged due to the growth of the fetus in the womb, it creates pressure on the bladder. The bladder hasn't got sufficient space to accumulate urine and expand, so just a little accumulation stimulates the desire for relief.

If frequent urination disturbs the woman's sleep, this is not good, as she needs her rest. Ayurveda suggests this simple home remedy: Eat a handful of white sesame seeds with about 1/2 teaspoon of jaggery or natural brown sugar. This mixture will pacify vata dosha; by soothing vata, it prevents the excess stimulation that contracts the bladder. In this way, frequent urination during pregnancy can be corrected.

Additional suggestions:

- Don't drink anything for at least 2 hours before going to bed.
- Don't drink anything with caffeine, such as coffee, tea, or cola, especially in the evening. Caffeine is a diuretic (it promotes urination) and is exactly what you don't need if you want to counteract frequent urination.
- For further recommendations, see "Urinary Incontinence."

Frigidity

See "Low Libido"

Gallstones

Gallstones are a kapha disorder associated with underactive thyroid and slow metabolism. Gallstones begin with stagnation of bile in the gallbladder. The bile becomes thick, accumulates, coagulates, and slowly leads to stone formation.

Prevention of gallstones, and what to do when gallstones are present, are two different lines of treatment. First let's consider what to do when gallstones have already developed.

TO ALLEVIATE THE PAIN. In general, gallstones are not painful. They may remain in the gallbladder for a long time without causing any pain; indeed, you will not know they are there. Pain occurs when the gallbladder tries to push the stones out of the gallbladder through the bile duct.

To reduce pain, put a warm castor oil pack on your abdomen. Castor oil produces a slow, sustained heat that is soothing and healing. Warm up about 3 tablespoons of castor oil and pour it onto a handkerchief or other soft cloth, spreading it equally on the cloth. Place this compress on the abdomen above the gallbladder (on the right side of your abdomen, above the line of your navel and below the ribs). If you have a hot water bottle, you may place it on top of the pack to keep it warm. (Electric heating pads are not recommended.)

FOR ACUTE ATTACK. During an acute gallstone attack, use this herbal formula:

musta 4 *parts*
trikatu 3 *parts*
guduchi 6 *parts*

Take 1/4 teaspoon of this mixture 2 or 3 times a day with honey. It will reduce the pain and ease the gallbladder attack.

LIVER FLUSH TO ELIMINATE THE GALLSTONE. When the pain is gone, you can do a liver flush to wash out the gallstone. This liver flush should not be done if the stone is large, so *before doing the treatment it is vital to get an ultrasound report on the exact size of the gallstone and consult with your physician about using the treatment.* If it is a small and recently formed stone, this treatment will help. If it is quite large, such as 3 to 4 mm. in diameter, then the flushing treatment will not be good.

Combine 8 ounces olive oil, 4 ounces lemon juice, a chopped fresh garlic clove, and 1/4 teaspoon cayenne pepper. Drink this entire mixture in the early morning (at about six o'clock) on an empty stomach. Don't eat anything until at least noon. If you feel thirsty, drink hot water or a little lime juice.

The treatment is a shock to the gallbladder, which contracts and squeezes the gallstone(s) out into the duodenum.

That night, take 1/2 teaspoon of *triphala* with warm water. The next day you will pass some green stuff in the stools. This is thick, coagulated bile containing the gallstone crystals.

> **TIME TO SEE THE DOCTOR**
>
> IMPORTANT: This liver-flushing treatment should *not* be done without the approval and guidance of your physician or the direct supervision of an Ayurvedic physician. Otherwise, you may damage the gallbladder and experience dangerous complications.

PREVENTION OF GALLSTONES. In order to prevent gallstone formation, one has to improve both thyroid function and metabolism. In general, the following formula is effective:

punarnava 5 *parts*
shatavari 4 *parts*
kutki 2 *parts*
chitrak 2 *parts*
musta 3 *parts*
shilajit 1/4 *part*

This mixture (1/4 teaspoon 3 times a day with honey), taken regularly for 2 to 3 months, will help to prevent gallstone formation.

YOGA POSTURES. Several yoga *asanas* are beneficial for prevention of gallstones. The Bow pose, Peacock pose, Spinal Twist, and Narayan pose (lying on the left side) will help to empty the gallbladder. (For illustrations of yoga postures, see appendix 4.) These postures will improve circulation in the gallbladder, helping to prevent the crystallization process.

DIET. Stay away from deep-fried food, dairy products such as yogurt and cheese, and all fatty foods, especially animal fat and any saturated fat. These accelerate coagulation of bile into gallstones.

Gas and Flatulence

No one under the sun is exempt from flatulence. Every person at some time or another gets gases and disturbances in the colon.

We are all vulnerable to this condition for several reasons. First, the colon is the main seat of vata dosha, the dosha that is derived from ether and air. If vata increases in the colon, due to eating vata-aggravating foods, cold weather, anxiety, insomnia, and other factors, gases may build up. Also, whenever we eat anything, we swallow a small amount of air, which increases vata. And any food we eat undergoes slight fermentation, which produces gases. These gases, in the segmented colon, create flatulence, distension, and discomfort.

Here are some effective ways to control flatulence.

GINGER REMEDY. Grate some fresh ginger root until you have about 1 teaspoon of pulp, and add 1 teaspoon of lime juice. Take this mixture immediately after eating.

LEMON JUICE REMEDY. Another simple method to reduce excess gas is to stir 1 teaspoon lemon juice and 1/2 teaspoon baking soda into 1 cup cool water. Drink it down quickly, right after meals, for best results! (It forms carbon dioxide, which facilitates digestion.)

CUMIN-FENNEL-CELERY SEED MIXTURE. Prepare a mixture of roasted cumin, fennel, and *ajwan* seeds (Indian celery seed) in equal proportions. (See pages 183–184 for suggested method of preparation of roasted seeds.) After each meal, take about 1/2 to 1 teaspoon of this mixture, chew well, and swallow with about 1/3 cup warm water.

CHARCOAL TABLETS. Another simple remedy is charcoal tablets, which you can buy in most health food stores. Swallow two tablets after lunch and dinner. The charcoal absorbs gases and helps to prevent flatulence.

HERBAL TABLETS. Ayurveda also suggests the herbs *shankavati* and *lasunadivati*. These herbs are useful for an aching stomach and are helpful to reduce flatulence. Take 1 tablet (available from most sources of Ayurvedic herbs) at night for 5 days.

DIETARY GUIDELINES. Flatulence is mostly a vata condition, so following a vata-pacifying diet can help prevent it. Avoid raw foods, cold food and drinks, and most beans. (See chapter 8 for guidelines.) Fermented foods also increase gases in the colon, so it's best to avoid them.

TRIPHALA. Finally, it is helpful to take the herbal compound *triphala*. At night before going to bed, steep 1/2 to 1 teaspoon *triphala* in a cup of boiling hot water for 5 to 10 minutes, then drink it.

Glaucoma

Increasing intraocular pressure, due to accumulation of kapha dosha in the vitreous humor (the viscous fluid inside the eyeball), is called glaucoma. When glaucoma is occurring in an eye, palpation will show a tenseness in that eye. If pressure in the eye becomes high, headaches may occur. Glaucoma may become a serious condition and can cause blindness, so one has to be very watchful.

In persons who lift heavy weights (either at work or for exercise), who strain in exercise, who have high cholesterol or high triglycerides, or who have diabetes or nicotine toxicity due to smoking, intraocular pressure has a tendency to increase and may lead to glaucoma.

If upon examination by an eye doctor it is determined that you have higher than normal intraocular pressure, these remedies may be helpful.

AN HERBAL REMEDY. In earlier stages of glaucoma, Ayurveda treats this problem with the following formula, which will help to relieve the tension in the eye:

punarnava 5 *parts*
jatamamsi 3 *parts*
shanka pushpi 3 *parts*

Boil 1 teaspoon of this mixture in a cup of water for a few minutes to make a tea. Drink twice a day.

***TRIPHALA* TEA EYEWASH.** To relieve the tension in the eye, wash the eyeball with *triphala* tea, which helps to regulate pressure in the eye. Boil 1/2 teaspoon *triphala* in 1 cup water for 2 minutes, strain it thoroughly (through cheesecloth double-folded, or through a coffee filter) so that no particles of *triphala* remain in the tea, cool it down, and wash the eye. (For more on *triphala,* see appendix 2.)

TREAT THE SOURCE OF THE PROBLEM. In addition, one has to determine and then treat the root cause of the glaucoma. If the problem is diabetes, follow the instructions in the section "Diabetes." If high blood pressure is the problem, then try to regulate the blood pressure (see "Hypertension"). If you have high triglycerides and high cholesterol, then you have to control that (see "Cholesterol").

REDUCE KAPHA. Follow a kapha-pacifying diet. Especially avoid coffee, white sugar, and dairy products.

BE CAREFUL OF EXERCISE. Strictly avoid heavy weightlifting and similar straining. When you do yoga postures, avoid inverted poses such as Headstand and Shoulder Stand.

Gum Disease

See also "Teeth and Gums—Ayurvedic Care"

Gum disease includes receding gums, bleeding gums, gingivitis, and swollen gums. From an Ayurvedic perspective, excess vata dosha leads to receding gums, while pitta dosha is responsible for bleeding gums, gingivitis, and swollen gums.

FOR GENERAL CARE. For general cleaning of the teeth and caring for the gums, Ayurvedic dentistry recommends the use of certain bitter and astringent herbs, particularly *neem,* which is bitter, and *lodhra, kushtha,* and *bilva,* which are all astringent. You can make an excellent cleanser for brushing your teeth by mixing the powdered form of these herbs. You can use *neem* plus any one of the other three, mixed in equal proportions.

Rinsing your mouth with a tea made from these herbs is also beneficial.

You can also buy any one of several commercial toothpastes with *neem* and other Ayurvedic herbs in natural food stores or by mail order (see Resources).

FOR RECEDING GUMS. Receding gums expose the roots of the teeth, and then both the gums and teeth become sensitive to cold and more susceptible to infection. To help with this problem, take a mouthful of warm sesame oil, and swish it around in your mouth for about 3 minutes before going to bed. Then massage your gums with your index finger. It is better not to rinse with water afterward; leave the oil residue in your mouth.

FOR BLEEDING GUMS AND GINGIVITIS. *Triphala* tea is effective for gingivitis and bleeding gums. *Triphala* has astringent qualities, and it is a hemostatic—that is, it stops bleeding. Gargling and swishing the mouth with *triphala* tea are helpful for both gingivitis and bleeding gums.

- One cup orange juice with 1/2 teaspoon natural sugar and a pinch of cumin will help bleeding gums.
- Drink the juice of 1/2 lemon squeezed into a cupful of water.
- Raw apples are also beneficial. Eating a raw apple about an hour after meals helps to clean the teeth and heal the gums. Pears are also effective.
- Eat some melon, chewing it slowly. (Again, at least an hour after meals.)
- Try eating about 10 to 20 raspberries 2 or 3 times a day on an empty stomach. (Don't combine them with any dairy products.)
- Massaging the gums with coconut oil can also help heal gingivitis and bleeding gums.

FOR INFECTED GUMS. Tea tree oil is effective for painful infected gums, as is clove oil. Both help to reduce pain and heal the infection. All you need is one drop of tea tree or clove oil directly at the site of the pain. A small piece of natural, edible camphor will also take care of pain in the gums. (Do not use synthetic camphor; it is poisonous.)

- Dental floss with tea tree oil will take care of infected pockets in the gums below the gumline. Some dental floss treated with tea tree oil is available commercially; otherwise, just dip the floss in the oil prior to flossing.

Hair Care Secrets

In Ayurveda, hair (along with nails) is considered to be a by-product of bone formation. The *dhatu* or tissue responsible for building bones *(asthi)* also gives rise to the hair. (For an explanation of the *dhatus,* please see page 31.)

Thus, proper nutrition of the bones is necessary for healthy growth of your hair. If you don't completely absorb calcium and magnesium, for example, not only will your bones be adversely affected, but your hair may become brittle, develop split ends, break easily, and even begin to fall out.

It is important to note that if your hair *is* unhealthy, it may be an indication that you are not absorbing these minerals effectively; this suggests that the health of your bones will be—or may already be—adversely affected. So the health of your hair (as well as your nails) is a good indicator of the health of your bones.

The following Ayurvedic secrets of healthy hair will help you keep your hair's natural strength and luster.

PROPER DIET. Healthy hair depends first upon eating nutritious food. Dairy products such as cheese, milk, and freshly prepared yogurt are good for bones and hair, as are white radish and daikon. Coconut, cooked apples, and cabbage are also beneficial.

TAKE A MINERAL SUPPLEMENT. You can improve the condition of your hair (and also strengthen your bones) by taking supplements of calcium, magnesium, zinc, and other minerals. An effective formula will contain a daily dose of about

calcium	1,200 mg.
magnesium	600 mg.
zinc	60 mg.

Oil Massage for Hair Health and Beauty

Rubbing a little oil on your scalp is beneficial for your hair. *Amla* oil, *bhringaraj* oil, and *brahmi* oil are all cooling, are quite favorable for healthy growth of your hair, and help maintain the hair's natural luster. These oils are fine for all body types. (Please see instructions on how to prepare these oils in appendix 2.)

Before going to bed, rub 2 teaspoons of the oil onto your hair. Note that the object here is to apply the oil to the *scalp,* not the hair. Gently massaging the scalp improves circulation at the root of the hair and thus increases the supply of nourishing minerals that support the roots.

First pour the oil into a small dish. (You may wish to warm it up a little.) Dip your fingertips into the oil, and then run your fingers through your hair, with the intention of getting the oil to the scalp, not oiling the hair. *Gently* massage from the center of your scalp (the crown of your head) down toward your ears. A rough or rapid application may disturb the roots of your hair.

SESAME SEEDS. Every morning, eat a handful of white sesame seeds. One handful of sesame seeds contains about 1,200 mg. of calcium and magnesium and promotes healthy growth of your hair.

COCONUT WATER FOR CALCIUM. Drinking coconut water (the "juice" inside the fresh coconut) also helps to provide essential calcium for hair growth. You can have 1/2 cup a day. Drinking coconut milk (made from coconut "meat" blended in water) is also helpful, but is a second choice.

NOTE: If you have high cholesterol, you may not want to use so much coconut, as coconut is high in saturated fat, which increases cholesterol in the blood.

STIMULATE YOUR HAIR BY COMBING. Gently combing your hair with a comb, a little in the opposite direction of its natural tendencies, helps to improve the circulation at the root of the hair and will make your hair healthier.

Vigorous brushing of the hair is not recommended.

YOGA FOR YOUR HAIR. Several yoga postures are effective for relieving pressure and tension in the neck, which will increase circulation to the scalp. These include the Shoulder Stand; the Camel, Cobra, and Cow poses; and the Spinal Twist.

NOTE: For strategies to combat hair loss, see "Baldness."

Hangover

The effects of overconsumption of alcohol—headache, dullness, inability to focus the mind clearly, nausea, dizziness, and so on—are all symptoms of excess pitta. Drinking too much alcohol may become toxic to the stomach and liver, which triggers pitta and can eventually lead to serious illness.

The following recommendations will help you get over the effects of drinking too much alcohol the night before and will help restore normal functioning.

• Drink a glass of water with about 1 teaspoon lime juice, 1/2 teaspoon sugar, and a pinch of salt added. Just before drinking, add 1/2 teaspoon baking soda. This will immediately take care of pitta aggravation, and you will feel much better.

• A glass of fresh orange juice with 1 teaspoon lime juice and a pinch of cumin powder can help with both alcohol and drug-induced hangover.

• If you are feeling drowsy and dull, with an aching head, a burning stomach and no appetite, try a cup of cool lassi. Blend 1 tablespoon of fresh yogurt with 1 cup of water and a pinch of cumin powder. Drink this 3 or 4 times in the day. It will be effective to prevent dehydration, relieve nausea, and soothe the burning in your stomach.

• You can also use this herbal formula:

shatavari 5 parts
shanka bhasma 1/8 part
kama dudha 1/8 part
jatamamsi 3 parts

Take $1/2$ teaspoon of this mixture 2 or 3 times in a day. Put it on your tongue, and wash down with warm water.

• Most of the time, drinking coconut water (the natural liquid inside the coconut) is beneficial for hangover.

• Doing *nasya* with *bhringaraj* oil or *brahmi* ghee may also be effective. (Instructions for preparing medicated oils and ghee are in appendix 2. To buy them already prepared, see Resources. Guidelines for *nasya* appear in appendix 3.)

• The herbal compound *tikta* is an effective antidote for alcohol toxicity. If you take $1/2$ teaspoon of the powder 3 times during the day that you need it, washed down with warm water, it should take care of the hangover. If you cannot locate *tikta*, you may substitute aloe vera, myrrh, or *sudharshan*.

Headaches

Headaches are a very complex phenomenon. Ayurveda speaks a great deal about the etiological factors behind headaches and the many ways headaches manifest.

Generally, headaches are classified as vata type, pitta type, and kapha type. In vata individuals, fear, anxiety, stress, nervousness, constipation, and physical overactivity can aggravate systemic vata, which can go into the skeletal, muscular, or nervous system and cause headaches. Vata-caused headaches will tend to be in the occipital area (the back of the head) or on the left side.

In pitta individuals, acid indigestion, hyperacidity, acidic pH of the saliva and stomach, excess pitta in the intestine and colon, and getting overheated, as well as a diet high in pitta-provoking food, can create a headache. That headache will be more in the temple or temporal area.

Because of a kapha-producing diet, systemic kapha in the stomach increases, enters into the general circulation, and can lodge in the sinuses and create kapha-type sinus headaches. Kapha headaches tend to be more in the frontal and nasal areas of the head.

Headaches can also be due to ear problems, eye problems, insomnia, food allergies, exposure to cold temperatures, tension in the neck, or working too long (for instance, in front of a computer) in a wrong position. Even using two pillows below the head for sleeping can cause headaches.

Clearly the causes are extremely varied. Remember that in Ayurveda, treatment is determined by the specifics of each situation. Thus in order to successfully treat your headache you need to know as much as possible about its cause.

FOR VATA-TYPE HEADACHES

These headaches are in the back (occipital) portion of the head. They are characterized by throbbing, pulsating, migrating pain that radiates from the back of the head and may go to the front. A vata headache may be associated with tension in the neck and shoulder muscles, back stiffness, constipation, and sciatica. This kind of headache is aggravated by high altitude. It gets worse when you move your body and subsides when you rest.

WARM WATER ENEMA. Vata headaches are often due to toxins accumulated in the colon. Ayurveda recommends using a warm water enema to relieve any constipation and taking *triphala* (1/2 teaspoon at night with 1/2 to 1 cup warm water) over several weeks to systematically detoxify the colon.

OIL ENEMA. Probably the best way to pacify vata is by oil *basti* (enema). Half a cup of warm sesame oil injected into the rectum and retained for at least 5 to 10 minutes helps to calm vata. (Detailed instructions for *basti* are in appendix 3.)

OIL MASSAGE. For tension in the neck and shoulders, massage the tight muscles there with sesame oil. Then take a hot shower.

GHEE NASYA. Putting 3 to 5 drops of warm ghee in each nostril will help reduce vata and will be effective for soothing your headache (see appendix 3).

NIGHTTIME FOOT AND SCALP MASSAGE. Before you go to sleep at night, rub some sesame oil gently on the top of your head and on the soles of your feet. This is one of the most effective ways to keep vata under control.

IN CASE OF DEHYDRATION. Vata headache is frequently associated with dehydration, especially if you have just gone to a higher altitude. If dehydration has occurred, make some homemade dextrosaline: Mix 1 tablespoon sugar, 1/4 teaspoon salt, and about 10 drops of lime juice in a pint of water and drink it. The moment the dehydration is corrected, a vata headache will disappear or at least be greatly reduced.

A SOOTHING PASTE. If, after this treatment, the headache does not subside, then take 1/4 teaspoon nutmeg powder in your palm, and add sufficient water to make a paste by rubbing your hands together. Apply the paste to your forehead. Leave it on for about half an hour and then wash it off. This should help to soothe a vata-type headache.

FOLLOW THE VATA-BALANCING DIET. Remember that if you are prone to vata headaches and other vata-related problems such as constipation and insomnia, following a vata-pacifying diet will help a lot (see chapter 8).

FOR PITTA-TYPE HEADACHES. Pitta headaches start in the temple area and go to the central part of the head. A pitta headache is characterized by shooting, burning, piercing, or penetrating pain, and it is worsened by bright light, hot sun, or high temperatures, or by eating sour fruits, pickles, or highly spicy food. It may be associated with nausea and/or burning of the eyes. The person may also become quite irritable. A pitta headache is often felt behind the eyes and may be associated with dizziness.

These headaches are related to the stomach and intestines.

ALOE VERA. If you have a pitta-type headache, take 2 tablespoons of aloe vera gel, up to 3 times in a day.

A COOLING TEA. Drinking cumin-coriander tea (equal amounts of each, about 1 teaspoon of the mixture per cup) can help to relieve a pitta-type headache. Let the tea cool to room temperature before you drink it.

A COOLING PASTE. This cooling paste may help to quickly relieve a pitta headache. Mix 1 teaspoon sandalwood powder with sufficient water to make a paste, and apply it to your forehead and/or temples. Leave it on your skin for about half an hour, then wash it off.

SOOTHING GHEE *NASYA*. A few drops of warm ghee placed in the nostrils will be beneficial for soothing a pitta-type headache.

EAT SOMETHING SWEET. Sometimes a pitta headache responds quickly if you just have something sweet to eat. Try a piece of sweet fruit, or some ice cream.

NIGHTTIME MINIMASSAGE. At night, rub a little *bhringaraj* oil or *brahmi* oil on the soles of your feet and on your scalp. Take precautions not to get oil on your pillow and sheets.

COVER YOUR HEAD. If you have a pitta-type headache—or are prone to getting them—don't walk or work in the sun without wearing a hat. A hat on your head protects against aggravating pitta and helps to prevent the headache.

FOR KAPHA-TYPE HEADACHES

If your headache occurs in winter or spring, strikes in the morning or evening, and gets worse when you bend down, it is a kapha headache. It is often associated with sinus congestion and clogging of the nose, and it often accompanies a cold or a cough. It may go along with hay fever and other allergies. The pain of a kapha headache is usually dull and deep-seated. It starts in the upper frontal area of the skull, moves down to the forehead, and sometimes comes down to the sinuses.

EUCALYPTUS STEAM. To immediately relieve a kapha headache, put 10 drops of eucalyptus oil in boiled water, cover your head with a towel, and inhale the steam. This helps to relieve the congestion and often completely takes care of the headache. Ginger steam—boiling fresh ginger or dried ginger powder and then inhaling the steam—is also effective.

USE THIS WARMING PASTE. A warming ginger paste can be quite helpful. Take 1 teaspoon ginger powder, mix together with sufficient water to form a paste, and apply it to your forehead. You can also put some of the paste across the bridge of your nose and over your cheekbones. A paste of *vacha* powder (calamus) is also helpful and is preferable for pitta individuals, as the ginger powder may burn their skin. Leave the paste on for about half an hour, then wash it off. *Be careful when washing off ginger paste:* Avoid getting any in your eyes.

NOTE: Ginger paste can sometimes create a burning sensation on the skin, especially in pitta individuals. It is not dangerous, but if you begin to feel an uncomfortable burning feeling, wash the ginger off with warm water.

A PASTE FOR SINUS HEADACHES. For sinus headaches (usually related to kapha), make a paste out of $1/2$ teaspoon cinnamon and sufficient water, and apply it locally.

SALTWATER REMEDY. For some individuals, a kapha-type headache can be quickly relieved by this simple remedy: Mix 1 teaspoon warm water and at least $1/8$ teaspoon salt to make a thick, concentrated solution. Put 3 to 5 drops of this salt water in each nostril. This greatly helps to drain and unclog the sinuses and relieve the headache.

TIME TO SEE THE DOCTOR

Generally headaches can be relieved using Ayurvedic remedies. However, if you have a headache that persists for more than a couple of days; if your headache is accompanied by a fever or stiff neck; if you also experience neurological symptoms such as blurred vision, difficulty with coordination or speech, memory loss, numbness, or weakness in your arms or legs; if you wake up at midnight with a headache; or if you are having headaches often that seem to be becoming more severe, then please see a doctor.

YOGA POSTURES FOR HEADACHES

Generally, a person having headaches should do the Moon Salutation. Certain yoga postures are also helpful, such as the Boat pose, Hidden Lotus, Bow pose, Spinal Twist, Palm Tree pose, and Standing on the Toes. (For illustrations of yoga poses see appendix 4.) Inverted poses such as Headstand, Shoulder Stand, and the Plow pose are not recommended.

Hearing Loss

Hearing is governed by an aspect of vata known as *prana* vata. In older people, *prana* vata tends to get debilitated, leading to what is known as conductive or nerve deafness: The person doesn't hear properly because the nerves become weak.

To improve hearing, try the following natural remedies:

TAKE *YOGARAJ GUGGULU*. This special compound of Ayurvedic herbs pacifies vata dosha and strengthens weakened nerves. Take 200 mg. of this compound 2 or 3 times a day with warm water, after meals. *Yogaraj guggulu* can be ordered in capsules from many sellers of Ayurvedic herbs. (See Resources for addresses.)

DIET. Avoid vatagenic foods such as popcorn, corn chips, beans, raw vegetables, and cold drinks. (Guidelines for the vata-balancing diet maybe found in chapter 8.)

KEEP OUT OF COLD DRAFTS.

TRY GARLIC OIL. Pour about 1 tablespoon of sesame oil into a small pan, and into it place 1 clove of garlic, well chopped. Cook till the garlic turns brown, then let it cool. While cooking, press the garlic into the oil. This helps the healing properties of the garlic ooze out and permeate the oil. The resulting mixture, which has an excellent fragrance, is called garlic oil. Place 5 to 10 drops (of body-temperature oil) into the ear. This will improve the hearing capacity of the auditory nerve.

NOTE: Oil should be used in the ear only when there is no infection.

YOGA POSTURES. The following yoga postures may improve hearing: Lion, Camel, Cobra, and Cow (see appendix 4). Alternate Nostril breathing may also be effective (see chapter 6).

TIME TO SEE THE DOCTOR

Ayurveda offers several recommendations to restore hearing or retard hearing loss. However, if these treatment suggestions don't result in any improvement after a couple of months, or if your hearing loss seems to be increasing rather than diminishing, seek a doctor's advice.

Heart–Ayurvedic Care

According to Ayurveda, the heart is the seat of *prana, ojas,* and mind. It is a most vital organ. In fact, a person is as old as his or her heart. So we have to take good care of this precious organ.

If a person has high blood pressure, high cholesterol, and high triglycerides, and in addition lives a stressful life, that person runs a great risk of heart problems. So to keep the heart healthy, it is important to control these factors as much as possible.

High blood pressure is discussed at length in a separate section ("Hypertension"), as is high cholesterol ("Cholesterol"). Please see those sections for more complete recommendations. A few suggestions follow:

DIET

In order to control cholesterol and triglycerides, it's important not to eat food with a high fat content, such as fatty fried food, ice cream, heavy meats, and cheese. Yogurt is also not helpful.

EXERCISE

To keep your heart healthy, you need some daily exercise, though the quantity of exercise and the degree of strenuousness depend on your age, level of fitness, and constitutional type. Kaphas need the most vigorous exercise, vatas the least, with pittas in the middle. (See page 60 for further guidelines.)

For most people, walking at least two

Cholesterol-Reducing Foods

Some foods may actually help to *reduce* cholesterol. These include:

- oatmeal
- corn
- apples
- fresh fruit juice, such as orange or grapefruit
- millet
- most fresh vegetables

Be sure to include some of these foods every day in your diet if you have high cholesterol.

miles a day is very beneficial. Some more vigorous aerobic cardiovascular exercise may also be beneficial, such as fast walking, gentle jogging, or jogging in place on a trampoline. (You don't need to use the large gymnastic trampoline; you can use the small variety, usually about 3 feet in diameter.)

STRESS MANAGEMENT

To keep stress levels low, here are two important recommendations.

DO SOME QUIET MEDITATION. Meditation is one of the best ways to relax, dissolve stress, and allow the body to heal. By meditating for 10 to 20 minutes twice a day, a person's heart may be healed. Please see chapter 7 for guidelines on how to meditate.

DO DAILY PRACTICE OF SAVASANA. *Savasana* is the yogic rest pose. While lying quietly, flat on your back with your arms by your sides, watch the flow of your breath. Inhale and exhale, inhale and exhale.... You'll notice that after exhalation (and before inhalation), there is a brief, natural stop. Similarly there is a natural stop after inhalation and before exhalation. In that stop, stay naturally quiet, silent, for just a few seconds. This practice brings tranquillity and rest, which are healing for the heart. Remain in *savasana* practicing this quiet breathing for 10 to 15 minutes.

OTHER REMEDIES

In addition to these recommendations for diet, exercise, and stress management, several other simple home remedies can help keep your heart healthy.

GOLD WATER. Gold is healing for the heart. It is good for the coronary artery and is said to gradually reduce cholesterol. For instructions on making gold water, see appendix 1.

HERBS FOR YOUR HEART. Certain Ayurvedic herbs are strengthening and healing to the heart.

• First is the herb *arjuna*. Take 1/2 teaspoon 3 times a day with honey and warm water. *Arjuna* does much the same thing as gold: It is a coronary vasodilator, it protects the heart, it strengthens circulation, and it helps to maintain the tone and health of the heart muscle.

• Ginger is also important for a healthy heart. Make fresh ginger tea by boiling a little grated or sliced ginger in a cup or two of water. Or grate a little ginger and add it to your rice and/or your soup. Eating a little bit of ginger every day will help to prevent heart attack.

• The following formula of four Ayurvedic herbs is good for the heart.

punarnava 4 *parts*
kutki 3 *parts*
gulwel sattva 1/4 *part*
shilajit 1/4 *part*

Steep 1/2 teaspoon of this herb mixture in a cup of hot water to make a tea. Drinking that tea twice a day after lunch and dinner will help your heart.

• Another simple domestic remedy to protect the heart and keep it healthy is to include a little garlic in your diet. Garlic reduces cholesterol, strengthens the circulation, and acts as a decongestant.

RUDRAKSHA. *Rudraksha,* the "tears of Shiva," are the dried seeds from the fruit of the *rudraksha* tree. An ancient story says that when Lord Shiva came out of deep meditation, a few tears dropped from his eyes and fell to earth, from which sprang up the *rudraksha* tree. The seeds are good for the heart both physically and spiritually; they are said to be good for meditation and for "opening the heart chakra."

You can wear a necklace of the beads externally, in front of the heart. Or soak a *rudraksha* bead overnight in water and drink the water in the morning. Drinking *rudraksha* water can reduce blood pressure and strengthen the heart.

YOGA POSTURES. *Unless there are acute heart problems,* Ayurveda suggests daily perfor-

Ancient Advice for a Healthy Heart

Charaka, one of the ancient sage-physicians who wrote down the principles and practices of Ayurveda thousands of years ago, gave the following advice for care of the heart:

"One who wishes to protect the heart, circulatory system and vital essence should avoid, above all else, those causes leading to mental stress and instability. One should regularly adopt measures that support the heart and vital essence, cleanse the blood vessels, increase knowledge and calm the mind.

"The practice of nonviolence is the best among life-promoting practices, conservation of vital energy among the strength-promoting, and acquisition of knowledge among the nourishing practices. Control of the sensory organs is best to achieve happiness, and knowledge of reality for pleasure. Among all of these, celibacy is regarded as the best.

"From the heart, as the root, ten great vessels carry *ojas* throughout the body. In its importance, the heart is to be regarded as the central supporting member of a house."

> TIME TO SEE THE DOCTOR
>
> IMPORTANT: If you have any heart problems, or you are over 40, it is wise to consult your physician before beginning any new exercise program.

mance of the set of yoga postures known as *surya namaskar,* the Sun Salutation. Do at least 6 to 12 cycles a day. That will help to strengthen the health of the heart and help to prevent heart attack.

If there are heart problems, the Sun Salutation may be too strenuous. In that case, substitute the following postures: Locust, Lotus, Bridge, Cow, Camel, Bow, and Cobra poses, Forward Bend, and Standing on One Leg—the Palm Tree pose. (Illustrations of yoga postures appear in appendix 4.)

BREATHING EXERCISE. A deep breathing exercise such as *ujjayi pranayama* will also be helpful (see chapter 6).

Heartburn and Acid Stomach

Although there are several rather strong medications on the market for heartburn and acid stomach, these conditions are usually quite easy to control with the following natural Ayurvedic home remedies:

ALOE VERA GEL. Take 2 tablespoons of aloe vera gel with a pinch of baking soda. This will have an immediate soothing effect.

INSTANT EFFERVESCENCE. You might also try this formula. Into 1 cup of water add

lime juice 10 drops
organic sugar 1/2 teaspoon
baking soda 1/4 teaspoon

Put the baking soda into the cup last. When you add it, an effervescent reaction will occur. Immediately drink the mixture to neutralize heartburn and acid stomach.

PAPAYA JUICE. For hyperacidity and indigestion, try drinking 1 cup papaya juice with 1 teaspoon organic sugar and 2 pinches cardamom.

NOTE: Pregnant women should not eat papayas, which contain natural estrogen and may create the danger of miscarriage.

FOLLOW THE PITTA-PACIFYING DIET. Generally, acid stomach can be controlled by a

> TIME TO SEE THE DOCTOR
>
> If your heartburn is not helped by the remedies recommended in this section or if it occurs often for no apparent reason, you should consult a doctor. If you feel you have heartburn and it is accompanied by vomiting, dizziness, chest pain radiating into your neck or shoulder, or shortness of breath, you need help *immediately*: You may be having a heart attack.

pitta-pacifying diet. Strictly avoid all hot spicy food. No pickles, and no fermented food. Minimize or cut out citrus fruit and sour fruit. And avoid overeating.

A SOOTHING BREATHING EXERCISE. The breathing technique known as *shitali pranayama* is also helpful. It is not only cooling (to combat the excess pitta) but also stimulates digestion.

Hemorrhoids

According to Ayurveda, there are two basic kinds of hemorrhoids, associated with vata and pitta imbalances.

- Vata hemorrhoids are small, dry, and irregular in shape and may be accompanied by fissures or cracking of the anus. They are rough and hard to the touch and look like raisins. Vata hemorrhoids may become active when the person takes antibiotics or does a lot of cycling or physical exercise.
- Pitta-type hemorrhoids tend to get red, irritated, and inflamed and to bleed. They may look like purple grapes and are painful—sometimes very painful—to the touch. When they burst, they bleed extensively.

There are also kapha hemorrhoids, which look like green grapes. They don't bleed, and people generally live with them without problems, so we won't consider them in this section.

We can also distinguish between "internal" and "external" hemorrhoids. The internal kind are usually of the kapha variety and are more like polyps. They are not painful and are generally not problematic.

In most cases, hemorrhoids can be completely healed by Ayurvedic treatment, but one must first understand the distinction between the two basic problematic types in order to treat them properly.

EFFECTIVE TREATMENT FOR VATA HEMORRHOIDS

- A person with vata hemorrhoids should follow the vata-pacifying diet. Especially, it is vital to keep away from the nightshade vegetables—potatoes, tomatoes, and eggplant—all of which aggravate hemorrhoids.
- Take *triphala guggulu,* 1 tablet 3 times a day.
- Another helpful herbal formula for vata-type hemorrhoids is a combination of these herbs:

hingwastak $^1/_8$ *part*
dashamoola *2 parts*

Take $^1/_2$ teaspoon 2 or 3 times a day with warm water.

- It is important to keep the stools loose and soft, as hard stools irritate the hemorrhoids. Taking 1 teaspoon of *sat isabgol* (psyllium husks) with a glass of warm milk at night is beneficial for vata hemorrhoids.
- Another way to help keep the stools soft is to take $^1/_2$ to 1 teaspoon of *triphala* powder at bedtime with warm water.
- Prepare a warm castor oil or sesame oil pack, and sit on it for a while. Both oils are warming; castor oil especially produces a slow, sustained heat that is soothing and

healing. Warm up about 3 tablespoons of oil, and pour it onto a handkerchief or other soft cloth, spreading it equally on the cloth (or dip the cloth in the oil).

EFFECTIVE TREATMENT FOR PITTA HEMORRHOIDS

• For pitta-type hemorrhoids, the first step is to follow the pitta-pacifying diet, especially avoiding spicy and fermented foods (see chapter 8).

• For hemorrhoids which become active and inflamed and start bleeding, one should prepare an herbal mixture of:

guduchi 1 *part*
neem 2 *parts*
kama dudha 1/8 *part*

Take 1/2 teaspoon of this mixture twice a day with warm water.

• If you have rectal bleeding from the hemorrhoid, drink a few ounces of cranberry juice and pomegranate juice (mixed half and half) between meals. That juice will act as a hemostatic, to stop the bleeding.

• Locally, you can apply coconut oil, which helps to control inflammation and irritation as well as bleeding.

• As in the case of vata hemorrhoids, it is important to keep the stool soft to avoid aggravating the condition. To accomplish this, take 1/2 to 1 teaspoon of *amalaki* at night with cool water. Or you can take 1 teaspoon of *sat isabgol* (psyllium husks) with a glass of warm milk at night.

• Steep *triphala* (1 teaspoon) overnight in a glass of water, and then the next day, early in the morning, after brushing your teeth, drink that tea.

GENERAL RECOMMENDATIONS

• All types of hemorrhoids respond well to aloe vera juice. Drink 1/2 cupful of the pure juice 3 times a day.

• Or you can add a pinch of ginger to 1 tablespoon aloe vera gel, and take it twice a day.

• Drink 1 cup carrot juice mixed with 2 teaspoons cilantro juice twice a day on an empty stomach for relief of hemorrhoids.

• Externally, you can also apply a mixture of 1/2 teaspoon turmeric and 1 teaspoon ghee directly to the hemorrhoid at bedtime. (But remember that the yellow color of the turmeric will stain whatever cloth it touches.)

• After each bowel movement, instead of using dry toilet paper, wash the anal orifice with warm water, and then apply some castor oil to the hemorrhoid. The dry paper may irritate the delicate mucous membrane and aggravate the hemorrhoid. It can also spread some fecal matter to the site of the hemorrhoid and lead to complications.

Herpes

ORAL HERPES

Herpes labialis comes through the oral contact of kissing, or drinking from the same cup or glass. It is essentially a pitta disorder that comes from *rakta dhatu* (blood) and breaks out on the skin, particularly in the corner of the mouth or on the upper lip.

Many people confuse herpes and canker

sores, which are somewhat similar in appearance. With canker sores, however, only one ulcer appears; herpes produces a rash consisting of numerous small blisters, possibly clustered around one central, larger bump. Also, canker sores are usually *in* the mouth, while herpes sores are on the outside.

• Externally, one can apply *tikta ghrita* (bitter ghee) directly onto the affected area. Aloe vera gel or ointment is also quite effective.

• You can also use 1/4 teaspoon *kama dudha,* mixed into 1 teaspoon dairy cream. Apply to the sore in the morning and at bedtime.

• Internally, use this Ayurvedic herbal mixture:

neem 3 parts
kama dudha 1/8 part
maha sudarshan 3 parts

Take 1/2 teaspoon of this mixture 3 times a day, either with 1 teaspoon *tikta ghrita,* if you have it, or with warm water.

• At night, take 1/2 teaspoon *triphala* in warm water. This will pacify systemic pitta and will help relieve the herpes.

GENITAL HERPES

Genital herpes is similar to oral herpes. But they are transmitted differently; oral herpes through kissing or drinking glasses, as mentioned above, and genital herpes through sexual contact.

• For internal treatment, use the same herbs and herbal formulas recommended above.

• Externally, *tikta ghrita* can also be helpful. Also, dry genital intercourse can sometimes aggravate the herpes, so apply some *tikta ghrita* to the glans penis and/or labia minora before intercourse.

TO NEUTRALIZE STRESS

One of the primary causes of herpes eruptions appears to be psychological stress. The virus lies locked in the neuromuscular cleft and comes out during times of stress. To minimize stress:

TAKE HERBAL TEA. Make some tea of chamomile, *jatamamsi,* and *brahmi.* Mix these herbs in equal proportions and use 1/2 teaspoon to make a tea; take it twice a day.

MEDITATE. Meditation is also effective to soothe the system and reduce stress. (See chapter 7 for meditation suggestions.)

NOTE TO MEN: If you know you are susceptible to herpes outbreaks, be careful shaving around your lips and the corners of your mouth. The lips form a delicate and sensitive muco-cutaneous junction that is easily injured. Any small cut or scratch can activate the herpes virus. To help prevent this from happening, apply some *neem* oil after shaving.

Hiccups

Hiccups are caused by ischemia, or lack of blood supply to the diaphragm. As a result, the diaphragm undergoes the spasmodic periodic movements that we call hiccups.

HOLD YOUR BREATH. The simplest remedy for hiccups is to hold your breath. Take a deep breath; hold the breath behind the belly button; then gradually exhale.

BROWN BAG REMEDY. If you find it difficult to do this, take a paper bag, open it, hold the edges near your nose, and breathe into the bag (both exhaling and then inhaling). This will force you to inhale your own carbon dioxide, which naturally relaxes the muscles of the diaphragm. Continue for 1 or 2 minutes. Your hiccups should quickly be relieved.

HONEY AND CASTOR OIL. If the above procedure doesn't stop the hiccupping, mix 1 teaspoon honey with 1 teaspoon castor oil. Every 2 or 3 minutes dip your index finger into the mixture and then lick your finger.

DEEP BREATHING EXERCISE. Another simple remedy is Alternate Nostril *pranayama,* slightly modified as follows:

1. Inhale through the left nostril while closing the right nostril with your thumb.
2. After inhaling, hold your breath for just a moment, then
3. *Swallow.*
4. Exhale through your right nostril while closing the left nostril with your ring and little finger.
5. Repeat steps 1 to 4, this time starting by inhaling through the right nostril.

You can do this breathing exercise for 5 minutes.

Time to See the Doctor

There are certain serious pathological hiccups, such as cardiac hiccups, which occur in persons having congestive heart failure; uremic hiccups, which occur due to renal failure (when the kidneys do not perform their function) and the resulting toxicity of uric acid in the blood; and cerebral hiccups, due to cerebral pathology. These serious hiccups require medical attention and treatment.

If the remedies in this section aren't helpful and your hiccups are continuing longer than two days, see your doctor.

CONSTIPATION MAY BE THE CAUSE. Hiccups can also occur due to chronic constipation, bloating, and gases in the colon. If this appears to be the situation, do *basti* (enema), using 1 cup warm sesame oil for the enema. Try to retain the oil for at least 2 to 3 minutes, longer if possible. The warm oil in the rectum will relax the diaphragm and internal muscles and help alleviate the hiccups.

- If your hiccups are still continuing after another half hour, do a regular warm water enema.

Hypertension

A healthy heart pumps the blood through the veins and arteries with a certain optimum amount of pressure. But sometimes, due to various causes, the pressure increases, and when it does, the person is at greater risk for heart disease and possibly paralyzing stroke.

Blood pressure will increase when there is increased viscosity of the blood, increased velocity, or constriction due to decreased diameter of the blood vessel.

TYPES OF HYPERTENSION

From the Ayurvedic point of view, high blood pressure falls under three categories, primarily vata and pitta but also kapha.

Vata is responsible for constriction of the blood vessels. This frequently happens in old age. Somewhere around 65, the walls of the blood vessels often become thicker and the passage becomes narrower, with the result that many individuals develop a type of hypertension known as essential hypertension. It is a vata condition and is different from the narrowing of the arteries that occurs as a result of fatty deposits on the artery walls, which is a kapha condition.

Pitta is responsible for the rushing of the blood with more force. Kapha is related to increased blood viscosity.

Physical and emotional stress, including anger and anxiety, constrict the blood vessels and can increase blood pressure for a time. Heavy responsibilities, or stressful situations such as public speaking, may send your blood pressure soaring. There is even a phenomenon known as "white coat syndrome"; when a person goes to the doctor, anxiety and tension may increase, with the result that blood pressure goes up. This is all quite common and quite physiological, and fortunately it is also usually temporary. But if blood pressure *stays* high, it can become dangerous.

Time to See the Doctor

If high blood pressure is temporary and related to a stressful situation, some rest and relaxation will generally take care of it. And even in the long term, just because pressure is high does not necessarily mean it has to be treated with medications. Entirely natural means, such as diet, exercise, herbs, meditation, and yoga, which have no negative side effects, may be quite sufficient to deal with hypertension.

However, high blood pressure does require a doctor's supervision. Hypertension is a potentially life-threatening condition. I do not recommend that you use the following treatments in place of standard medical care.

Rather, try these Ayurvedic remedies—preferably with your doctor's knowledge and approval—as an adjunct to your medical care, and ask your doctor to monitor your progress. If the remedies are successful, he or she will find less and less need to supervise your condition and keep you on medications. At the least you should be able to gradually reduce the dosage of your medicines.

FOODS FOR HYPERTENSION

Several foods can help you control hypertension:

- Drink 1 cup mango juice, followed about an hour later by 1/2 cup warm milk, with a pinch of cardamom, a pinch of nutmeg, and 1 teaspoon ghee. (*Note:* If your cholesterol level is high, skip the ghee.)
- Mix orange juice and coconut water (the natural juice inside a fresh coconut) in a ratio of 2 parts orange to 1 part coconut. Drink 1/2 to 1 cup 2 or 3 times a day.
- Add 1 teaspoon coriander and 1 pinch cardamom to 1 cup freshly squeezed (not canned) peach juice. Drink this as many as 2 or 3 times a day to help with high blood pressure.
- Eat some watermelon with a pinch of cardamom and a pinch of coriander added. This will act as a mild diuretic and will help to regulate blood pressure.
- Try some cucumber raita with your meal. Cucumber is a good diuretic. Raita is a yogurt-based condiment often used in Indian cooking. (See the recipe in the accompanying sidebar.)
- Mung dal soup, made of mung dal with cilantro, cumin, and a pinch of turmeric, is good for persons with hypertension.
- Honey water can also help. Add a teaspoon of honey and 5 to 10 drops of apple cider vinegar to a cup of hot water, and drink it in the early morning. This drink helps to reduce cholesterol, maintains vasodilation, and helps to regulate blood pressure.

Cucumber Raita

2 cucumbers
3 tablespoons ghee
1/2 teaspoon black mustard seeds
1/2 teaspoon cumin seeds
1 pinch hing
4 curry leaves
1 pinch cayenne or 1/2 small chili, chopped
1 small handful fresh cilantro leaves, chopped
1/2 cup plain fresh yogurt

Skin and grate the cucumbers. Pour off and discard any excess juice.

Heat the ghee in saucepan over medium heat, and add the mustard, cumin, hing, and curry leaves. Cook a moment until seeds pop.

Add the cayenne or chili and the cilantro, shake the pan, and remove from heat.

Stir the yogurt and grated cucumber together in a bowl.

Add the cooled spices to the yogurt mixture, mix well, and serve.

Serves 4–6 as side dish (1–2 spoonfuls per person).

NOTE: This recipe is from Vasant Lad and Usha Lad, *Ayurvedic Cooking for Self-healing* (Albuquerque: Ayurvedic Press, 1994), page 138.

AVOID PITTA-PROVOKING FOOD. Persons with hypertension should not eat salt, fatty fried foods, or hot spicy food.

HERBS FOR HYPERTENSION

Ayurveda suggests the following mixture of herbs for hypertension:

punarnava 1 part
passion flower 1 part
hawthorn berry 2 parts

Steep $^1/_2$ teaspoon of this mixture in a cup of hot water for 5 to 10 minutes, and drink the tea after lunch and dinner.

Another formula of Ayurvedic herbs is also effective for regulating blood pressure:

jatamamsi 2 parts
musta 2 parts
tagar 1 part

Use as above: $^1/_2$ teaspoon steeped in a cup of hot water for 5 to 10 minutes as a tea, after lunch and dinner.

OTHER REMEDIES AND RECOMMENDATIONS

KEEP COOL. Working hard under the hot sun should be avoided by anyone with high blood pressure, as that may promote hemorrhage in the brain. Be cautious about this.

MAGNETIC WATER. You may be able to keep your blood pressure under control by drinking magnetic water. Put a cupful of water (preferably in a glass container) next to the north pole of a magnet. Let it sit for 2 hours. Drink a cupful of magnetic water twice a day.

Charging the water in this way increases its diuretic properties and thus helps bring down high blood pressure, in the same way as several widely used current hypertension medications, which are diuretics.

RUDRAKSHA. Soak 1 or 2 *rudraksha* beads in a cup of water overnight, and the next day drink that water. This is beneficial for regulating blood pressure.

Deep Relaxation to Help High Blood Pressure

Tension and stress increase high blood pressure. A wonderful and effective way to relax is the yogic rest pose, *savasana*.

Lie quietly, flat on your back with arms by your sides. Observe the flow of your breath. You will notice that after exhalation there is a brief, natural stop, and another natural pause after inhalation and before the next exhalation. In that stop, stay naturally quiet for just a few seconds. This practice will bring you deep relaxation, a natural antidote for hypertension. Remain in *savasana* practicing this quiet breathing for 10 to 15 minutes.

MEDITATION. Meditation is excellent for regulating blood pressure. (See chapter 7 for guidelines to help you meditate.) Several research studies, including a study funded by the National Institutes of Health, have shown that meditation can be as effective as medications in controlling hypertension, and it produces none of the negative side effects often associated with hypertensive drugs.

BREATHING EXERCISE. Some gentle *shitali pranayama* can help control blood pressure. Make a tube of your tongue, and inhale through that tube into the abdomen. Hold the breath for a few seconds and then breathe it out through your nose.

YOGA POSTURES. Effective yoga *asanas* for helping control hypertension include Yoga Mudra and the Moon Salutation. (See the illustrations in appendix 4.)

EXERCISE AND WORK WITH CARE. No one with elevated blood pressure should practice the Headstand or engage in weightlifting or vigorous exercise without a physician's guidance.

> IMPORTANT NOTE: As mentioned above, hypertension may lead to serious complications. Although these Ayurvedic recommendations are time-tested, safe, and effective, it would be wise to use them in conjunction with the advice and care of your physician.

Hypoglycemia

Hypoglycemia (low blood sugar) is a very common condition. If you are late to eat at your regular mealtime and you feel light-headed or dizzy while standing up, or experience palpitations, tremor, nausea, drowsiness, sweating, nervousness, or mental confusion, all these indicate hypoglycemia. In some serious cases of hypoglycemia, a person can even have convulsions and fall into coma.

The brain uses blood sugar (glucose) as its sole food, and it depends on it for the necessary energy for its activity. If the brain doesn't receive sufficient blood sugar, it goes into crisis; it will create tremors, headache, sweating, nausea, drowsiness, and the other symptoms mentioned because it is starving for blood sugar.

According to Ayurveda, hypoglycemia is common in persons with pitta *prakruti* (a pitta constitution) or pitta *vikruti* (a present pitta imbalance). Increased pitta stimulates the secretion of insulin, which lowers the blood sugar level and creates hypoglycemia. Hypoglycemia in turn induces the secretion of adrenaline, which causes rapid heartbeat and tremors.

An unduly large dose of insulin taken by a diabetic person may lead to hypoglycemia. This condition is also common among alcoholics.

Hypoglycemia is a disorder that needs careful attention. To maintain their blood sugar level, pitta individuals should eat regular meals—breakfast, lunch, and dinner—and also have some fruit or another snack between meals or whenever they feel hypo-

> **Time to See the Doctor**
>
> Reactive hypoglycemia may indicate a pancreatic tumor. When a middle-aged person craves sugar about 90 minutes after a full meal, it may mean that he or she has, or is going to develop, a pancreatic tumor. This is a serious health concern and requires medical attention.

glycemic symptoms. Emphasize proteins and complex carbohydrates for main meals; they digest more slowly, so the rises and falls in blood sugar will be less rapid.

Hypoglycemia can be classified into two types: fasting and reactive. Fasting hypoglycemia simply results from not eating, which is why people with a tendency toward low blood sugar need to eat regular meals. In addition, some individuals choose to fast, whether for religious reasons or for cleansing purposes. If they do too much prolonged fasting, hypoglycemia may result.

Reactive hypoglycemia occurs when the pancreas, often in response to a large intake of sugar, secretes too much insulin, which then reduces the blood sugar level. This is also called postprandial (after-eating) hypoglycemia. About 90 minutes after eating, the blood sugar level drops, and the person craves something sweet.

To deal with reactive hypoglycemia, one should treat pitta dosha.

DIET. Follow the pitta-pacifying diet (outlined in chapter 8). Stay away from hot spicy foods, fermented food, sour and citrus fruits, and alcoholic drinks. Smoking cigarettes should be curtailed or eliminated, as cigarettes also aggravate pitta.

LICORICE TEA. Drink licorice tea. When you are feeling lightheaded or faint or have some other hypoglycemic symptoms, make a cup of licorice (*yashti madhu*) tea, using 1 teaspoon of licorice root per cup of water. This tea will safely increase your blood sugar level. (However, individuals with hypertension should use licorice tea only sparingly; it increases water retention and may raise blood pressure.)

HERBAL REMEDIES.

- The best herbs to take are *brahmi, jatamamsi, shanka pushpi,* and licorice. These herbs are brain tonics; they nourish the brain and allow it to function on limited sugar. Mix these herbs together in equal proportions and use the mixture to make a tea. Steep 1/2 teaspoon of the herbs in 1 cup hot water, and drink after lunch and dinner.
- If the problem is postprandial hypoglycemia due to gastrojejunostomy, Ayurveda suggests using

  guduchi 5 parts
  shanka bhasma 2 parts
  kama dudha 2 parts

  Take 1/2 teaspoon twice a day (after lunch and dinner) with some water.

- If there is a suspicion that reactive hypoglycemia may lead to pancreatic tumor (see "Time to See the Doctor"), see your doctor. In addition, use *shilajit,* a nervine tonic that is rejuvenating for the pancreas. A good formula for using *shilajit* is the following:

shilajit 1 part
shardunika 1 part

Take $^1/_2$ teaspoon of this mixture after lunch and dinner with some water. This formula will also help to prevent adult-onset diabetes (diabetes mellitus).

YOGA POSTURES. Some yoga *asanas* to strengthen the pancreas and help prevent hypoglycemia include the Peacock, Camel, and Locust poses, and the Elevated Lotus, as well as *nauli* (an abdominal exercise explained in appendix 3). Individuals susceptible to hypoglycemia should do these yoga exercises and Alternate Nostril breathing.

NASYA. *Brahmi* ghee *nasya*, 5 drops in each nostril, will quickly relieve nausea, sweating, and mental confusion (see appendix 3).

FOR DROWSINESS. Drowsiness can be corrected by taking some sweet juice, such as pomegranate or sweet orange juice.

Impotence

See also "Low Libido"; "Premature Ejaculation"

Impotence, which is a man's inability to have or to maintain an erection, may have several causes. Many people think it is always an emotional or psychological issue, but it can also be due to stress or to certain physical problems.

For example, when a person has high cholesterol, the fat and plaque may get deposited on the coronary arteries, blocking the flow of blood to the heart and triggering a heart attack due to the insufficient blood supply. Similarly, the plaque may get deposited in the blood vessels leading to the penis, resulting in a "penis attack"—in which the blood supply to the penis is insufficient to create or sustain an erection, resulting in impotence.

MASSAGE TO IMPROVE CIRCULATION. A simple and effective remedy is to massage the pubic area (the lower part of your abdomen) and the root of the penis with a few drops of *mahanarayan* oil. This massage will improve the circulation and may be sufficient to eliminate the problem.

APPLY SOME HERBALIZED OIL. You can also apply some *bala* oil or *ashwagandha* oil directly to the penis.

MASSAGE THE PROSTATE AREA. Massaging above the prostate gland (midway between the scrotum and the anus) with any of the three oils mentioned above will also be beneficial. If you do not have these oils, you can just use a little plain ghee. First rub in a circular motion, then finish with strokes from the anus toward the base of the penis. Use a light pressure. Like the massage of the pubic area, this will help improve circulation.

STRENGTHENING HERBAL FORMULA. For internal use, make a mixture of equal proportions of the following herbs:

ashwagandha
bala
vidari

and take 1 teaspoon of this mixture twice a day in warm milk, continuing for 3 months. While the milk is heating, add a few pieces of chopped fresh garlic. The garlic improves the blood supply and increases the dilation of the blood vessels. The combination of the garlic with these strengthening herbs will help alleviate the problem.

MILD APHRODISIAC DRINK. Every night, drink a cup of warm milk with a pinch of saffron added. Saffron is an aphrodisiac and also increases sperm count.

RELAX WITH TRANQUILLITY TEA. If the cause of impotence is psychological, such as fear or anxiety, you may be able to correct the problem by drinking some Tranquillity Tea, an herbal compound that contains *jatamamsi, brahmi,* and *shanka pushpi* in equal proportions. Make a tea from 1/2 teaspoon of this mixture, and drink it about an hour before going to bed. It will definitely help with the emotional and psychological stress that may be at the root of the problem.

YOGA POSTURES. Certain yoga exercises may also help. The Rooster pose, which involves sitting in such a way that pressure is applied on the prostate gland, is particularly beneficial. Also try the Elevated Lotus, Vajrasana, Chakra Asana, and the Bow pose. (For illustrations, see appendix 4.)

Incontinence, Urinary

See "Urinary Incontinence"

Indigestion

As discussed in chapter 3, the effectiveness of your digestion depends on the strength of your digestive fire (agni). If your food intake is large in quantity and heavy, very liquid, or quite dense in quality, these properties are antagonistic to the properties of gastric fire and can inhibit the normal function of the agni, leading to indigestion.

Emotional eating—eating for emotional reasons when the system is not in need of food or is given too much to comfortably digest—is another potential cause of indigestion. A third major causative factor is wrong food combining. Eating bananas and milk, melon and grains, and other incompatible food combinations adversely affects the digestive fire, leading to indigestion. (See chapter 8 for a chart of incompatible food combinations.)

These various factors promote excess secretion of acid, leading to acid indigestion, heartburn, nausea, or even diarrhea; fermentation of the food in the stomach or intestines may also occur, leading to gas, bloating, and a possible stomachache, depending on the severity of the cause.

So one has to deal with indigestion first by avoiding these causative factors, and second by using the herbal treatments recommended below.

FOUR WAYS TO INCREASE YOUR DIGESTIVE FIRE

The first key to prevention of indigestion is to enhance the digestive fire. Here are several suggestions:

GINGER. One of the best herbs to kindle agni is ginger. Before each meal, chop or grate a little fresh ginger, add a few drops of lime juice and a pinch of salt, and chew it up. Alternatively, you can simply cut a thin slice of ginger, put on a pinch of salt, and chew that.

GARLIC AND *TRIKATU*. Here is another before-eating stimulant for your digestion. Make a mixture of 1/4 teaspoon garlic powder, 1/2 teaspoon *trikatu,* and a pinch of rock salt. (*Trikatu* is composed of ginger, black pepper, and Indian long pepper in equal proportions.) Take it before lunch and dinner.

HERBAL MIX. A similar mixture is 1 clove of fresh garlic, chopped up with 1/4 teaspoon cumin powder, a pinch of rock salt, a pinch of *trikatu,* and 1 teaspoon lime juice. Take before meals.

BAY LEAF. Enliven your gastric fire with the common spice bay leaf. Steep 1/2 teaspoon crushed or ground-up bay leaf in a cup of hot water for about 10 minutes to make a tea. Add a pinch of cardamom, and drink after eating.

FASTING

Fasting can be beneficial to dispel indigestion. Fasting not only kindles the digestive fire, it also gives the digestive system a rest. When you have indigestion, you can either observe a complete fast, or try this: Drink 1 cup of sweet fresh pineapple juice with a pinch of ginger, a pinch of black pepper, and 1/2 teaspoon organic sugar. Take this 3 times a day.

WHEN YOU HAVE INDIGESTION

To relieve a case of indigestion:

ONION JUICE. Take 1/4 cup of fresh onion juice with 1/2 teaspoon honey and 1/2 teaspoon black pepper.

GARLIC. Or chop up a clove of fresh garlic, add a pinch of salt and a pinch of baking soda, and eat it.

LIME JUICE. For acute indigestion, squeeze the juice from 1/4 lime in 1 cup warm water. Just before drinking, add 1/2 teaspoon baking soda, and then drink it down quickly.

FOR CHRONIC INDIGESTION

For people with chronic poor digestion (that is, weak agni), prepare this herbal mixture:

trikatu 1 part
chitrak 2 parts
kutki 1 part

Take 1/4 teaspoon of this effective formula before meals, with a little honey and fresh ginger juice. If you don't have fresh ginger, just use honey. This mixture will strengthen the digestive fire.

TEN TIPS TO PREVENT INDIGESTION

- Don't eat unless you are really hungry.
- Don't eat emotionally. Emotional eating can affect the digestive fire adversely.

• Eat only two or at most three meals a day: breakfast, lunch, and dinner. Avoid snacking between meals.

• Avoid cold and iced drinks, especially during or after meals. They cool the digestive fire. For best digestion, take small sips of warm water during a meal.

• Fill your stomach to one-third of its capacity with food and one-third with liquid, leaving one-third empty. This aids in proper digestion and promotes mental clarity.

• Chew your food well to make sure the saliva is well mixed in. Saliva plays a major role in digestion.

• You can finish your meal by drinking a cup of lassi. This is made by blending 4 teaspoons of yogurt with 2 pinches each of ginger and cumin powder in 1 cup of water.

• Yoga postures that can be helpful for improving digestion include Leg Lifts and the Peacock pose. (See illustrations in appendix 4.)

• You might also want to try the Ayurvedic procedure known as *nauli* (see appendix 3).

• The *pranayama* (breathing exercise) called Breath of Fire will help to stoke your digestive fires (see chapter 6).

Ingrown Toenail

See "Toenail Infection"

Insomnia

Insomnia is an uncommonly common disorder in the modern world, caused primarily by an increase of vata dosha in the mind or nervous system. Insomnia is a cause or a complicating factor in many other problems. It may be related to constipation. It may be a result of stress or being overtired, or it may create fatigue and lead to greater stress. It may be a symptom of depression, or it may intensify depression. So we have to deal with it effectively.

DIETARY REMEDIES

WARM MILK. It's definitely true that drinking a cup of warm milk before going to bed helps bring on a peaceful sleep. You can have it plain if you prefer, but the following suggestions will make it more delicious as well as more effective:

• Add a pinch (up to 1/8 teaspoon) of nutmeg.

• Add some crushed almonds (blanched is better), a pinch of nutmeg, and a pinch of cardamom. You can prepare the almonds in a nut grinder or coffee grinder.

• Try garlic milk. Mix together 1 cup milk, 1/4 cup water, and 1 clove of fresh, chopped garlic. Boil gently until 1 cup of liquid remains.

TRY CHERRIES. Cherries are good for mental fatigue and stress, both of which can contribute to insomnia. Eating 10 to 20 cherries daily may help relieve these conditions and help you sleep.

TOMATO JUICE. Here's a use for tomato juice you probably never thought of. Drink 1 cup with 2 teaspoons natural sugar and 2 pinches of nutmeg. Drink the juice between four and five in the afternoon; have dinner between six and seven. That evening you should get a sound sleep.

HERBAL REMEDIES

HERBAL FORMULA. An effective herbal formula to help you sleep is:

tagar 1 *part*
valerian root powder 1 *part*
chamomile 1 *part*

Take 1/4 teaspoon of this powdered mixture with a little warm water just before going to bed.

CHAMOMILE TEA. Justly famous around the world, a cup of chamomile tea at bedtime is truly beneficial for inducing sleep.

ADDITIONAL REMEDIES AND RECOMMENDATIONS

WARM OIL MASSAGE. One of the simplest and most effective ways to induce sleep is to rub some oil on the scalp and the soles of the feet before going to bed. Use sesame oil, *brahmi* oil, or *jatamamsi* oil, and massage gently for a few minutes. Slightly warming the oil before applying is helpful.

NUTMEG. Using this common spice can help induce sleep. A fine paste made of nutmeg powder mixed with an equal amount of ghee can be applied around your eyes and on your forehead before bed to help you fall asleep.

TAKE A HOT BATH. A hot bath or shower at bedtime helps to soothe vata and promote sound sleep.

TRY YOGA MEDITATION. Sleep disturbances are often due to worries and anxieties that keep the mind agitated at night. To help dissolve those anxieties, meditate for a while before going to sleep. Sit comfortably on your bed and put your attention on the "third eye" (the area on your forehead between your eyebrows). Follow your breath in and out, or do the traditional *So-Hum* meditation: Inhale while thinking the syllable "*So*" and exhale with "*Hum.*" (Further guidelines are in chapter 7.)

Then lie on your back. Watch your breath, and continue the *So-Hum* meditation, focusing your mind gently on the "third eye." You will sleep like a child.

Irritable Bowel Syndrome

According to Ayurveda, irritable bowel syndrome is due to vata pushing pitta into the colon. To help correct the situation, combine the following herbs:

shatavari 1 *part*
kama dudha 1/8 *part*
shanka bhasma 1/8 *part*
arrowroot 2 *parts*

Take 1/2 teaspoon of this mixture a couple of times a day with a little warm water, just after eating.

• You can also take 1 teaspoon of *sat isabgol* (psyllium husks) with 1/2 cup of fresh yogurt 1 hour after dinner.

• To create another simple remedy, boil 1 teaspoon of flaxseed in a cupful of water to make a tea, and drink it at bedtime.

• In certain chronic cases of irritable

bowel syndrome, Ayurveda recommends introducing 1/2 to 1 cup of warm sesame oil into the rectum. If you use this enema treatment, try to retain the oil for 5 minutes. Once the colon is well lubricated with sesame oil, irritable bowel syndrome will be controlled. You can do this oil enema *(basti)* once or twice a week, as needed. (For more about *basti*, see appendix 3.)

Jet Lag

Jet lag is essentially a condition of excess vata in the body. Traveling on a jet at a tremendous speed induces a light, mobile, and spacy quality in the system, which aggravates vata. To prevent jet lag, Ayurveda suggests the following three-part strategy:

1. *An hour before flying,* swallow 2 capsules (00 size) of ginger, with a cup of water.
2. *While on the plane,* drink at least 2 to 3 cups of water, at intervals of 1 to 2 hours. Flying creates a slight dehydration of the body, which can be corrected by drinking sufficient liquid. Dehydration increases vata. Don't drink coffee or any other caffeinated beverage; caffeine also provokes *vata.*
3. *When you reach your destination,* rub a little warm sesame oil on your scalp and on the soles of your feet. Also, drink 1 cup of hot milk with a pinch each of nutmeg and ginger. These two simple actions will help pacify vata.

If you reach your destination before nightfall, you can drink a tea made of equal proportions of chamomile, mint, and *jatamamsi* (1/3 teaspoon each), steeped in a cup of hot water for 10 minutes.

If you don't expect to have herbs available where you are going, you can mix them at home and take them with you in a small plastic sandwich bag or other convenient container.

Kidney Problems

See also "Kidney Stones"

Congestion, high pitta, or crystal urea in the kidney, as well as kidney stones, can all create tightness and pain in the lower back area. For these problems, Ayurveda suggests the following simple remedies.

First, prepare a mixture of these herbs:

punarnava 1 part
gokshura 1 part
fennel seed 1 part

Take 1 full teaspoon of this mixture 2 or 3 times a day after meals, washing it down with warm water.

Another simple, natural treatment for kidneys is cumin-coriander-fennel tea. Prepare the tea by mixing equal amounts of these herbs, boil in water, and drink 2 or 3 times a day. (Use about 1/4 teaspoon of each herb per cup of water.)

For another effective remedy, combine about 1/2 teaspoon of the Ayurvedic herb *musta* with 1/2 teaspoon fennel, steep in a cup of hot water for 10 minutes, strain, and drink. This drink will strengthen the kidneys.

Kidney Stones

There are different types of kidney stones, corresponding to vata, pitta, and kapha dosha.

• Calcium stones are kapha stones. They are generally soft and painless, though they may become painful when they start leaving the pelvis of the kidney and enter the ureter. An individual with an underactive thyroid or parathyroid gland can develop calcium stones.

• Phosphate stones are rough; they irritate the bladder and cause pain because of their rough quality. They are primarily caused by increased phosphates in the system, due to excess eating of nightshade plants (potatoes, eggplant, tomatoes).

• Oxalate stones are sharp. They are pitta stones. They irritate, burn, and create bleeding, and they may create a great deal of pain from loin to groin. A diet high in oxalic acid promotes formation of pitta stones. Thus individuals who eat spinach, potato, tomato, and rhubarb, which are rich in oxalic acid, have a tendency to form stones. These food items should be strictly avoided by anyone concerned about preventing the formation of kidney stones.

HERBAL REMEDIES. If you already have a kidney stone, to decrystallize the pelvis of the kidney Ayurveda suggests *punarnava guggulu* and *gokshuradi guggulu.* Take one tablet of each twice a day after lunch and dinner.

If you have begun to pass a kidney stone and are having a great deal of pain, prepare the following herbal formula:

punarnava 1 part
mutral 1 part
coriander 1 part

Take 1 teaspoon of this mixture twice a day, with a can of beer. Beer, which is essentially fermented barley soup, is a diuretic. It accelerates the passing of the kidney stone and, in combination with the herbs, effects a decrystallization of the kidney. You will pass the stone more easily, without much pain. NOTE: You can use nonalcoholic beer if you prefer, or you can heat up regular beer in a saucepan and the alcohol will quickly evaporate.

Another effective herbal remedy is this formula:

punarnava 5 parts
gokshura 3 parts
mutral 2 parts
shilajit 1/8 part

Taking 1/2 teaspoon of this mixture twice a day with a can of beer can help the kidney stone pass with less discomfort.

Again, if you don't like to drink beer, you can substitute nonalcoholic beer, or drink barley tea or barley soup instead. All are diuretic and will accomplish the same action.

HOT AND COLD APPLICATIONS. Another way to ease the pain of passing a kidney stone is to alternate hot and cold applications to the kidney area. Use a hot water bottle or hot compress, and an ice bag or a bag of frozen vegetables. Alternate them every 30 seconds to 1 minute, until the pain subsides.

WATERMELON JUICE. Try drinking a cup of watermelon juice with 1/4 teaspoon coriander power. Watermelon is a diuretic (as is coriander), so this mixture will give the kidneys a good flushing and help to remove small stones and crystals. Use this 2 to 3 times a day.

Low Libido

Libido is the desire for pleasure and satisfaction. According to Ayurveda, this desire derives from *shukra dhatu,* the male reproductive tissue, and *artava dhatu,* the female reproductive tissue. When there is weakness or debility in the male or female reproductive tissue, libido is low.

Low libido is a symptom that many people have in middle age or even earlier. In addition to weakness in the reproductive tissue, emotional factors and high stress are the primary causes of a reduced sex drive. It can be effectively treated with Ayurvedic programs and remedies that reduce stress and strengthen the reproductive system.

But as always in Ayurveda, the question arises, What is the total context of the situation? Low libido can be a problem that affects one's marriage or partnership. On the other hand, reduced sexual desire may sometimes be a healthy response by the body, shutting off excess loss of the health-giving vital fluid. From this perspective, low libido may be seen as an expression of the body's intelligence.

Intentional celibacy is quite different from low libido. In celibacy there is incredible sexual power, but the person consciously *controls* that sexual energy and transforms it into supreme bliss or supreme intelligence.

In cases of low libido, that energy is simply lacking. In this section we will explore several ways to increase it.

FOR MEN

A simple but effective technique is to gently press the glans penis (the head or tip of the penis) with the top of your index finger. Specifically, press on the groove about one inch behind the tip of the penis. A *marma* point is located at the center of that groove. (See glossary for a brief explanation of *marma* points.) Gently press for a minute or two, then release. This technique will also help remedy premature ejaculation. (See further suggestions under "Premature Ejaculation.")

- You can also gently massage the glans penis with *bala* oil or *shatavari* ghee. Or apply a little castor oil or *brahmi* ghee. (See appendix 2 for guidance in preparing herbalized oils and ghees.)
- Internally, taking the herb *ashwagandha* is effective. Add 1 teaspoon *ashwagandha* and 1/2 teaspoon *vidari* to a cup of warm milk, and drink it at night. This formula is strengthening for men with low libido. NOTE: It is better to cook the herbs in the milk for a few minutes than to just mix the powder in the cup.

FOR WOMEN

A similar herbal formula is helpful for women, but use *shatavari* instead of *ashwagandha.* Mix 1 teaspoon *shatavari* with 1/2 teaspoon *vidari,* and take it with a cup of warm milk at night before going to bed.

• You can also gently massage the pubic bone with *bala* oil, *shatavari* ghee, castor oil, or *brahmi* ghee.

FOOD REMEDIES FOR BOTH MEN AND WOMEN

ALMONDS. Eat 10 raw (unroasted) almonds for breakfast. Soak them overnight in water, and the next morning peel off the skins before eating.

• Make this strengthening almond drink: As above, soak 10 raw almonds in water overnight, and peel off the skins the next morning. But then put the almonds in a blender, and add:

warm milk 1 cup
ghee 1 teaspoon
natural sugar 1 teaspoon
nutmeg a pinch
saffron a pinch

Blend thoroughly. It is yummy, and excellent for combating low libido!

DATES. Soak 10 fresh dates in a quart jar of ghee. Add:

ginger 1 teaspoon
cardamom 1/8 teaspoon
saffron 1 pinch

Cover, and keep in a warm place for at least 2 weeks. Then eat 1 date daily, in the early morning. These dates taste delicious and help to remedy low libido and sexual debility as well as chronic fatigue.

APPLE DESSERT. Another delicious and strengthening concoction is the following apple dessert. Remove the skins and core from 5 raw apples. Blend or mash them to make a pulp, and mix thoroughly, adding some honey according to your taste. Then add:

powdered cardamom 1/8 teaspoon
saffron 1 pinch
nutmeg 1 pinch
rose water 10 drops

Enjoy 1/2 cup of this dessert at least an hour after meals.

NOTE: Avoid milk, yogurt, and fish for at least 4 hours before and after eating this apple dessert.

FIGS AND HONEY. After breakfast, eat 3 figs with 1 teaspoon honey. An hour later, take a glass of lassi. (See page 190 for lassi recipe.) This will help restore sexual energy.

GARLIC AND ONIONS. Adding some more garlic and onions to the diet is helpful. However, these foods are not considered good for meditation as they are somewhat dulling to the mind, so if that is a concern of yours, you can skip this and the following two recommendations.

• Garlic milk is said to have aphrodisiac qualities. Mix together 1 cup milk, 1/4 cup water, and 1 clove chopped garlic. Boil gently until only 1 cup of liquid remains, and drink at bedtime.

• Take 1 tablespoon onion juice mixed with 1 teaspoon fresh ginger juice twice a day.

OTHER REMEDIES FOR MEN AND WOMEN

HERBAL REMEDY. Low libido can be effectively treated with this herbal formula:

shatavari 1 part
vidari 1 part
nutmeg 1/8 part
tagar 1/2 part

Take 1 teaspoon of this mixture in the morning and another teaspoon in the evening, with warm milk. Continue taking it twice a day for 1 month.

LOW LIBIDO AND CONSTIPATION. These two conditions are often found together. To easily overcome constipation, take *triphala* daily, 1/2 teaspoon at night with warm water. Brew the *triphala* powder in about a cup of hot water, let it steep for 10 minutes, strain, and drink.

FOR PSYCHOLOGICAL AND EMOTIONAL ISSUES. If stress and psychological problems such as anxiety or hostility are contributing to your state of low libido, it will be helpful to meditate regularly, practice yoga *asanas*, and do breathing exercises. Particularly helpful *asanas* include *Vajra*, Rooster, Camel, and *Nataraj*. (Guidelines for yoga postures are found in appendix 4.)

Memory Problems

Everyone has occasional episodes of forgetfulness. Forgetting a name, date, or other information that seems to be on the tip of the tongue can make a person frustrated. One may forget where one has parked the car or left one's keys. Such experiences are common to everyone. On the other extreme, a severe form of forgetfulness happens in Alzheimer's disease, in which one may fail to recognize one's wife, husband, children, friends, or family members.

Memory problems are often the result of an inadequate supply of nutrients to the brain. Also, as age advances, memory frequently becomes poorer. Alcohol destroys brain cells, so memory loss among alcoholics is quite common. Memory problems may also be due to the use of drugs such as LSD, marijuana, and cocaine, as well as to alcohol abuse. All these can damage the brain tissue and memory will be affected.

According to Ayurvedic principles, memory is recorded on the sensitive film of the nerve cells within the brain, which are of a kapha nature; memory is enlivened and brought back at a proper time by means of vata. Most memory problems are due either to stagnation of kapha or to aggravation of vata dosha, with its light, airy, even spacy qualities. Thus, in order to improve memory, we need to control vata and kapha. Pitta, on the other hand, is sharp and penetrating and supports good memory.

The following recommendations will help you improve your memory and prevent memory loss.

MEMORY FOODS

CARROTS. Carrots, which contain carotene, are good for memory. Carrots also enhance pitta, which brings sharpness of recall. Drink carrot or beet juice, both of which are blood builders and will help improve memory.

KITCHARI FAST. Kitchari is a simple, nourishing dish made essentially of 50 percent basmati rice and 50 percent split yellow mung dal, with some spices usually added for flavor. A five-day kitchari fast, using plain kitchari with just some chopped cilantro leaves added, will cleanse the system and help to strengthen memory. (For more delicious kitchari recipes, use your imagination or consult a cookbook such as *Ayurvedic Cooking for Self-Healing* by Usha Lad and Vasant Lad; see Bibliography.)

Simple Kitchari Recipe

1 cup basmati rice
1 cup yellow split mung dal
1 small handful cilantro leaves, chopped
6 cups water

Wash the rice and mung dal twice, using plenty of water. If you have time, let the mung dal soak for a few hours before cooking, to help with digestibility.

Add rice, dal, and cilantro to the water.

Bring to a boil, and boil 5 minutes uncovered, stirring occasionally.

Turn down heat to low, and cover, leaving the lid slightly ajar. Cook until tender, about 25 to 30 minutes.

FRUIT FAST. A 3- to 5-day fruit fast, with *triphala* at night (1/2 teaspoon steeped for 5 to 10 minutes in a cup of hot water), will sharpen the nervous system and make the brain more capable of investigating deeply into the memory. *Note:* A fruit fast should not be attempted by anyone who tends to get hypoglycemia.

The following fruits are recommended for the fast:

For vata	Papayas, prunes, mangoes
For pitta	Grapes, pomegranates, apples
For kapha	Apples, cranberries, pomegranates

OTHER FOODS. Additional foods that are helpful for improving memory include sweet potatoes, tapioca, okra (frequently used as a brain tonic), and spinach, which promotes pitta and stimulates memory. *Sattvic* foods in general are good for memory. Foods traditionally considered most *sattvic* include fresh fruits and vegetables, almonds, oranges, ghee, and milk. One food that is particularly bad for memory is heavy meat. This should be strictly avoided by anyone with memory problems.

HERBS FOR MEMORY

• Ginkgo and gotu kola have recently been touted as good for improving memory, and indeed they are truly beneficial. Both of these herbs serve to dilate the cerebral blood vessels, increasing circulation to the brain, and are good memory tonics.

• In Ayurveda there are specific herbs known as *medhya* herbs. *Medhya* means "that which improves memory." The first and foremost is *brahmi* (which is similar to gotu kola). Also, *jatamamsi, bhringaraj,* and *shanka pushpi* are valuable for the brain and memory. You can use these herbs separately, or mixed together in equal proportions to make a tea.

brahmi
jatamamsi
bhringaraj
shanka pushpi

Steep 1 teaspoon herbs in 1 cup hot water for 10 minutes, and drink it on an empty stomach in the morning and evening. Continue taking this tea for 1 month to help improve circulation to the brain and eliminate memory problems. If it seems to be beneficial, you can continue using it indefinitely.

• Drink *brahmi* milk—$1/2$ teaspoon *brahmi* boiled for a couple of minutes in a cup of milk—at bedtime. It will improve your memory remarkably. Add a pinch of saffron for increased benefit. You can drink *brahmi* milk every day for a month, or continue indefinitely.

• A teaspoon of *brahmi* ghee, taken 5 to 10 minutes before breakfast and before dinner, also helps.

• Aloe vera gel (1 tablespoon) with a pinch of black pepper and $1/4$ teaspoon *bhringaraj* powder, taken 2 or 3 times a day, is also beneficial.

PRACTICAL TIPS FOR GOOD MEMORY

WRITE IT DOWN. Write down important information in order to remember it. Then you can go over it, and over it. Also, make a list of things you want to do or buy. Then you won't forget the milk or bananas!

DEVELOP A POETIC ATTITUDE. Think in rhymes and rhythms. In the oral traditions of India and other countries, students memorize vast amounts of knowledge that is usually set in rhyme and rhythm.

ASSOCIATE. Use association to aid memory. Suppose somebody tells you his name. Try to associate that name with something familiar. You might even imagine a picture to go along with the sound.

MEDITATION ON FORGETFULNESS. There is an ancient Vedic technique to recapture a lost memory: If you forget something, just sit quietly and stay in the forgetfulness. Breathe into the forgetfulness, and try to dig out the memory. Suddenly it will come back!

OTHER REMEDIES

EXERCISE. Daily walking, especially fast walking if you are fit for it, improves circulation and helps strengthen memory. Walk for half an hour, 5 times a week, Monday to Friday.

YOGA POSTURES. Yoga postures are helpful, especially the inverted poses (Shoulder Stand, Headstand, Plow pose, and Camel pose), which help to bring more blood to the brain. The Bow and Cobra poses are also helpful, as is Savasana, the yogic rest pose. Also do the Sun Salutation, 12 cycles a day.

OIL MASSAGE. *Brahmi* oil rubbed on the soles of the feet and on the scalp stimulates cerebral neural receptors under the skin, which send messages to the brain cells and can activate memory.

NASYA. The nose is the doorway to the brain and memory. Nose drops of warmed-up *brahmi* ghee, 5 drops in each nostril, can help to improve memory. (See appendix 2 for instructions on how to make medicated oils and ghees.)

PRANAYAMA. Alternate Nostril Breathing helps to improve cerebral circulation (see chapter 6).

MEDITATE FOR BETTER MEMORY. Memory problems may be caused by stress, anxiety, and worries. Regular meditation is beneficial for relieving stress. Try the Empty Bowl or *So-Hum* meditation explained in chapter 7.

AVOID TOXIC SUBSTANCES. A person who has memory problems should avoid alcohol and marijuana. Also, strictly avoid drugs that will directly affect the brain, such as LSD. Smoking cigarettes can also adversely affect memory, as nicotine toxicity constricts the cerebral blood vessels, which will damage the brain cells. Some research indicates that certain commonly prescribed medications, such as diazepam (Valium), may also seriously impair memory.

These do's and don'ts will be effective in protecting and improving your memory.

Menopause Problems

Menopause is a natural phenomenon. The body stops producing female hormones, and menstruation ceases. In addition to their reproductive and other functions, female hormones are necessary for regulation of bone metabolism. That is why some women may end up with osteoporosis. This is particularly true of vata and pitta individuals. (See "Osteoporosis" for suggestions on preventing this condition.)

Some women may experience menopausal syndrome, characterized by hot flashes, retention of water, and mood swings. Some may have insomnia. The following recommendations will help you move through this natural stage of your life gracefully and comfortably.

DIETARY GUIDELINES. The main dietary recommendation for menopause is to follow the vata-pacifying diet (see chapter 8). This is true for all constitutions but is especially crucial for vata types.

ALOE VERA. Taking fresh aloe vera gel (1 teaspoon 3 times a day) will help prevent and relieve uncomfortable symptoms.

MINERAL SUPPLEMENTS. It is important to take some mineral supplements. Specifically, take a formula of calcium, magnesium, and zinc that provides a daily amount approximately as follows:

calcium	1,200 mg.
magnesium	600 mg.
zinc	60 mg.

Natural Hormone Sources

It has become commonplace for modern medicine to prescribe hormone replacement therapy for menopausal women. Ayurveda has long recognized the value of female rejuvenating herbs at this stage of life, to prevent and/or alleviate menopausal syndrome. However, these herbs, rather than being a synthetic formula, provide your body with natural food precursors of estrogen and progesterone.

The herbs *shatavari* and wild yam (which is similar to the Ayurvedic herb *vidari*) are most effective. A mixture of the two will be strengthening and healing to your system.

vidari or wild yam ½ teaspoon
shatavari ½ teaspoon

Take this formula twice a day after lunch and dinner during the entire menopausal stage, with a few sips of warm water or ½ cup of aloe vera juice.

Take these supplements at night. They should help with menopausal symptoms such as hot flashes, and they can also help prevent osteoporosis.

FOR HOT FLASHES. Try drinking 1 cup of pomegranate juice with 1 teaspoon rock candy powder or organic sugar and 5 to 10 drops of lime juice. You can drink this 2 or 3 times per day, as needed to relieve hot flashes.

FOR VAGINAL DRYNESS. To alleviate vaginal dryness, you can pour some sesame oil on a piece of sterile cotton, mold it into a tamponlike shape, and insert it into the vagina at night. Use a sanitary pad to catch any leakage of the oil. (Consider tying a clean thread or string to the cotton to help you remove it in the morning.)

HELPFUL YOGA POSTURES. Certain yoga *asanas* are beneficial. Do the Sun Salutation at least 12 cycles per day, as well as postures that will strengthen the lower abdominal area, such as the Lotus, Locust, Bow, Boat, and Spinal Twist. Leg Lifts and the Chest-Knee pose are also helpful. (See appendix 4.)

Menstrual Difficulties

See also "PMS"

TYPES OF DYSMENORRHEA

According to Ayurvedic theory, painful or difficult menstruation (dysmenorrhea) can be divided into three types: vata, pitta, and kapha. It is important to know as specifically as possible what the problem is (vata, pitta, or kapha) in order to treat it effectively. Please note that these difficulties are independent of one's *own* constitutional type. That is, somebody with a pitta constitution could be having vata-type menstrual problems. So read the following descriptions carefully and compare them to your own experience.

- *Vata.* More pain before the onset of menstruation, bloating, lower abdominal pain, lower back ache, constipation, cramps, and insomnia are associated with vata-type dysmenorrhea. Menstrual flow tends to be scanty.
- *Pitta.* Congestive dysmenorrhea is a pitta problem. Pitta creates congestion, inflammation, and irritation. The breasts become tender, the bladder becomes sensitive, and there can be a burning sensation while passing urine. There may be hot flashes and irritability. It may lead to profuse menstrual flow.
- *Kapha.* In kapha-type menstrual difficulties, there is also congestion, and pain occurs more in the later part of the menstrual period, associated with white discharge, bloating, water retention, feelings of heaviness, lethargy, and drowsiness. The woman feels like sleeping during the daytime.

TREATMENTS FOR DYSMENORRHEA

Now for some effective treatments for each type of disorder.

VATA. For vata-type menstrual discomfort, make an herbal compound of

ashwagandha
vidari
tagar

Mix equal proportions of these herbs together, and take 1 teaspoon of the mixture with warm water after lunch and dinner.

Also effective for relieving vata-type cramps and discomfort is applying castor oil on the lower abdomen.

Take 1 tablespoon of aloe vera gel with 2 pinches of black pepper 3 times a day until the cramps subside.

PITTA. Women with pitta-type symptoms should use

shatavari 2 parts
kama dudha 1/8 part
musta 1 part

This formula is effective for pitta-type menstrual pain. Take 1/2 teaspoon of this mixture twice a day with warm water, after meals.

You will also find application of some coconut oil on the lower abdomen quite soothing.

KAPHA. Kapha-type menstrual problems can be effectively treated by using a mixture of

punarnava 1/2 part
manjistha 1/2 part
trikatu 1/8 part

Take about 1/2 teaspoon of this mixture twice a day, after lunch and dinner, washed down with warm water.

Application of mustard oil and castor oil (half and half) to the lower abdomen will also help with kapha-type menstrual discomfort.

NOTE: This may be a good time to remind you of an important Ayurvedic principle. If you are finding that your self-treatment is not working or even appears to be making the condition worse, you may have made a mistake in your diagnosis of the problem.

Don't give up! Remember, you are not a trained Ayurvedic diagnostician. Simply reassess the situation and try a different line of treatment.

FOR ALL BODY TYPES

HERBAL REMEDIES. Ayurvedic medicine includes a series of powerful herbal compounds based on the herb *guggulu*. In addition to other healing qualities, these compounds are especially good for regulating menstruation. For vata-type pain, use *triphala guggulu* or *yogaraj guggulu*. Pittas may use *kaishore guggulu*. Kaphas will do best with *punarnava guggulu*. In each case, take one tablet twice a day. These tablets are generally available from sources of Ayurvedic herbs (see Resources).

• Another universal remedy that should bring some relief from menstrual pain is to roast some cumin seeds in an ungreased pan until they smell pungent. (It will just take a few minutes.) When they are cool, chew about 1 teaspoon slowly, and follow with one tablespoon aloe vera juice.

FOR EXCESSIVE MENSTRUAL FLOW. A tea made of raspberry leaves and hibiscus flowers (equal amounts, 1 to 2 teaspoons of herbs per cup of water) is often quite effective.

• You might also try drinking a cup of coconut water (the natural juice inside a fresh coconut) with $^1/_2$ teaspoon rock candy powder or natural sugar added.

• Eating about 10 to 20 fresh raspberries on an empty stomach, up to 2 or 3 times a day, may be helpful.

STRATEGY TO PREVENT MENSTRUAL PROBLEMS

Perhaps more important than all these pain remedies is a strategy to *prevent* menstrual problems. You can follow this strategy quite easily, effectively, safely, and inexpensively.

ALOE VERA GEL. For the entire week before you expect your period to start, take 1 tablespoon of aloe vera gel, 3 times a day. This will help prevent all types of menstrual pain and discomfort.

DIETARY GUIDELINES. Throughout the month, follow the dietary guidelines for your constitutional type (see chapter 8).

YOGA POSITIONS. Throughout the month, spend a few minutes every day on the yoga postures recommended for your body type (see page 60). Yoga *asanas* are not recommended during the menstrual period. Just rest, read, and relax as much as possible.

If you follow these recommendations, your menstrual problems may soon be nothing but a memory.

Migraine

See also "Headaches"

Although migraine headaches can result from a vata, pitta, or kapha imbalance, they most frequently occur when systemic pitta moves into the cardiovascular system, circulates, and affects the blood vessels around the brain. The hot, sharp quality of pitta dilates the blood vessels and creates pressure on the nerves, causing this painful condition.

FOLLOW THE PITTA-PACIFYING DIET. To treat migraine headaches, it is vital first to take care of pitta with a proper pitta-soothing diet. (See the dietary guidelines in chapter 8.) Especially avoid hot, spicy foods, fermented foods, and sour or citrus fruits. Carefully following a pitta-soothing diet is effective both for migraine relief and as a preventive measure.

PREVENTIVE BREAKFAST. Certain individuals get migraines at midday, which then subside later in the evening. For such individuals, try this preventive method. It may sound too simple, but it is effective. First thing in the morning, take 1 ripe banana. Peel it, chop it into pieces, and add 1 teaspoon warm ghee, 1 teaspoon date sugar, and a pinch of cardamom on top. This is delicious, and it will help to reduce pitta and prevent a headache from arising.

HERBAL REMEDY. The following herbal compound will be beneficial:

shatavari 5 *parts*
brahmi 4 *parts*
jatamamsi 3 *parts*
musta 3 *parts*

Prepare this mixture, and take 1/2 teaspoon twice a day, morning and evening, after breakfast and dinner, with a little lukewarm water. This formula is designed to pacify the aggravated pitta and help relieve migraine headaches.

AVOID DIRECT SUN. Because migraine headaches are predominantly a pitta disorder, they are affected by the hot sun. When the sun rises, its hot, sharp, penetrating rays increase pitta in the cardiovascular system and cause the dilation of the blood vessels in the brain, which results in the painful headaches. So it is important to avoid direct exposure to the sun, and if you do go out in the sun, wear a hat.

SOOTHING NOSE DROPS. Once a headache has developed, putting about 5 drops of warm *brahmi* ghee in each nostril will help relieve the pain.

RECOMMENDED YOGA POSTURES. Generally, a person having migraines should do the Moon Salutation (see appendix 4). Helpful yoga postures include the Hidden Lotus, Boat pose, Bow pose, Spinal Twist, Palm Tree pose, and Standing on the Toes.

A COOLING *PRANAYAMA*. You will also find a cooling breathing exercise such as *shitali* helpful (see chapter 8).

A HEALING YAWN. When you have a migraine, gently squeeze your earlobes, pulling the ear down, and do the act of yawning. That will relieve the pressure on the blood vessels and help to pacify the headache.

See "Headaches" for a detailed analysis of vata, pitta, and kapha headaches and their proper treatment.

Morning Sickness

Early in pregnancy, morning sickness—nausea and vomiting in the early morning, immediately or soon after waking up—is quite common. This condition is due to aggravation of pitta and is especially common among pitta individuals. It usually occurs from approximately the sixth to the tenth week of pregnancy.

Some medical researchers have said that the level of estrogen in the blood rises during pregnancy. Estrogen is pittagenic. The higher estrogen level in the blood triggers pitta in the stomach and increases acid secretion, so that the stomach becomes more acidic. In the early morning, when the stomach is empty and acidic, morning sickness can occur.

Also, certain odors can trigger nausea and vomiting at any time of the day or night, but sensitivity to smell is greatest in the morning. During pregnancy, a woman's sense of smell becomes unusually sensitive. The reason is interesting. According to Ayurveda, the earth element is particularly prominent during pregnancy, because the fetus is building and growing and the earth element is responsible for solidity and structure. The earth element is also associated with the sense of smell. (In Ayurveda, the senses are related to the elements like this: Space = touch; Air = hearing; Fire = sight; Water = taste; Earth = smell.)

Ayurvedic literature talks poetically about morning sickness, saying that it is common among women whose babies will develop a copious head of hair after birth.

START THE DAY WITH A LITTLE FOOD. Believe it or not, the first thing to do upon waking up in the morning is to put something in your stomach. Have a little light food. You might try some crackers with a slightly salty taste. Salt is generally pitta-provoking, but a small quantity of salt stimulates salivary secretion and helps to reduce pitta. Fresh lime juice is also helpful, with a little salt and sugar.

EAT OFTEN. If you are troubled by morning sickness, eat small frequent meals, as many as five or six in a day. An empty stomach has more acid secretion, and irritation and nausea easily follow.

COCONUT WATER. Add 1 teaspoon of lemon juice to a cup of coconut water (the natural juice inside a fresh coconut), and take a sip every 15 minutes to settle your stomach.

EFFECTIVE HERBAL REMEDY. The following herbal formula is effective for settling morning sickness:

shatavari 5 parts
shanka bhasma 1/8 part
kama dudha 1/8 part

Take 1/2 teaspoon of this mixture with lime juice or lemon juice in the early morning and at bedtime to reduce acid secretion in the stomach and relieve nausea.

TRY ALMONDS. Soak 10 raw (unroasted) almonds overnight, and next morning peel off the skin and eat them. In addition to providing a high-quality protein, almonds are a good source of calcium. Pregnant mothers need both. And they settle the stomach.

WALK IT OFF. Sometimes walking in the fresh morning air helps with morning sickness, because fresh cool air reduces pitta. It also helps to relieve stress. It sometimes happens that a pitta woman, working for a demanding boss and coming home to a criticizing husband, develops some unresolved anger. Stress builds up in the solar plexus and manifests as morning sickness. It is important for her to reduce her stress level by doing some early morning walking or other appropriate exercise.

MINIMASSAGE. In the morning, before taking a shower, warm up 3 to 5 ounces of sesame oil (for vata constitutions), coconut oil (for pittas) or sunflower oil (for kaphas), and rub it over your body for 5 to 10 minutes. Be sure to get some on your scalp and feet. Then take a nice warm shower. This soothing oil massage (called *abhyanga*) will minimize stress and help with morning sickness.

MILK WITH ROSE WATER. Buy some rose essence or rose water. When you are feeling nauseated, put 1 drop in a cupful of milk, boil the milk, and then drink it warm. (You can just as well use 5 fresh rose petals from your garden to boil in the milk.) This will help to eliminate the nausea. As a preventive measure, taking a cup of this rose milk with a teaspoon of ghee at bedtime will pacify pitta and help to control morning sickness.

DRINK A LOT. Vomiting can lead to dehydration, so you need to drink extra liquid to compensate. Better still, make some homemade dextrosaline by adding 2 teaspoons sugar, the juice of 1/2 lime, and a pinch of salt to 1 pint of water. Drink 1 cup every 2 hours to eliminate dehydration and help the nausea and vomiting subside.

PEACOCK FEATHER ASH. This remedy might sound strange, but it is quite effective. Ayurvedic literature says that morning sickness can be remedied by using peacock feather ash. Burn a peacock feather in such a way that you can collect the ash. The smell of the burning feather is quite awful, so someone else should burn the feather, not the pregnant woman. Take just a pinch of the powdery ash with a teaspoon of honey. This can immediately stop morning sickness.

EFFECTIVE HERBAL FORMULA. No matter what your constitutional type is, this formula will be beneficial for you:

shatavari 5 parts
kama dudha 1/8 part
shanka bhasma 1/8 part
moti bhasma 1/8 part

Take 1/2 teaspoon 2 or 3 times a day with ghee. Or, if you don't want to use ghee, use warm water. Sometimes during pregnancy women may not feel like taking ghee.

Muscle Cramps and Spasms

While running, walking, riding a bicycle, standing up for a long time, doing yoga stretches incorrectly, or even sleeping, a person can get muscle cramps. Any muscle—upper arm, forearm, leg, calf, or even a toe or the baby finger—can undergo sudden spasm.

Muscle cramps and spasms have numerous causes. They may be due to insufficient blood supply to the muscle or, in some cases, to excess blood supply, as in the case of "writer's cramp." Muscle spasms can be due to lack of calcium in the diet or malabsorption of calcium, since calcium plays a significant role in relaxing the muscle. A related problem is hypoparathyroidism (underactive parathyroid), in which the person loses calcium; this may also cause the muscles to undergo spasm. Exposure to cold and poor circulation may also be responsible.

The Ayurvedic understanding is, in simplest terms, that muscle spasms are caused by vata dosha. Vata, increased by mobile, cold, or rough qualities, makes a muscle stiff and hard, and it undergoes spasm.

FOR IMMEDIATE RELIEF. Whenever a muscle is under spasm

- Grab hold of it.
- At the same time, press your index finger deeply into the "belly" of the muscle (the bulging central part of the muscle) for 15 to 20 seconds. A *marma* point (like an acupressure point) is located in the center of the muscle; pressing on it helps the muscle relax.
- Take a few deep breaths.

This procedure will increase circulation, and the muscle will relax.

ANOTHER PRESSURE POINT REMEDY. A *marma* point is located at the midpoint of both the lips. If there is a spasm in the upper body, such as in the arms or fingers, grab hold of your upper lip, in the middle, between your thumb and index finger. If the spasm is in the legs or the lower part of the body, grab the lower lip.

These energy points on the lips send messages to the brain, which in turn relays a signal to the motor system to relax the muscles. Just grabbing the lips for 30 seconds should help relieve the spasm. Press fairly strongly, but not hard enough to be painful.

CONTRACT AND RELAX THE MUSCLE. Repeatedly alternate contraction and relaxation of the muscle. This will improve circulation and help to release lactic acid, which will relax the muscle.

MASSAGE. Another approach is to apply a little oil to the muscle belly and gently massage. *Mahanarayan* oil is best if you have it; otherwise, some sesame oil or other oil will do. Gentle massage of the painful cramped muscle will relax the muscle fibers, improve the circulation, and pacify the vata. That will help relieve the spasm.

After rubbing in the *mahanarayan* oil, apply a little heat. For best results, use a hot water bottle (not an electric heating pad).

Winter, with its dry, cold weather, is vata season. During winter season, when vata individuals get exposed to the cold, their muscles may cramp. Rubbing the muscle with *mahanarayan* oil (or sesame oil) and hen applying heat will be soothing and healing.

SOAK IT. For a cramp in your foot, soak the foot in a bucket of warm water that contains salt (1 or 2 tablespoons).

A hot ginger powder–baking soda bath (2/3 cup baking soda and 1/4 cup ginger per tubful of water) is also effective for muscle relaxation.

HERBAL RELAXANTS. Make yourself a cup of chamomile tea, *jatamamsi* tea, or comfrey tea. Or, even better, you can make a tea using equal amounts of all three of these herbs (1/3 teaspoon of each per cup). It will help to relax your muscles.

FOR PREVENTION. As a preventive measure against future cramping, drink some *dashamoola* tea—1/2 teaspoon of *dashamoola* powder steeped for a few minutes in 1 cup hot water. Have a cup or two of *dashamoola* tea every Saturday.

MINERAL SUPPLEMENTS. Getting repeated muscle cramps suggests that you either have a calcium deficiency or are not absorbing enough of the calcium in your food. First, take some supplements of calcium, magnesium, and zinc. Your formula should contain approximately 1,200 mg. calcium, 600 mg. magnesium, and 60 mg. zinc. Take these supplements at bedtime.

Second, to improve absorption, take *triphala* every night or in the very early morning. Use about 1/2 teaspoon *triphala* powder per cup of boiling water.

YOGARAJ GUGGULU. *Yogaraj guggulu* tablets (200 mg. per tablet), taken 2 or 3 times a day for 1 month, are effective for pacifying vata in the muscles, which is the root cause of muscle cramps.

EFFECTIVE HOME TREATMENT FOR ABDOMINAL CRAMPS. Muscle cramps and cramps in the stomach may be related. Muscle pain can happen anywhere in the body, in the skeletal muscles as well as in the smooth muscles of the abdomen. As with spasm in the arm or leg, abdominal cramps may have many causes, such as eating too big a meal, or lifting too heavy a weight, which strains the abdominal muscles. Gases in the stomach, constipation, or acid indigestion can also create cramps in the stomach or abdomen.

- For painful cramps in the abdominal muscles, take the herbal compound *shankavati* (one 200-mg. tablet after dinner).
- This antacid formula may also be effective:

shatavari *1/2 teaspoon*
guduchi *1/4 teaspoon*
shanka bhasma *pinch*

Take this entire amount once or twice a day, after meals.

- Warm milk is helpful for abdominal muscle cramps. Its alkaline property helps pacify acidity, and it is also a good source of calcium, which helps muscles to relax. One cup of warm milk taken at bedtime will help to dispel acid irritation and spasm of the stomach.

• *Lasunadivati* (garlic compound) is effectively used for smooth muscle spasm as well as skeletal muscle spasm. Take 1 tablet after dinner for 5 days. You can also buy odorless garlic tablets; take them as directed on the package. Garlic relaxes the muscles, calms down vata dosha, and helps to take care of muscle cramps.

• *Hingwastak churna,* 1/4 teaspoon taken twice a day after lunch and dinner, will also help relieve abdominal muscle pain. It may also create some gas, however.

• *Triphala* is very effective in relieving gases, promoting proper elimination, and facilitating absorption of calcium and other key minerals. Take 1/2 teaspoon of *triphala* daily at bedtime with warm water. It will minimize your chances of getting muscle cramps in the stomach.

Nasal Crust

Some individuals, when their systemic kapha dosha becomes high (perhaps due to eating too many kapha-increasing foods), become sensitive to pollen, dust, ragweed, cat hair, dog hair, and other allergens, as well as to cold temperatures. As a result, they may develop rhinitis, with nasal congestion and nasal discharge. Even in the absence of infection, dryness in the atmosphere may dry up the mucous membranes and nasal passage; to compensate for that, the body will produce more mucus. Then, due to continuing dry heat in the environment, the nasal discharge becomes thick, dry, and crusty. This is known as nasal crust.

People with deviated nasal septum can also accumulate nasal discharge, and because of dryness in the air it may form a crust. Nasal crust can create stuffy nose, sinus headache, and difficulty breathing. It can be one of the causes of snoring and of sleep apnea. Nosebleeds may also be due to nasal crust.

Ayurvedic medicine offers a number of effective remedies:

STEAM IT. The simplest remedy is to inhale steam. You can use plain water, water with some ginger boiled in it, or a tea of the following ingredients:

ginger
ajwan (Indian celery seed)
turmeric

Put equal amounts of each of these herbs in a pint of water, and boil it up. Then turn off the fire, put a towel over your head, and inhale the steam. This will ease out the discharge. The crust will come out, and you will breathe freely. Though simple, this is an effective remedy.

MENTHOL AND EUCALYPTUS. Rubbing menthol on the forehead and on the sinus area will help. Placing a few drops of *mild* eucalyptus oil in the nose will also help.

NOTE: Do not use pure eucalyptus oil. Dilute a few drops of eucalyptus oil with sesame oil or some other mild oil so that it doesn't burn your skin or the sensitive tissue in the nose.

USE AN ONION. Chop up an onion, and sniff its fragrance. Onions contain ammonia, which is a powerful decongestant. It brings tears to the eyes and promotes sneezing. The tears from the eyes will pass through the tear ducts and into the nasal passage, which will lubricate and loosen the crust; then the sneezing will help the crust to be eliminated.

LUBRICATE THE NOSTRILS. Putting a few drops of *brahmi* ghee or saline solution into the nose will also lubricate the nasal passage and facilitate removal of the crust. You can make an effective saline solution by adding $^1/_8$ teaspoon salt to $^1/_2$ cup water.

BURN IT OUT. A meal of spicy food will also help. For example, a hot soup or vegetables spiced with cayenne pepper, curry powder, or chili pepper (within your limits of comfort!) will increase circulation and help to eliminate stuffy nose and nasal crust.

USE A HUMIDIFIER. At night, run a humidifier so that the room will be warm and moist. If possible, don't use an ultrasound humidifier. A hot-water type is best.

VITAMINS AND HERBS. Finally, take some or all of the following:

- Vitamin C—1,000 mg. (1 gram) twice a day
- *Amalaki* (a good source of vitamin C)—1 teaspoon at bedtime in warm water. (Don't use it if you are already taking *triphala* at night; *amalaki* is one of the ingredients of *triphala*.)
- Zinc—60 mg.
- *Sitopaladi churna*—$^1/_2$ to 1 teaspoon, with 1 teaspoon honey and 1 teaspoon ghee.

Nausea and Vomiting

See also "Morning Sickness"

Nausea and vomiting have numerous possible causes, including excess acid secretion, toxins in the liver, pregnancy, worms in the colon, food poisoning, and flu. (For suggestions on reducing nausea and vomiting during pregnancy, see "Morning Sickness.")

In the event of food poisoning or excess acid secretion in the stomach, vomiting occurs as a protective response of the body to get rid of toxins. With flu also, excess bile may build up in the stomach, and vomiting occurs to cast it out. In such cases vomiting is a sign of health, of the body taking care of itself.

But when vomiting becomes persistent, it may lead to dehydration or other problems, and it has to be stopped. Morning sickness, for example, may adversely affect the flow of nutrition going to the fetus.

Ayurveda recommends quite a few effective ways to relieve nausea and put a stop to vomiting.

PACIFY PITTA. Nausea and vomiting indicate high pitta in the stomach, with increased acid secretion irritating the gastric mucous membrane. Therefore, it is good to follow a pitta-soothing diet, especially abstaining from hot, spicy food or fermented food.

TRY FASTING. Fasting gives a healing rest to the digestive system. Don't eat for a day—and drink 1 cup of sweet fresh pineapple juice with a pinch of ginger, a pinch of black pepper, and $^1/_2$ teaspoon organic sugar. Take this 3 times during the day.

• Alternatively, you can drink cranberry juice or pomegranate juice on your fast.

EIGHT WAYS TO SETTLE NAUSEA AND VOMITING. Here are eight simple and effective suggestions to help you soothe nausea and vomiting:

• To 1 cup of water, add 10 drops of lime juice and $^1/_2$ teaspoon sugar. Last, add $^1/_4$ teaspoon baking soda. Stir and drink. This can immediately stop nausea and vomiting.

• An effective remedy is to chew 1 or 2 cardamom seeds.

• A mixture of 1 teaspoon ginger juice (or freshly grated ginger pulp) and 1 teaspoon onion juice will help to settle nausea and vomiting.

• Make a mixture of equal parts lemon juice and honey. Dip your index finger into the mixture and lick it, consuming the mixture slowly.

• Try stirring $^1/_2$ teaspoon honey and 2 pinches of cardamom into half a cup of plain yogurt.

• A tea made from 1 teaspoon cumin seeds and a pinch of nutmeg steeped in a cup of hot water will be quite soothing.

• Drinking sugar cane juice can also be helpful, as is cranberry juice with a little lime juice added.

• Ayurveda also recommends the following herbal formula to quickly stop nausea and vomiting:

rose petal powder $^1/_2$ *teaspoon*
sandalwood powder $^1/_4$ *teaspoon*
rock candy powder $^1/_2$ *teaspoon*
lime juice 10 *drops*

Take this entire mixture in room temperature water.

Vomit for Healing

Most people find vomiting a rather unpleasant experience, but there are times when one might want to induce vomiting. When someone has a flu or a bad cold, excess kapha may build up and the person suffers from persistent headache, congestion, and coughing. Mother Nature may bring on vomiting to remove the kapha, but if that doesn't happen, Ayurveda suggests taking matters into your own hands.

Drink a glass of water with $^1/_4$ teaspoon salt dissolved in it. The salty water itself is emetic (provokes vomiting), but you can also rub the back of the tongue to stimulate the "gag" reflex and vomit out the water. The moment vomiting occurs, fever will generally come down, the headache will disappear, congestion in the chest will be greatly relieved, and you will feel much better.

FOR NAUSEA IN CHILDREN. Try giving the child some coconut water. Add 1 teaspoon lemon juice to a cup of coconut water (the natural juice inside a fresh coconut), and have the child take a sip every 15 minutes or so to settle the stomach.

FOR WORMS. Nausea and vomiting may also be a sign of worms. If a person has a history of passing worms in the stool and gets repeated attacks of nausea and vomiting, use the following strategy:

- Take the herb *vidanga*, about $\frac{1}{2}$ teaspoon twice a day with a little warm water.
- Keep the colon clean by taking $\frac{1}{2}$ teaspoon *triphala* at night for several weeks. Mix the *triphala* into $\frac{1}{2}$ cup of warm water, let it steep for 10 minutes, then strain and drink.

TO DETOXIFY THE LIVER. Nausea and vomiting may be a sign that there are excess toxins in the liver. To detoxify the liver, the following formula is effective:

kutki $\frac{1}{4}$ *teaspoon*
shatavari $\frac{1}{2}$ *teaspoon*
shanka bhasma *pinch*
kama dudha *pinch*

Take this mixture 2 or 3 times a day with water to relieve nausea and vomiting.

Nightmares

Nightmares are quite common in children up to the age of 12 but are more rarely found in adults. The main causes of nightmares in adults are (1) fears, anxieties, worries, and other psychological stresses, and (2) eating too much food too late at night. There may be other physical causes, such as problems with adenoids, or sleep apnea, or nasal crust that doesn't allow adequate breathing. Whenever there is cerebral hypoxia—lack of oxygen and *prana* to the brain—the person can get nightmares. This can occur even due to insufficient fresh air in the room.

TREATING NIGHTMARES IN CHILDREN

The main cause of nightmares in children is psychological—fear and anxiety based on frightening images they have seen or scary stories they have heard. So it is important not to feed the child's imagination with disturbing images. Keep children busy with creative play; don't let them watch violent or horrifying television programs or read frightening stories.

The child's room should be pleasant and filled with sweetness, with nice music and perhaps some tinkling bells. Bells have a happy sound that children like. You can tell the child, "When there is a bell, monsters won't come." And they'll sleep peacefully.

Rather than watching frightening or violent movies, tell children positive, uplifting stories, such as from the *Ramayana*, about baby Krishna, or any other beautiful, happy story.

Give the child a mini–oil massage before bed. Rub some oil, especially *brahmi* oil or *bhringaraj* oil, on the soles of the feet and on the scalp. This will help relax the child. (See appendix 2 for instructions on making herbalized oils.)

Sometimes nightmares come as a result of bedwetting. To help prevent this, see that the child doesn't drink much for at least two hours before going to sleep. Some cumin-coriander-fennel tea (again, not just before bedtime) can help prevent bedwetting.

REMEDIES FOR ADULTS AND CHILDREN

TRANQUILLITY TEA. Make a tea from equal proportions of

jatamamsi
brahmi
ginkgo
yashti madhu (licorice root)

Drinking a cup of this tea (made from 1 teaspoon of the herbal mix steeped in 1 cup hot water) before going to bed will help create a more peaceful mind and body. This tea is good for children as well as adults.

• You can also make a similar tea of equal amounts of *jatamamsi* and *shanka pushpi.*

HERBS FOR ALLERGIES. If allergies are the cause of the nightmares, you can help remedy them with *sitopaladi* and *yashti madhu.* Mix them in equal proportions, and take 1/2 teaspoon of each with honey twice a day. For children, use 1/4 teaspoon of each.

JATAMAMSI. If you sew an ounce or two of the herb *jatamamsi* inside a small silk bag and place it under the pillow, its fragrance will help create a tranquil night.

NASYA. Doing *nasya* will help. Put 2 to 3 drops of warm ghee or any Ayurvedic nose drops (such as *brahmi* ghee) in each nostril,

Are Your Dreams Vata, Pitta, or Kapha?

To eliminate nightmares, it can be helpful to know if they are the result of a doshic imbalance of kapha, pitta, or vata, so that the imbalance can be corrected. By analyzing the nature and content of the dreams, it is usually possible to find out.

• Vata dreams. Vata dreams are active and hyper. They are plentiful, and the dreamer may well forget them in the morning. Horror, fear, running, jumping, flying high in the sky, falling deep down into a valley, being attacked or pursued, being locked up—these are vata dreams.

• Pitta dreams. These dreams can be rather violent. In addition to such themes as teaching, studying, trying to solve a problem, or failing at an examination, pitta dreams may involve fire, war, nuclear weapons, fighting, killing, and murder.

• Kapha dreams. Kapha dreams are generally mild and romantic. Water figures prominently, such as swimming in the ocean. Seeing gardens, lotus flowers, swans, and elephants and eating candy are all characteristic of kapha dreams. Drowning, or seeing oneself as dead, are "negative" aspects of the kapha dream repertory.

and inhale (see appendix 3). *Nasya* is equally effective for children.

EAT EARLY. Eat dinner before seven o'clock. Eating too late at night may create nightmares.

CUT DOWN ON STRESS. Yoga *asanas,* regular exercise, Alternate Nostril *pranayama,* and meditation morning and evening help to relax the nervous system and reduce stress. (You will find instructions for *pranayama* in chapter 6 and guidelines for meditation in chapter 7.)

CRYSTALS. Wearing crystals, or putting some amethyst crystals on the four corners of the bed, may also help. You can tell your child, "Look, I've put these crystals around your bed; it will keep the ghosts and monsters away." They will feel comfortable and will sleep well.

The root cause of nightmares is wrong thinking: negative imagination, loneliness, isolation, fear, disturbed relationships. That is why prayer, positive thinking, positive affirmations, and positive imagination are the best medications for nightmares.

Nosebleed

Nosebleed has many possible origins. Trauma to the nose, extreme dryness of the nasal passage so that the nasal mucous membranes crack and bleed, allergies, rhinitis, a nasal polyp, or high blood pressure may all cause nosebleed. Going to a high altitude or consuming excess alcohol are also possible causes.

Usually we don't have any time to investigate the cause; we need to treat it immediately. Here are several effective remedies:

DRINK COOL WATER. This alone will stop many nosebleeds.

USE A COLD COMPRESS. Dip a handkerchief or any clean soft cloth into cold water, and place it on the forehead and the nose. Then *gently* blow the nose so that the clot, if there is one, comes out. (If there is a dry nasal crust, it will irritate the nasal passage and cause bleeding.)

SNIFF COLD WATER. Take a little cool water in your palm, inhale it up into the nose, and gently blow the nose.

SQUEEZE YOUR NOSE. If the cold water doesn't stop the bleeding, then pinch the nose with your thumb and index finger, as if you were about to dip under water. Hold for 2 or 3 minutes, breathing normally through the mouth. That should stop the bleeding.

GHEE OINTMENT. If the bleeding still doesn't stop, another simple remedy is to put a couple of drops of lukewarm ghee in each nostril. Dip a cotton swab into a jar of ghee, and apply it to the nose. Ghee is hemostatic—that is, it stops bleeding.

STAND OR SIT UPRIGHT. Don't lie down, which will encourage bleeding. Also don't do any inverted yoga postures such as Headstand, Shoulder Stand or Plow. Remaining upright will minimize bleeding.

HUMIDIFY YOUR SURROUNDINGS. Many nosebleeds are due to a dry nose, caused by hot, dry air. So as a preventive measure in dry climates or in winter when heating the house can create a lot of dry air, be sure to humidify your bedroom, workroom, or the entire living space. It is better not to use an ultrasound humidifier; a hot water unit is best.

HERBAL REMEDY. Orally, take a mixture of:

manjistha 1/3 *teaspoon*
kama dudha 1/8 *teaspoon*

Take this mixture with a little warm water twice a day.

JUICE CURE. To stop or prevent nosebleeds, you can drink cranberry juice, pomegranate juice, or a half-and-half mixture of the two.

POMEGRANATE NOSE DROPS. When making the pomegranate juice, if you pick up a few drops of the fresh juice in an eyedropper and place them in your nostrils, it should instantaneously stop the bleeding.

FOLLOW THE PITTA-PACIFYING DIET. According to Ayurvedic principles, even though nosebleed has some vata symptoms, such as dryness and cracking of the nasal passages, it is essentially a pitta disorder, in which pitta becomes hot and sharp and causes the bleeding. So when you have a nosebleed, don't eat hot and spicy foods, abstain from alcohol and cigarettes, and don't work under the hot sun. These are all pitta-provoking.

> **TIME TO SEE THE DOCTOR**
>
> If, after trying these remedies, your nose is still bleeding, or if you have repeated nosebleeds over a couple of weeks, see your doctor. You may have a serious health problem. The bleeding may be due to high blood pressure, which needs to be cared for. Or it could possibly be caused by leukemia, a type of blood cancer.

Obesity

Obesity is a condition in which an individual is significantly overweight, and an excessive amount of body fat has accumulated under the chin and on the breasts, belly, buttocks, and/or thighs. Though it is not a serious disease in itself, it may shorten the span of life, as well as create diminished efficiency and a predisposition to diabetes, hypertension, low libido, and arthritis. Ultimately, obesity reduces happiness.

To a great extent, obesity is due to the socioeconomic problems of an affluent society. A prosperous life, a sedentary job, and lack of exercise are the major contributors to obesity. From an Ayurvedic point of view, the main causes of this condition are eating too much, sitting too much, and doing too little.

Obesity is a kapha disorder. In obese individuals the gastric fire is strong, but the cellular fire in the tissue is relatively low.

Whatever excess food or calories a person consumes are not burned and instead turn into adipose tissue, leading to overweight and obesity.

There are numerous other potential causes. Certain hereditary factors of the endocrine system, such as excess production of growth hormone, may contribute to the condition. When women are pregnant, they may eat too much and be unable to lose the weight afterward. Stress may induce repeated emotional eating, leading to significant weight gain. Frequent munching between meals is also detrimental to maintaining a healthy weight. Certain drugs, including steroids and oral contraceptives, can change the metabolism and produce weight gain, as can insulin. Addictions, including alcohol and cigarettes, are often associated with obesity. But the main factor is usually eating too much, along with insufficient exercise.

Habitually drinking cold drinks and eating fatty fried foods, dairy products such as cheese, yogurt, and ice cream, and consuming excess sugar and carbohydrates are all causative factors.

WATCH YOUR DIET. In treating obesity, the first step is to control what you eat. Follow the kapha-pacifying diet (see guidelines in chapter 8). Avoid habitually drinking cold drinks and eating fatty fried foods. Minimize dairy products such as cheese, yogurt, and ice cream. Be sure to include salad (without creamy dressings) and beans in your meals. Drink hot water instead of ice-cold drinks. Obese people generally hate hot water, but they should drink it, either plain or in herbal teas such as ginger, mint, or cinnamon.

If you like to eat meat, you can have some fish or chicken once a month, but no beef, lamb, or pork.

GET ADEQUATE EXERCISE. Do some regular exercise. A daily walk of at least half an hour is essential. And do some aerobic exercise, such as gentle jogging. Obese people hate jogging, but they should at least walk fast, carrying 2.5-pound hand-held weights. Swimming is also good exercise.

Lift weights to reduce body weight. Do some gentle weight lifting, using 5-pound weights to get started. This will help to burn adipose tissue. Also, muscle tissue burns calories more quickly than fat.

If you want to lose weight, you must understand some simple arithmetic. When you take in more calories than you burn off, you will gain weight. In order to lose weight, you *must* burn off more calories than you take in. In practical terms, this means two things: reducing your caloric intake, and increasing your output in the form of exercise. Follow the kapha-reducing diet, and increase the amount of exercise you do every day.

YOUR POSTEXERCISE PRESCRIPTION. Immediately after exercise, kapha individuals will feel hungry and thirsty and will want to rush to the restaurant to have a cold drink and a bite to eat. But the cold drink will slow down the metabolism, defeating the gain from the exercise. And we know that the eating will be counterproductive. So after exercise heavy and obese people should skip snacks and stay away from cold water and other cold drinks, and choose hot drinks such as herbal teas.

EAT YOUR BIGGEST MEAL EARLY IN THE DAY. According to Ayurveda, the best policy regarding meals, if you are overweight, is to skip breakfast entirely (maybe have some hot herbal tea), then take your biggest meal at noon. Supper should be light. Don't snack between the two meals.

If you can't seem to skip breakfast, take your main meal then, early in the day. Have a light lunch and a lighter supper; skip supper entirely if you can.

DROP ALCOHOL AND TOBACCO. Quit drinking alcohol and smoking. These emotional habits unduly stimulate *jatar agni* (gastric fire) and make a person hungry.

LISTEN TO MUSIC. While eating your meals, listen to soft music and chew your food more, so that moderate eating gradually becomes habitual.

LEARN TO LOVE YOURSELF. Most obese people do not love themselves. This is significant because there is a deep relationship between food and love. Food is the food of the body; love is the food of the soul. When an individual is missing love in a relationship, he or she may try to find love through eating, and food will become a substitute for love. When a woman misses her husband or a man misses his wife, they frequently begin to eat too much.

Obese people also hate how they look, and they hate looking in the mirror because they don't like what they see. When people hate their body, they become anxious and worried; then suddenly they become hungry and need to eat. This is not real hunger; it is false, emotional hunger. (See "Eating Disorders" and "Overeating" for further discussion of emotional eating.)

To help develop more love for yourself just as you are, try this technique. Go into your bathroom and remove all your clothes, or wear some shorts. Then take a good look at the person you see in the full-length mirror. Look at that image, starting at the head, the eyes, cheeks, lips, and neck; look at your chest, your belly, and so on.

As you look at the image in your mirror, at the same time look within. Ask yourself, do you like those eyes of yours? Do you love your nose? Don't you have some affection toward your own lips, your own chest?

In this way, gradually, by looking outside, into the mirror, and at the same time inside at your own inner observer, two things will happen. First, you will begin to feel that you are beyond your body, that you are something higher, nobler, greater, and more beautiful, that you are pure existence. Second, this process will also bring greater acceptance, and you will start feeling more love for yourself. So look at yourself in the mirror, and love that person that you see.

A second important factor in loving your-

TIME TO SEE THE DOCTOR

If you are very heavy and have not exercised for a long time, and especially if you are over 40, you *must* see your doctor before you start an exercise program more strenuous than walking.

self is to stop judging, comparing, and criticizing yourself. What you are is unique, and it is divine. Stopping judgment, criticism, and comparison is the beginning of self-love.

These two exercises will really help.

DRINK HOT WATER AND HONEY. Whenever you become hungry, drink a cup of hot water with 1 teaspoon honey and 10 drops of lime juice added. This will be a good substitute for eating and will help to melt the fat.

HERBAL HELPERS. Here is an herbal formula that will help you lose weight.

kutki *3 parts*
chitrak *3 parts*
shilajit *2 parts*
punarnava *5 parts*

Take 1/2 teaspoon of this mixture twice a day with 1 teaspoon honey, before meals.

• In addition, take 1 tablet of the following herbs all together, with warm water, 3 times a day after meals: *triphala guggulu*; *chitrak-adhivati*; *punarnava guggulu*.

• It will also be helpful for you to take *triphala* every night. At least 1 hour after dinner, pour 1 cup of boiling water over 1/2 to 1 teaspoon *triphala*; let it steep for 10 minutes, and drink.

SNACKS YOU CAN AFFORD TO EAT. In between meals, if you like to munch, eat raisins, which are a mild laxative. Don't eat corn chips, which are salty and fatty and difficult to stop eating; don't eat popcorn either. You might also try celery sticks or carrot sticks.

USE HOT SPICES. Use spices in cooking. The kapha-pacifying diet uses many spices, such as cumin, coriander, fennel, cardamom, ginger, cinnamon, and garam masala: These spices are good for kindling the gastric fire. (See chapter 8 for details of the kapha diet.)

HAVE COMPANY WHEN YOU EAT. It is better to eat with friends, particularly with skinny people and people with good eating habits! You'll be happy to be surrounded by them. But don't compare, thinking, "All my friends are thin, and I'm chubby." Be in the company of slim people, and be active with them. That will help to reduce your weight.

HELPFUL YOGA POSTURES. Certain gentle yoga *asanas* are helpful, including the Palm Tree pose and the Triangle pose. Also, while sitting on the floor, bend forward as far as you comfortably can, with the goal of eventually touching your head to your knees. (You'll have to work up to this one gradually.) The Fish, Camel, Cobra, and Cow poses are simple, helpful postures you can easily perform. Remember, don't try to do them perfectly right away. (See the illustrations of yoga postures in appendix 4.)

BREATHE AWAY FAT. *Bhastrika pranayama* (Breath of Fire) will increase the rate at which your body burns off fat. Right Nostril breathing (*surya bhedi*) will also be helpful (see chapter 6).

DON'T NAP IN THE DAYTIME. Obese people frequently like to take siestas, but this is not a helpful practice. Don't sleep during the day. Daytime sleep slows down agni (metabolism) and increases kapha dosha. Rather, do some hard physical work, and watch less TV. Generally I find that obese people get fixed to the couch, watch TV, and drink soda pop.

If you follow these suggestions, you can definitely take control of your weight problem. Don't try to lose a lot of weight all at once. That almost never brings long-term improvement. Kapha individuals are noted for their ability to make steady, determined, consistent progress. So be persistent, and over time you will be successful.

Osteoporosis

Osteoporosis is a thinning and increasing porosity of the bone due to increased vata. Bones are normally porous, but because of increasing vata—a normal occurrence as a person grows older—the porosity increases. Sometimes the individual loses so much bone that weak spots develop in the skeletal structure. Then the hips, forearms, or even the spine can fracture quite easily. The bones may crack under the body's own weight, or a minor injury may be enough to create a fracture.

Osteoporosis is more common in women than men. Women lose bone rapidly after menopause. This is because the postmenopausal body produces little or no estrogen, which is necessary for maintaining bone metabolism utilizing calcium, magnesium, zinc, and other materials for building the bone. So it is during the postmenopausal years that women may have a tendency toward osteoporosis.

Men also need estrogen to maintain strong bones, but testosterone and prostatic secretions also play an important role. However, men may lose bone mass due to heavy drinking, heavy smoking, chewing tobacco, and taking steroids.

Lack of exercise can also reduce bone mass. To some extent, people need some stress to the body, in the form of exercise. Research has shown that if a person is confined to bed for several weeks, the bones become significantly weaker. Once the ill effects of lack of exercise became clear, exercise programs were designed even for astronauts in space. Exercise is a food for the bones.

For women, the combination of increased vata simply from growing older (see chapter 2, where we talk about the stages of life), plus the menopausal cessation of estrogen, may have a powerfully deleterious effect on bone mass.

EXERCISE. Gentle, daily exercise for 30 minutes a day, 5 days a week, can help to treat osteoporosis. Walking is excellent and quite sufficient, but you may do swimming, gentle jogging, or whatever suits your constitution and level of fitness, and the condition of your bones.

Some people recommend weight-bearing exercise, even including weight lifting, for building bone. While this is good in general, for a person with osteoporosis it can be quite dangerous; as mentioned above, even a slight injury may crack the fragile bones of a person with osteoporosis. Therefore a good, safe way to begin an exercise program is to do some underwater exercise. As the bones become stronger, weight-bearing exercise, even including some gentle weight lifting, may be acceptable and effective.

CALCIUM. It is important to get a plentiful supply of calcium from natural food sources, such as sesame seeds, soybeans, soy milk, cow's milk, cheese, carrots, and coconut. Calcium supplements, such as from oyster shells, may also be helpful. Your daily dose should include about 1,200 mg. calcium, along with 600 mg. magnesium and 60 mg. zinc for maximum absorption and effectiveness.

Almond milk also contains a significant amount of calcium. Soak ten almonds overnight in water. In the morning, peel them and blend in the blender with a cup of warm milk. (You can use goat's milk or soy milk if you prefer them to cow's milk.) Pour into a cup or glass, and add a pinch each of ginger, cardamom, and saffron. Drink twice a day, before breakfast and before bedtime.

Daily chewing a handful of white sesame seeds in the morning provides at least 1,200 mg. of natural calcium. These seeds won't create clogged arteries, as dependence upon calcium from dairy products may. This is an effective way to help prevent osteoporosis in menopausal women.

However, merely taking calcium may not be sufficient. Along with it you need to bring some physical stress to the system through exercise.

BE CAREFUL WITH YOGA POSTURES. If osteoporosis has begun to develop, yoga exercises should be done gently, with great care, as there is a real danger of breaking a bone.

HERBAL HELPERS. Certain herbs can help to make up for estrogen in the metabolic cycle. Try the following formula:

shatavari 5 parts
vidari 3 parts
wild yam 2 parts

These herbs are food precursors of estrogen and progesterone. To this formula you can add 1/8 part each of *shanka bhasma* (conch shell ash) and *kama dudha* (coral shell ash). They contain a natural source of calcium bicarbonate, which can help to prevent osteoporosis.

Take 1/4 teaspoon of this mixture twice a day with warm milk, whether cow's, goat's, or soy milk. Treat this as a daily maintenance dose, and take it indefinitely to help prevent osteoporosis.

Overeating

See also "Obesity" and "Eating Disorders"

Because of hard work, especially physical labor, some people need to eat a large amount of food to replenish the body. In such individuals, overeating may occasionally occur. But most overeating takes place because of emotional factors, and that is what we will be considering here.

Food nourishes the body; love nourishes the soul. When you are with a loving friend or close family members, you can become so happy that you forget to eat. You feel no need for food at that time because you receive a higher food—love.

But when a person doesn't receive that love or feel that happiness, he or she becomes lonely or has a feeling of rejection or of not being loved. Food may become the substitute for love. So eating, in order to suppress feelings of loneliness, grief, sadness, or depression, is the emotional, psychological cause of overeating. Statistically, overeating happens more in women than in men.

From an Ayurvedic perspective, due to emotional factors and stress, *prana* vata stimulates *jatharagni,* the gastric fire, and this stimulation activates the stomach. The stimulation is translated or experienced as hunger, and that is the reason people may eat more food.

There are many ways to deal with the problem of overeating. With a little care, it can be overcome.

EXPRESS YOUR FEELINGS. First, you have to let go of your feelings of loneliness and not being loved. Write about your feelings. Express them. That way, the energy that is blocked in the solar plexus starts releasing, and emotional hunger will begin to subside.

MEDITATE AND BREATHE. Whenever you feel emotionally hungry, sit quietly and pay attention to your breath. Or do 10 to 15 minutes of *So-Hum* meditation (see chapter 7).

Shitali pranayama (making a tube of the tongue and inhaling through that tube into the belly) will also be quite helpful. (See chapter 6.)

• Or take 12 deep breaths, then drink a cup of warm water. This will help dissolve the emotional hunger, and overeating can be avoided.

YOGA. Yoga exercises such as the Moon Salutation, Camel pose, Cobra pose, and Spinal Twist will help you control overeating due to emotional factors (see appendix 4).

WALK OFF THE CRAVINGS. Whenever you have emotional cravings for food, take a brisk walk for 20 minutes in the fresh air. That will help reduce the cravings.

EAT LIGHTLY. If you feel you must eat, then eat some light food. Try some light crackers, or some cereal or grains such as millet or rye. Or drink some fruit juice. Follow a low-fat diet. (See the guidelines for the kapha diet in chapter 8.) That way you won't have to deny yourself when you feel like eating, but the light food won't put on weight or fat.

TRY BANANAS. Eating 1 ripe banana, chopped up with 1 teaspoon ghee and a pinch of cardamom, is effective for pacifying emotional, obsessive eating habits.

TEST YOUR HUNGER. When you are hungry, here is one way to find out whether it is an emotional craving or a real biological need. Drink some licorice tea, chamomile tea, or mint tea. If it was emotional hunger, the warm soothing tea will take care of it, and you will feel better. If you are really hungry and need some food, the tea won't diminish your appetite.

FOR HYPERTHYROIDISM. If your overeating is due to hyperthyroidism, which is a metabolic disorder, Ayurveda suggests using *kaishore guggulu.* This herbal compound helps to regulate metabolism and pacifies overactive thyroid.

DRINK *BRAHMI* MILK. When you feel hungry, drinking 1 cup of warm milk boiled with 1/2 teaspoon of *brahmi* will help you control overeating.

IF YOU HAVE ALREADY EATEN TOO MUCH. Roast 1 teaspoon coriander seeds and 1 teaspoon fennel seeds on a heavy iron pan, without any oil. (Stir constantly to avoid burning.) Add a pinch of salt, let the mixture cool, and eat it. It will help with indigestion.

Another aid to indigestion from overeating is to drink a cupful of water into which you have added the juice of half a lemon; just before drinking, add a pinch of baking soda, stir, and drink quickly.

Overweight

See "Obesity"

PMS

See also "Menstrual Difficulties"

TYPES OF PMS

Premenstrual syndrome or PMS is classified in Ayurveda in three types: vata, pitta, and kapha.

- Vata type is characterized by low backache, lower abdominal pain, distention, anxiety, fear, insomnia, and mood swings.
- Pitta-type PMS symptoms include tenderness in the breasts, urethritis, hives, hot flashes, irritability, and sometimes a burning sensation when passing urine.
- Kapha-type PMS involves water retention (breasts become enlarged and tender) and drowsiness, so that the woman loves to drink coffee!

PMS can be cared for successfully using the following Ayurvedic remedies and preventive measures.

IMPORTANT: In all cases, start the preventive program one week before the anticipated start of your period.

FOR VATA-TYPE PMS

- Drink *dashamoola* tea (1/2 teaspoon *dashamoola* steeped in a cup of hot water for 10 minutes); you can add a little honey for taste. Take twice a day.
- Eat about 10 cherries daily on an empty stomach for a week before the onset of menstruation.
- Use *kaishore guggulu* or *yogaraj guggulu,* 1 tablet twice a day.
- You can also take 1 tablespoon aloe vera gel with a pinch of black pepper, 3 times a day before food.

FOR PITTA-TYPE PMS

- Take the following herbal mixture:

shatavari 2 parts
brahmi 1 part
musta 1 part

Take 1/2 teaspoon of this mixture twice a day with warm water.

• Aloe vera gel (1 tablespoon) taken with a pinch of cumin powder is also effective.

FOR KAPHA-TYPE PMS

• Make this herbal mixture:

punarnava 2 *parts*
kutki 1 *part*
musta 2 *parts*

Take 1/2 teaspoon of this mixture twice a day with a little warm water.

• Eat about 10 cherries daily on an empty stomach for a week before the expected onset of your period.

• You can also take 1 tablespoon aloe vera gel along with a pinch of *trikatu* (a traditional Ayurvedic formula consisting of equal amounts of black pepper, *pippali,* and ginger).

FOR ALL BODY TYPES

• Warm ghee nose drops (5 drops in each nostril) stimulate natural hormones and help regulate balance of the system.

• When there is abdominal bloating and cramps, all constitutional types can put a warm castor oil pack on the lower abdomen. One of the qualities of castor oil is that it produces a slow, sustained heat that is soothing and healing. Warm up about 3 tablespoons of castor oil, and pour it onto a handkerchief or other soft cloth, spreading it equally on the cloth. Place this compress on the lower abdomen. If you have a hot water bottle, you may place it on top of the pack to keep it warm. An electric heating pad is not recommended.

NOTE: A warm castor oil pack will also help relieve the congestion and discomfort of endometriosis.

FOR PREVENTION

• Be sure to get regular exercise during the month, including half an hour of walking or other aerobic exercise at least five days a week. Yoga stretching is also helpful. However, Ayurveda recommends no exercise or yoga during the actual menstrual period. As much as possible, rest, read, and relax!

• To maintain health and balance, follow the dietary guidelines for your constitutional type (see chapter 8).

Premature Ejaculation

See also "Impotence"

For the man who repeatedly ejaculates prematurely, sex can become a nightmare. He may run away from his partner out of fear that his sexual performance is inadequate, causing serious difficulties in the relationship.

Premature ejaculation is primarily caused by aggravated vata. Vata, with its qualities of quickness and heightened sensitivity to the sense of touch (as pitta brings greater sensitivity to light), gives a predisposition toward faster ejaculation; in general, persons with a vata constitution cannot sustain sex for very long. When vata is unduly increased in a vata individual, premature ejaculation is common.

A psychological, emotional factor of nervousness, fear, or anxiety may also be involved, but this too is due largely to the aggravated vata dosha. Thus the main avenue of treatment is to balance vata dosha.

Another possible cause is high cholesterol (and the related situation, high triglycerides). In men who have this problem, cholesterol deposition takes place in the blood vessels of the penis and the entire reproductive system. These blood vessels become thick and narrow (ischemia), so that the blood supply to the muscles of the penis and prostate is insufficient, causing lack of sphincter control and leading to premature ejaculation.

Premature ejaculation can be brought under control. Here are some effective ways to deal with it.

MASSAGE THE PENIS. Do a gentle massage of the penis. To 1 ounce of sesame oil, add 5 to 10 drops of mustard oil. The diluted mustard oil has a heating effect, which will dilate the blood vessels and improve the circulation of blood to the penis.

> IMPORTANT: Do this massage about 1 hour before intercourse, and be sure to wash the penis thoroughly beforehand, or your partner's delicate skin may feel burned by the hot mustard oil. You can also use castor oil, which will improve the tone of the sphincter muscles.

• Certain medicated ghees, such as *brahmi* ghee, *shatavari* ghee, or *ashwagandha* ghee, can also be used for massaging the pubic bone and the glans penis before making love.

PRACTICE. Practice stimulating the organ up to the point of ejaculation, but don't ejaculate. Then sit up straight (in a Lotus posture, if you can), and raise the energy by doing Ashwini Mudra, pulling or sucking the anus inward in a series of tense-release movements. Do about 10 repetitions of the Ashwini Mudra. This way you train your organ to be ready but not to ejaculate. To succeed at this, you have to practice with great care.

Do this exercise about 1 to 2 hours before making love.

> IMPORTANT: This is not masturbation, nor an endorsement of masturbation.

• You can also learn to control ejaculation by contracting the muscles of the buttocks.

• Locate the *marma* point (an energy center like an acupressure point) at the center of the glans penis, on the underside. Gently press that point, and at the same time suck the anus inward and hold for five seconds. Release. Do this 10 times. This will improve the blood supply to the penis and will help to maintain the erection. Do this about 1 hour before sex.

YOGA POSTURES. Helpful yoga *asanas* include the Bow, Fish, and Camel poses, Elevated Lotus, and Vajrasana.

DIET SUGGESTIONS. As mentioned, premature ejaculation is a vata disorder, so a man with this problem should adhere to a vata-soothing diet (see guidelines in chapter 8). If you have high cholesterol, follow a low-cholesterol diet. And if you have diabetes, keep your sugar intake low. Most diabetic men suffer from premature ejaculation.

EFFECTIVE HERBS. Make an herbal formula, mixing equal amounts of the following herbs:

ashwagandha
bala
vidari

Take 1/2 teaspoon of this mixture twice a day with warm goat's milk. Cow's milk is acceptable if you can't find goat's milk, but goat's milk is more effective.

• Ginseng is also helpful. It has properties similar to the Ayurvedic herb *ashwagandha*. Take 1/2 teaspoon after lunch and dinner with warm goat's milk. Again, cow's milk is acceptable if you can't locate fresh goat's milk.

ALMOND MILK. Soak 10 almonds overnight in water. In the morning peel off the skin, put the almonds in a blender, and add 1 cup hot cow's milk and a pinch each of ginger, cardamom, and saffron. (Saffron is a mild aphrodisiac.) Drink almond milk every morning. You can also make a second cupful in the evening.

HEAL THE PROSTATE. Premature ejaculation often accompanies prostate problems such as prostatitis, or it may be a warning of developing problems. To help with this, massage the area of the prostate gland with castor oil. Apply a small amount of the oil (sesame oil is also beneficial) to the perineum, the area in between the anus and testicles. First rub in a circular motion, then finish with strokes from the anus toward the base of the penis. Don't press hard; use light strokes.

Prostate Problems

In middle-aged men, it is uncommonly common for the prostate gland to become enlarged, resulting in a number of uncomfortable symptoms. For example, the man may wake up several times during the night to pass urine. He may have difficulty urinating, so that it may take some moments for the flow to start, or the flow may be slow, or it may "dribble" at the end. He may find that the need to urinate occurs rather suddenly, or that he feels a frequent need to go. This happens when the bladder does not empty completely during urination; even though there may not be much urine left in the bladder, the residual fluid creates the sensation of needing to go.

Another problem that sometimes develops is prostatitis (inflammation of the prostate), which has many of the same symptoms described above but also is characterized by a burning sensation while passing urine.

HERBAL REMEDIES

A number of herbal remedies are effective in treating prostate problems.

• Make this formula of Ayurvedic herbs:

punarnava 2 parts
shilajit 1/8 part
gokshura 2 parts

Take 1/4 teaspoon twice a day, after meals, with a little warm water. Continue to take it until your symptoms resolve.

• You can also use ginseng, hibiscus, or horsetail tea, available in packages or as bulk herbs in most natural food stores. These teas can be drunk several times daily, as desired. Follow the directions on the package, or if

> TIME TO SEE THE DOCTOR
>
> Since prostate cancer is a possible diagnosis based on the above symptoms, you should see a medical professional to determine the source of your problem. If the cause is benign, the following remedies may be effectively used for self-treatment.

you use bulk herbs, add about 1 teaspoon of mixture to a cup of boiling hot water, steep 5 minutes, cool, and drink.

• Cumin-coriander-fennel tea will help relieve the burning sensation and other symptoms as well. Mix the herbs in equal amounts, and steep 1 teaspoon of the mixture in a cup of hot water for 5 to 10 minutes. Drink 2 or 3 times a day.

• Another Ayurvedic herbal compound that is helpful for enlarged prostate is *punarnava guggulu.* Take 1 tablet twice a day.

• Make a mixture of equal amounts of *vidari* and *ashwagandha,* and take 1/2 teaspoon 2 or 3 times a day, washed down with warm water.

OTHER HELPFUL REMEDIES

OIL MASSAGE. A gentle massage of the prostate area is also helpful. Apply a small amount of castor oil or sesame oil to the perineum (the area in the middle between the anus and testicles). First rub in a circular motion, then finish with strokes from the anus toward the base of the penis. Don't press hard; use light strokes.

FROM THE YOGA TRADITION. It will be helpful if you perform what is known in yoga as the Ashwini Mudra: pulling or sucking the anus inward in a series of tense-release movements. Do about 10 repetitions of the Ashwini Mudra morning and evening. They should be done while you are sitting.

The Kukutasana, or Elevated Lotus pose, is also helpful for prostate problems. (See illustration in appendix 4.)

Rashes and Hives

Skin rashes and hives indicate excess pitta or heat in the body; the Ayurvedic approach is to provide a cooling effect from both the inside and outside.

FOR IMMEDIATE RELIEF. Whatever the cause of the rash, whether allergies, an insect bite, or something else, cilantro juice will be immediately effective. Wash fresh cilantro, chop it into pieces, put it into the blender, add 1/3 cup of water, and blend. Drink the juice, and apply the pulp directly onto the skin.

TOPICAL SOLUTIONS. The following remedies applied directly to the skin will help soothe and heal rashes and hives:

• If you have a fresh coconut, break it open and apply the coconut water to the rash.

• Melon can also be soothing to rashes and hives. Eat some melon, and rub the remaining rind (not the outer tough skin) over your skin. With watermelon, eat the red part and rub the white part of the rind onto your skin.

• For rashes, hives, and other high-pitta conditions such as nausea, steep 1 teaspoon coriander, 1/2 teaspoon cumin, and 1 teaspoon natural sugar in 1 cup hot milk. Drink once or twice a day.

• You can also use a paste made of sandalwood and turmeric powders mixed in goat's milk. This paste is healing for the skin. The formula is simple:

turmeric *1 part*
sandalwood powder *2 parts*

Mix up about a teaspoon of powder in this proportion, add sufficient goat's milk to make a paste, and apply it to the affected area. Cow's milk is acceptable, but goat's milk is more effective. PLEASE NOTE: Your skin will look yellow for some time—up to 3 or 4 days—after you use the paste.

FOR INTERNAL HEALING. Here is an effective formula to help restore health to your skin from the inside:

coriander *2 parts*
cumin *1 part*
raw natural sugar *2 parts*

Steep 1/2 teaspoon of this mixture in a cup of hot milk, and drink it once or twice a day until the condition is healed.

Rectal Bleeding

See also "Hemorrhoids"; "Bleeding, Internal"

Numerous factors can give rise to rectal bleeding. These include hemorrhoids; inflammation of the rectal area due to aggravated pitta; anal fissures or polyps; passing dry, hard stools, which hurt the mucous membrane of the rectum; straining due to constipation; excessive pressure on the rectal veins due to liver cirrhosis; and congestive heart failure. In the last stage of pregnancy, prolonged pushing of the child during labor exerts pressure on the rectal blood vessels and leads to bleeding. Rectal bleeding is also common among people who eat refined foods containing little fiber. Eating hot spicy food may tend to produce constipation and rectal bleeding.

Whatever the cause, the following recommendations will be helpful.

WASH WITH COOL WATER. After each bowel movement, wash the anal orifice with cool water. This will help stop the bleeding, and if there is irritation, itching, and cracking, it will help to minimize it.

APPLY GHEE OR CASTOR OIL. This will help to soothe the irritation of the blood vessels.

DRINK CRANBERRY JUICE OR POMEGRANATE JUICE. These are both hemostatics (they stop

Time to See the Doctor

If these remedies do not stop your rectal bleeding in a week to 10 days, it would be wise to see your doctor. If the bleeding is profuse, go sooner. The bleeding could be a symptom of a serious illness.

bleeding) and will be helpful. Drink 1 cup twice a day.

AVOID HOT SPICY FOOD. Follow the pitta-pacifying diet (see chapter 8). Also avoid fermented food, sour fruit, citrus fruit, and alcohol.

KEEP THE STOOLS SOFT. This will help to minimize irritation and bleeding. Here are three ways to keep stools soft:

- Drink a cup of warm milk with 1 teaspoon plain ghee at bedtime. (This is a very mild laxative.)
- Take 1 teaspoon of *amalaki* or 1/2 teaspoon *triphala* at bedtime in warm water. Steep the herb in hot water for 5 to 10 minutes, then when it has cooled down, drink it.
- Take 1 teaspoon psyllium husks (*sat isabgol*) at night in 1 cup of warm water. This bulk laxative will keep the stools soft and avoid pressure on the rectal blood vessels.

USE VITAMIN K. If the bleeding is serious (that is, profuse or repeated), take vitamin K supplements according to the dosage recommended on the package. Also, you can buy vitamin K cream at most health food stores. Apply this cream to the anal orifice to stop the bleeding.

PACIFY PITTA. To reduce pitta, take vitamin E supplements, and drink cranberry juice and/or parsley juice.

PREVENTIVE MEASURES. To avoid rectal bleeding in the future, follow these recommendations:

- Strictly follow the pitta-pacifying diet: no sour fruit, citrus fruit, fermented food, or hot spicy food.
- Avoid hard physical labor if possible.
- Do abdominal yoga exercises such as *nauli* (see appendix 3 for instructions).
- The following yoga postures should improve elimination and help to prevent rectal bleeding: Camel, Cobra, Cow, and Spinal Twist.
- Take this herbal formula:

shatavari 5 *parts*
kama dudha 1/8 *part*
gulwel sattva 1/8 *part*

This herbal mixture (1/2 teaspoon with warm water), taken twice a day for 1 month, will help to prevent future rectal bleeding.

Rectal Itching

Rectal itching has several possible causes. One is worms and parasites, such as roundworms and pinworms. Itching may also be caused by hemorrhoids, inflamed ulcers, a yeast infection, or a fungal infection. Excess toxicity—ama in the colon—can also create itching of the anus.

FOR WORMS. If worms are the problem, you may be able to eliminate them entirely with this herbal formula:

vidanga 5 *parts*
shardunika 2 *parts*
trikatu 1/8 *part*

Use 1/4 teaspoon of this mixture twice a day washed down with warm water after meals.

• Also, take 1/2 teaspoon *triphala* every night in a cup of warm water. (Steep 5 to 10 minutes before drinking.)

FOR YEAST INFECTION. If there is a yeast infection, apply a little yogurt to the anal orifice, then wash the anus with water.

FOR HEMORRHOIDS. If the problem is hemorrhoids, take a baking soda bath, soaking the hemorrhoids in warm water with 1/3 cup baking soda added. Then apply *neem* oil to the hemorrhoids. (See also "Hemorrhoids.")

FOR FUNGAL INFECTION. Mix a little tea tree oil and *neem* oil together, and apply it directly to the anal area to heal the rectal itch.

PREVENTIVE DIET. Avoid hot spicy foods, fermented foods, and yeast-containing bread. Stay away from alcohol entirely.

Sinus Problems

The sinuses are air-filled cavities located on either side of the nose. There are ten sinus cavities, five on each side, all connected to the nose. They are covered with a superfine mucous membrane. The sinuses drain constantly into the nose; their chief function is to keep the nasal cavity moist. They also serve to amplify the voice when we speak.

Due to allergies, colds, or bacterial infections, the sinuses in both adults and children sometimes get clogged or infected. This is a condition of excess kapha that can be aggravated by many factors, including cold drinks, dairy products, and smoking.

Sinus problems can create complications of various kinds, from sinus headaches, snoring, and difficulty breathing to bad breath, ear infections, and sleep apnea. In serious cases, sinus infections can lead to brain infection, meningitis, or osteomyelitis.

HERBAL DECONGESTANT. When the sinuses become clogged and congested, it is important to drain them. A mixture of fresh ginger juice (or freshly grated ginger pulp) with 1 teaspoon honey taken 2 or 3 times a day will be quite helpful.

You can prepare this safe, effective decongestant formula:

sitopaladi 5 *parts*
trikatu 1/8 *part*
mahasudarhan churna 2 *parts*

Take 1/4 teaspoon of this mixture 2 or 3 times a day with warm water after meals.

HERBAL ANTIBIOTICS. To help prevent secondary infection, mix equal amounts of the following antibacterial herbs:

goldenseal
osha
turmeric
neem

Fill some 00-size capsules with the herbal mixture, and swallow 2 capsules twice a day.

NOSE DROPS AND NASAL WASH TO DRAIN THE SINUSES. Make a mild saline solution by dissolving 1/2 teaspoon salt into 1/2 cup lukewarm water. Instill 5 drops of the solution into each nostril with a dropper, or take a little in the palm of your hand and snuff it into

Use Medicated Steam to Clear up Your Sinuses

You will be amazed at how effective this simple method is to help clear up painful, congested sinuses.

Heat up about a cupful of water, and add 3 to 5 drops of eucalyptus oil. Turn off the flame, cover your head with a towel, lean over the pot, and inhale the steam.

You can also use ginger in the same way. Take 1 inch of fresh ginger, chop it into pieces, and boil it in about a cup of water. Then cover your head and inhale the ginger steam. It will be effective for draining the sinuses. (You can use powdered ginger as a backup if you don't have fresh.)

your nostrils. Repeat as often as needed to keep sinuses clear. (Several times a day is fine.)

Here is a more powerful remedy that you can use for severe sinus congestion and pain. You may not enjoy doing this, but it works. Use a garlic press to squeeze out some fresh garlic juice. With an eye dropper, pick up some juice and insert just a few drops into each nostril. Keep your head tilted back for about five minutes to let the juice work, then sit up and let it drain out onto a tissue. You will be surprised at how clear your sinuses feel. Do this once a day as needed; for a severe sinus attack, you may do it up to three times, in the morning, afternoon, and evening.

FOR A SINUS HEADACHE. Try mixing 1/2 teaspoon cinnamon with enough water to make a paste, and apply locally.

STRATEGIES FOR PREVENTION. Here are several ways you can help save yourself from future sinus problems.

- Avoid dairy products, especially cheese, yogurt, and ice cream.
- Avoid cold drinks.
- Avoid exposure to cold weather.
- Do not smoke cigarettes.
- Once a day, instill a little warm ghee in each nostril and sniff. You may use an eyedropper or use a clean finger dipped in ghee.
- Take this herbal formula on a regular basis:

sitopaladi 5 parts
mahasudarshan churna 3 parts
abrak bhasma 1/8 part

Take 1/4 teaspoon of this mixture 3 times a day, after meals. Wash down with warm water. Take it for 3 months.

Skin—Ayurvedic Care

Ayurveda has many wonderful suggestions for maintaining the health and beauty of your skin. Some you will find here. Others you will find, along with remedies for various skin problems, in the sections on "Acne,"

"Dandruff," "Dry Skin," "Rashes and Hives," and others.

The following suggestions will help you keep your skin healthy, glowing, and beautiful.

OIL MASSAGE. Daily oil massage over your whole body is very effective for keeping your skin healthy and beautiful. If you are vata or have a vata imbalance, use sesame oil. If you are pitta or have a pitta imbalance, use sunflower oil. If you are kapha or have a kapha imbalance, use corn oil or canola oil. Gentle oil massage maintains the beauty and texture of the skin.

TAKE TURMERIC. To have beautiful skin, take a capsule of turmeric daily. Ayurvedic tradition states that if a pregnant woman takes turmeric regularly, her child will have gorgeous skin!

GET ENOUGH IRON IN YOUR DIET. If your skin looks pale, it may be a sign of anemia. Drink some carrot juice, and eat cooked beets. This will give you natural iron and should improve skin color. (See further suggestions under "Anemia.")

SOAK UP SOME SUN. Apply the appropriate doshic oil to your skin (sesame for vata constitutions, coconut or sunflower for pitta, corn for kapha), and lie in the sun for a little while—10 to 15 minutes, or at the most half an hour. This will improve the circulation and strengthen skin tone.

NOTE: Sunbathing should be done either before noon or in the late afternoon (after three o'clock), when the rays are not as direct. Also, the danger of sunburn is greater at high altitudes, so take care to limit your exposure when you're in the mountains.

USE HERBALIZED OILS. For a wonderful face lotion, apply some *neem* oil or *brahmi* oil to your face. These oils are acceptable for all constitutions.

***SHIKAKAI* SHAMPOO.** For washing your hair, use a shampoo that includes the herb *shikakai.*

***NEEM* SOAP.** Use a *neem* or sandalwood soap for bathing.

BE SPARING WITH SOAP. As a general rule, it is beneficial to use soap on your skin only once or twice a week, not on a regular everyday basis. In a tropical climate, where people sweat a lot and their sweat contains salts and minerals that lodge in the skin, they have to take a soap bath every day. But in colder countries, where there is not much sweating, so much soap bathing is usually not necessary.

Of course, it depends on a person's job. Someone who does hard physical work and sweats a lot needs some kind of soap. But to maintain softness and luster, it's important not to wash off the sebaceous secretions that maintain the oiliness of the skin. If we apply soap daily, the oil will be washed off and the skin will become dry.

Pitta constitutional types may need soap a little more often, perhaps three times a week, both because they tend to perspire more and because pitta skin tends to be more oily.

MATCH WATER TEMPERATURE TO YOUR CONSTITUTION. Generally, washing in cool water is recommended for pitta, warm water for kapha, and hot water for vata. Vata individuals often have poor circulation, and hot water will improve circulation and help to keep skin healthy and beautiful.

GENTLE TOWEL MASSAGE. After bathing, gently rub your towel over the skin of your

Home Face-lift

You can do your own home facial massage and face-lift by applying gentle pressure from the chin to the forehead.

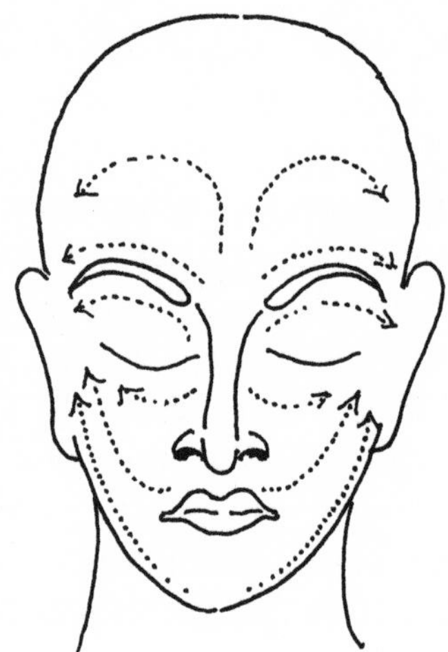

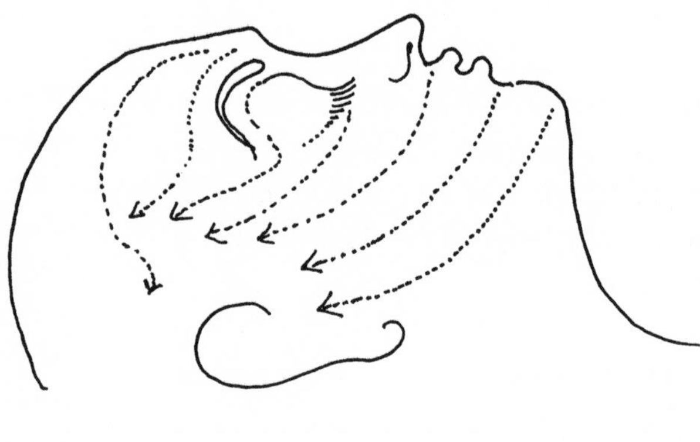

Face-lift Massage

Put your two index fingers together, and your two thumbs. Place the two index fingers between your lower lip and your chin, and the two thumbs just under the chin. Then, pressing lightly with your index fingers, sweep along the jawbone, with your thumbs underneath. When you reach the ears, go up in front of them, letting the thumb trail. Keep going up until your thumbs are just behind the temple area, above the ear. A *marma* point is located there. When you reach this point press lightly, with a lifting motion, for about 30 seconds. This procedure will stimulate the nerves that control the facial muscles, and it will improve the tone of those muscles and help remove wrinkles from the facial skin. Repeat seven times once a day, preferably in the morning.

face and body. This improves cutaneous circulation, removes dead skin, and helps your skin look young.

FRESH CHERRY MASK. Apply a pulp of fresh cherries to your face at night as a mask, before going to bed. Leave it on for 15 minutes. This will relieve dry skin and give you a beautiful complexion.

YOUR SMILE HELPS YOUR SKIN. Keeping a smile on your face will help maintain the tone of your facial muscles and skin; people may say you look ten years younger than you are!

Sleep Apnea

Apnea is a temporary suspension of breath. Sleep apnea is a brief interruption in breathing during deep sleep—sometimes numerous interruptions in a single night—that is quite common in young children but also occurs in some adults. It may also happen at high altitudes. Sleep apnea is often accompanied by loud snoring and an abnormal breathing pattern.

Apnea in older children and adults is less life-threatening. But because the person's sleep is briefly interrupted each time the breathing stops, sometimes dozens of times in a night, it can be physically exhausting. It strains the cardiovascular system and respiratory system and may create excess carbon dioxide in the blood. It may lead to drowsiness and irritability during the wakeful state and an inability to concentrate, due to insufficient sleep.

In Ayurvedic terms, sleep apnea occurs because *tarpaka* kapha is blocking *prana* vata. So treatment centers on controlling excess kapha.

TO CONTROL KAPHA. The first remedy is *pippali.* Take 1/4 teaspoon with 1 teaspoon honey and 1 teaspoon ghee on an empty stomach in the morning and evening.

- Instead of *pippali,* you can substitute *trikatu churna* (which consists of equal amounts of *pippali,* black pepper, and ginger).
- For an effective decongestant, take 1/2 teaspoon *sitopaladi* along with 1/4 teaspoon

Sleep Apnea in Premature Babies

Premature infants sometimes have sleep apnea. Because the respiratory center in the hypothalamus has not fully matured in these babies, from time to time the child may completely stop breathing and can turn blue or purple.

If this happens, don't panic, but act quickly: *If you tickle the soles of the feet, or sprinkle cool water on the belly at the diaphragm, the baby will start breathing again.*

This condition may cause SIDS, sudden infant death syndrome. It is a serious condition that needs prompt medical care. But when the breathing control center becomes mature, the baby's sleep apnea should go away.

yashti madhu in 1 teaspoon honey, twice a day. This will help both as a congestion remedy and as a preventive measure.

NASYA. Instill 5 drops of warm *brahmi* ghee or plain ghee in each nostril in the morning and before going to bed.

FOR OBESITY. One of the primary causes of sleep apnea is being significantly overweight. If that is the problem, you can treat obesity with this herbal formula:

kutki 1 part
chitrak 1 part
shilajit 1/8 part

Take 1/4 teaspoon of this mixture 2 or 3 times a day before breakfast, lunch, and dinner with warm water.

• Regular walking or other exercise will also help the obese person to breathe better. Be careful not to undertake exercise that might be too much for you if you are very heavy and have not exercised in some time. Stick to walking, or consult with your doctor if you want to do more.

CHANGE YOUR SLEEPING POSITION. Anyone with sleep apnea would do well to experiment with different sleeping positions to see if the condition eases. In particular, obese people, who are often in the habit of sleeping on their chest or on their back with their hands on their chest, might try sleeping on their left side. Just this one shift could remedy or at least reduce the problem.

KEEP THE HOUSE HUMIDIFIED. Sometimes dry, hot air creates a choking sensation in the nose and can be the cause of sleep apnea. A warm, comfortably humid atmosphere will be best. Preferably, use a hot water humidifier; ultrasound humidifiers are not recommended.

PANCHAKARMA. Under the supervision of an Ayurvedic physician, it would be helpful for a person with sleep apnea to undergo *panchakarma* purification therapy (see chapter 4). This includes *abhyanga* (oil massage), *virechana* (purgation therapy), and *nasya* (nasal administration of medications) among others. This procedure is cleansing and rejuvenating.

Smoking

See also "Addictions"

Addiction to smoking has two main causes: nicotine toxicity and stress. Once a person becomes a smoker, he or she has to achieve just the "right" amount of nicotine toxicity to maintain proper functioning of the brain as well as normal digestion and elimination. Also, at times of pressure or emotional disturbance, smokers habitually reach for a cigarette. So two parallel strategies are needed: detoxifying the nicotine toxicity and dealing with the stress.

HERBAL CIGARETTE. To gradually wean yourself from smoking, Ayurveda suggests that you prepare the following herbal mixture. It will help both with reducing your stress level and with detoxifying your body. Mix together equal amounts of:

brahmi
jatamamsi
rose petal powder

Remove 1/3 of the tobacco from a few of your cigarettes (at the end you light) and replace it with this mixture. When you feel like smoking, light and smoke the herbal mixture. When you reach the tobacco, stop. Soon you will see that the desire to smoke begins to diminish.

OVERWHELM YOURSELF. Here's another helpful procedure: Place a few drops of *brahmi* ghee directly on the cigarette, then light up. The smoke produced will be so strong, it will eliminate your desire to smoke.

EFFECTIVE HERBAL TEA. At times of stress, instead of smoking a cigarette, prepare and drink a tea made of equal proportions of *jatamamsi*, chamomile, and *brahmi*.

jatamamsi 1 part
chamomile 1 part
brahmi 1 part

Steep 1 teaspoon of this mixture in a cup of hot water, and drink. Take it slowly, sip by sip, to help relieve the desire to smoke.

CHEW INSTEAD OF SMOKING. Whenever the desire for a cigarette arises, chew one or two small pieces of dried pineapple instead, mixed with 1/2 teaspoon honey.

REDUCE STRESS BY MEDITATING. For stress management, spend some time every day meditating. If you know a practice, use it! Or try the Empty Bowl meditation explained in chapter 7. Most people find that when stress is reduced, their desire to smoke spontaneously decreases.

YOGA POSTURES. Yoga postures are helpful. Try the Moon Salutation sequence, as well as the Locust pose, Bow, Shoulder Stand, Plow, and Palm Tree. (Illustrations of yoga *asanas* are found in appendix 4.)

BREATHING EXERCISES. The *pranayama* (breathing exercise) known as Breath of Fire will also help you in your effort to quit smoking. It is explained in chapter 6.

Sore Throat

A sore throat is caused by irritation and inflammation of the throat. This condition is generally quite easy to remedy using Ayurvedic methods.

GARGLE. Perhaps the simplest remedy, and one that is quite effective, is gargling. Ayurveda recommends using 1 cup of hot water (not so hot that it might burn your throat) with 1/2 teaspoon turmeric and 1/2 teaspoon salt mixed in. Gargle with this mixture morning and evening.

TURMERIC MILK. Drinking 1 cup of hot milk boiled with 1/2 teaspoon turmeric is also helpful for sore throat.

SOOTHING HERBAL TEA. Another remedy that works well is ginger-cinnamon-licorice tea in the following proportions:

ginger 2 parts
cinnamon 2 parts
licorice 3 parts

Steep 1 teaspoon of the herbal mixture in water for 5 to 10 minutes, and drink up to 3 times a day.

> **Time to See the Doctor**
>
> If your sore throat persists for more than a few days even though you are trying these remedies, see a medical professional.

FOODS TO AVOID. When you have a sore throat, it is important not to eat dairy products such as cheese, yogurt, and ice cream. Also avoid fermented foods.

NOTE: A cup of warm turmeric milk, as recommended above, is an exception. Do stay away from *chilled* dairy products, which are mucus-forming and will exacerbate your sore throat.

YOGA POSTURES. The yoga posture known as the Lion pose is traditionally recommended for sore throats. The Yoga Mudra is also effective. (See yoga illustrations in appendix 4.)

BREATHING EXERCISE. You can also practice *bhramari* (Humming Breath), which is described in chapter 6.

Spastic Colon

For help with spastic colon, you can use the remedies suggested under "Irritable Bowel Syndrome." In addition, try the following Ayurvedic herbal formula:

shatavari 4 parts
hingwastak churna 1/8 part
ajwan 1/4 part
chitrak 1 part

Take about 1/4 teaspoon of this mixture 3 times a day with warm water, after meals.

Sprains and Strains

Stepping off the curb in a wrong way, losing your balance when walking (especially easy to do when you wear high-heeled shoes), falling on an outstretched hand—all of these can lead to a sudden twisting of an ankle, wrist, or hip joint, resulting in a sprain or strain.

Although sprains and strains are similar, there is a difference. A *sprain* affects ligaments and is a pitta condition. It is caused by excessive stretching or even tearing of the ligament and involves pain, swelling, and blackish-bluish discoloration. A *strain* affects muscle, is due to vata, and does not produce bruise discoloration, although there is pain.

WRAP IT UP. Whenever there is a strain or sprain, as soon as possible wrap the area in an elastic bandage.

DRINK SOME JUICE. Then drink some pineapple or pomegranate juice. These juices contain an enzyme that acts as an anti-irritant and anti-inflammatory. This helps to pacify pitta and accelerates the healing process.

SOAK IT. For ankle sprain, soak your foot in a pot of hot water with a homemade mustard seed tea bag. Make the bag by tying up 2 teaspoons of brown mustard seeds in a handkerchief, some cheesecloth, or other light cloth. Immerse the bag in the hot water.

To relieve the swelling, soak the foot for 15 minutes in hot water with 2 tablespoons of salt per gallon of water.

APPLY A HEALING PASTE. Make a paste out of 1/2 teaspoon turmeric and 1/2 teaspoon salt, with enough water to form the paste. Use cool water. Applying it to the injury will help reduce swelling.

If it is a strain rather than a sprain, use a *hot* paste of turmeric and salt to help pacify the vata.

HERBAL REMEDY. If you can't tell whether it is a strain or a sprain, take capsules of *kaishore guggulu* (200 mg. twice a day); this herbal formula will help heal both conditions.

> SUGGESTION: If you want to avoid sprained and strained ankles, don't wear high-heeled shoes.

Stomachache

See also "Indigestion"

Stomachache is a very ambiguous symptom. Many causes are possible: acid stomach, acid indigestion, constipation, eating the wrong kind of food, even toxicity in the liver. All these, and other factors, can create abdominal aches and pains.

To treat a stomachache intelligently and effectively, first we have to rule out the serious causes, such as appendicitis, enteritis, gastritis, and colic. You may need a physician's help to determine the cause. But for a common tummy ache, Ayurveda offers numerous simple, natural, and effective home remedies.

HERBAL REMEDIES

- Mix together 1/3 teaspoon cumin powder, a pinch of hing (asafetida), and a pinch of rock salt. Chew well; wash down with warm water.
- For stomachache associated with diarrhea, rub a little fresh ginger juice on your stomach, around the belly button.
- Try the Ayurvedic herb *shankavati.* It ordinarily comes in tablets; just take 1 pill twice a day, morning and evening. It will take care of an aching stomach.
- If you don't find *shankavati,* take *lasunadivati,* 1 tablet twice a day after food.
- Another helpful herb is *ajwan* (Indian celery seed), which you can usually buy from an Indian grocery shop. Mix 1/2 teaspoon with 1/4 teaspoon baking soda, chew the mixture, and drink it down with a little warm water.
- If this doesn't relieve your stomachache, mix together some roasted fennel, roasted cumin, and roasted coriander seed, and chew on about 1/2 teaspoon of the mixture. (Roast these seeds individually—that is, one type at a time—in a heavy cast iron pan, stirring constantly so they don't burn. Then mix them together.)
- To relieve indigestion, take 1/4 cup of fresh onion juice with 1/2 teaspoon honey and 1/2 teaspoon black pepper.

TWO HERBAL TEAS

• Make some cumin-coriander-fennel tea. Mix the three herbs in equal proportions, and use 1/2 teaspoon per cup of water. Drink 2 to 3 times a day to help soothe an aching stomach.

• Another simple tea can be made of equal amounts of the common Western herbs angelica, chamomile, and comfrey. Mix them together, and steep about 1/2 teaspoon of the mix in hot water.

THE MASTER KEY TO PREVENT STOMACHACHE

Most of the time, a stomachache is due to indigestion and low agni (digestive fire). Here are four ways you can kindle agni:

• One of the best herbs to strengthen digestive fire is ginger. Before each meal, chop or grate a little fresh ginger, add a few drops of lime juice and a pinch of salt, and eat the mixture. Or just cut a thin slice of ginger, put on a pinch of salt, and chew that.

• Ginger tea will also increase the gastric fire and reduce the stomachache. Boil a little fresh ginger (grated, chopped, or sliced), or use powdered ginger to make a tea, and drink it 2 or 3 times a day.

• *Draksha* (Ayurvedic herbal wine) before meals will help to kindle the digestive fire. Use 2 to 4 tablespoons mixed with an equal amount of water. Or take a few sips of port or another sweet wine.

• Another simple way to enliven your gastric fire is to use the common spice bay leaf. Steep 1/2 teaspoon of crushed or ground bay leaf in a cup of hot water for about 10 minutes to make a tea. Add a pinch of cardamom, and drink after eating.

ADDITIONAL REMEDIES AND RECOMMENDATIONS

EAT LIGHTLY. If your stomach hurts, avoid eating any heavy meals, beans, meat, and heavier grains like wheat. It is better to be on a diet of kitchari, a combination of rice and dal that is easy to digest. (See page 52 for a basic kitchari recipe). Between meals, take some fruit juice.

FOR CHRONIC INDIGESTION. For chronic poor digestion and frequent stomachaches, prepare this herbal mixture:

trikatu 1 part
chitrak 2 parts
kutki 1 part

Take 1/4 teaspoon before meals, with a little honey and fresh ginger juice. If you don't have fresh ginger, just use honey. This mixture will help strengthen the digestive fire.

TAKE A BREAK FROM EXERCISE. When you have an upset stomach, Ayurveda recommends that you just rest, read, and relax as much as you can until the condition clears. Exercise, including yoga *asanas,* is not recommended.

Stress

Stress is a psychosomatic disorder that has many causes in our day-to-day life. We may get stressed when traffic is jammed, when we have to stand in a long line, or when we deal with a difficult work situation. An all-too-common cause of stress is the feeling that we have too much to do and too little time to do it. Unemployment is another potential source, as are pollution and crime. Even watching crime stories day after day on television builds up stress. An unhappy relationship, a dominating spouse, faulty plumbing, school exams, burn-out at work—the list of causes is virtually endless.

Stress, in turn, may trigger allergies, asthma, herpes, high cholesterol, and hypertension. It may even lead to a heart condition. It can induce an imbalance of vata, pitta, or kapha, depending on the individual's *prakruti* (constitution).

Generally, vata individuals are likely to develop vata-aggravated stress reactions, such as anxiety or fearfulness, even phobias or anxiety neurosis. Pitta individuals increase in pitta during stressful situations and typically react to stress in the form of anger. They may also suffer from hypertension, peptic ulcer, ulcerative colitis, and other pitta disorders. Kapha individuals under stress can develop underactive thyroid function, slow metabolism, and even increased blood sugar, leading to a prediabetic condition. They tend to eat and eat and eat and become chubby.

TAKE A RELAXATION BREAK. To prevent the buildup of stress, the first line of defense is to stay calm and cool during potentially stressful circumstances. Take long, deep breaths, and breathe out your stress. Relax. Have a massage, or give yourself an oil massage by rubbing a few ounces of warm oil on your body, from head to toe. Vata individuals should use sessame oil, pitta individuals sunflower oil, and kapha individuals corn oil. After your massage, take a hot shower or a hot tub bath. Mental techniques such as positive imagery, prayer, singing and chanting, and meditation, as well as regular yoga exercises, are all effective to minimize and remedy stress.

ANALYZE YOUR STRESS. Separate the things in your life that you find stressful into two categories: things you can do something about, and things you can't. If you can do something about it, then do it! If there's nothing you can do, then surrender to it. Accept it. When there's nothing I can do about a situation, I have to surrender to it, and in accepting it, there is peace.

MONITOR YOUR NEGATIVE THINKING. Stress is often the result of fear that is based largely on imagination. Look at your negative thinking, and replace it with positive thinking. Just changing your thinking or your attitude can alleviate much stress.

EXAMINE YOUR ROLE AND YOUR GOAL. Find the right match between your job and your personality. Job stress is a terrible burden on many people when work and personality are not appropriately matched. If you love what you are doing, there is no stress. If you don't love what you are doing and you still have to do it, that is very stressful. So you have to discover your true role and your goal.

A SOOTHING BATH. A ginger–baking soda bath is quite soothing. Add 1/3 cup ginger and 1/3 cup baking soda to a hot bath for greater relaxation and healing.

OILS FOR RELAXATION. Rub a little *brahmi* oil on the soles of your feet and on your scalp at bedtime.

- Put one drop of pure castor oil (with no preservatives) into each of your eyes, and rub a little on the soles of your feet for a calming, soothing effect.

USE MEDICATED NOSE DROPS. Do *nasya* with *brahmi* ghee or plain ghee. Put 5 drops of the ghee into each nostril. (Refer to the *nasya* instructions in appendix 3.)

STRESS-REDUCING TEA. A tea made from equal proportions of the herbs chamomile, comfrey, and angelica will be relaxing. So will *brahmi* tea, which you can make by adding a cup of boiling water to 1/2 teaspoon *brahmi*. Or try a tea made from equal amounts of these herbs:

brahmi
bhringaraj
jatamamsi
shanka pushpi

Steep 1/2 teaspoon in 1 cup of hot water for 10 minutes. You can drink this tea 2 or 3 times a day for stress management.

YOGA STRETCHING. Certain specific *asanas* are effectively used for management of stress, especially the Shoulder Stand, Plow pose, Spinal Twist, and Locust pose. The Lion pose is also effective for relieving stress. (*Asana* illustrations appear in appendix 4.)

MEDITATION. Sit in the Lotus pose or the Easy pose (legs comfortably crossed) facing east, and meditate. Just observe the inflow and outflow of your breath, or do the *So-Hum* meditation (described in chapter 7).

BREATHE AWAY STRESS. *Ujjayi pranayama* is deeply calming and helpful for relieving stress. You can do it sitting up, or try lying on your back in Savasana (the "corpse" or rest pose) and doing this breathing exercise. (See instructions in chapter 6.)

LET YOURSELF CRY. If you have a lot of grief and sadness, it will help to cry out your stressful feelings. Crying is an excellent release for emotions.

LAUGHTER IS GOOD MEDICINE. Laughter is another good way to relieve stress. Try it, even if it is forced at first. Just start laughing! Soon real laughter will come and with it the release of tension and stress.

START YOUR WEEK WITH MEDITATION. Many people experience extra stress on Monday. They have to travel a long distance to work and start another week at a job they don't enjoy. It's a fact that heart attacks are more common on Mondays. To help you reduce stress at this crucial time, keep in mind that Monday is the day of the moon, and the moon represents the mind. So begin Monday morning—and your week—with 15 to 20 minutes of meditation before going to work. Regular daily meditation, morning and evening, is one of the best things you can do to keep your stress level low.

Sunburn

Sunburn is an acute inflammatory condition of the skin cells due to overexposure to ultraviolet radiation from the sun (or a solar lamp). The inflammation may be mild or serious, depending on the degree of exposure.

Something more may also be involved, however. Many people use large amounts of chemical products on their skin, as well as internally—chemical deodorants, chemical soaps, chemical perfumes, cough medicines, and numerous other medications. These substances all weaken the skin. When a person who uses a large number of these products lies in the sun, he or she is more prone to burn.

Also, according to Ayurveda, people of pitta constitution, who are generally more fair-skinned, are more susceptible to sunburn.

When sunburn is severe, the person may have many symptoms, including dizziness, nausea, blisters, undue sensitivity to light, and peeling of the skin. Repeated sunburn may create premature aging and wrinkling of the skin, and the person looks old, like a roasted potato!

Ayurveda has numerous recommendations both to prevent sunburn and to treat it effectively if it happens.

TOPICAL REMEDIES TO SOOTHE SUNBURN

- Apply aloe vera cream to the site of the burn. You can also use some pure aloe vera gel (with no preservatives added), or if you have access to an aloe plant, lightly rub a piece of the plant on the sunburned area.
- Coconut oil is also effective for soothing sunburned skin.
- Take a gauze pad, dip it into cool milk (either cow's milk or goat's milk), and apply it directly to the sunburn. If you have no milk available, use a cloth dipped in cool water, but milk is better.
- Apply *tikta ghrita* (bitter ghee) topically.
- Pulverize some lettuce and apply the pulp directly to the sunburn.
- Place an icebag or a bag of frozen food (like corn, peas, or beans) on the affected area to cool the skin. But don't leave ice touching your skin for more than a minute or two without a break.
- Apply a little fresh cream (from milk) directly on the sunburned skin.
- Make a paste of sandalwood and turmeric by mixing equal amounts of these herbs with a little cool water. Apply gently to the sunburned area. It will have a cooling effect. *Note:* This paste will stain your skin yellow for at least a couple of days and will also stain any clothing it touches.

TO PREVENT SUNBURN

- Avoid or minimize exposure to sunlight from 10 A.M. to 3 P.M. Those are the peak hours of the sun's strength.
- Limit your time in the direct sun to no

more than half an hour. At high altitudes, even this may be too long.

• Before going into the sun, apply *neem* oil to the exposed parts of the body. *Neem* is a good sun blocker that will help protect your skin.

NOTE: As always in this book, "*neem* oil" does not mean pure *neem* extract, but a few drops of *neem* mixed with sesame oil or another mild oil. This is the way *neem* oil is commercially sold.

• Drink coconut water or coconut milk.

• Follow a pitta-soothing program. Don't take saunas or get overheated. Eat pitta-pacifying foods, especially avoiding spicy and fermented foods (see chapter 8).

• Before and after showering, apply *neem* oil to your skin. Coconut oil is also helpful.

Swelling (Edema) During Pregnancy

See also "Edema"

During pregnancy, the enlarged uterus exerts pressure on the pelvic blood vessels and constricts them, which leads to swelling of the feet. Swelling may also be due to lack of protein, lack of iron, or lack of exercise. Or it may be due to high blood pressure or poor circulation. Whatever the cause, it is important to treat it.

EFFECTIVE HERBAL REMEDIES

DRINK CUMIN-CORIANDER-FENNEL TEA. Mix equal proportions of these three herbs, and use $^1/_4$ to $^1/_2$ teaspoon of each herb per cup of hot water. Drink 2 or 3 times a day.

USE A DIURETIC TEA. If the swelling is severe, certain herbal teas made of diuretic herbs can help to stimulate the kidneys. Make a tea of *punarnava* or *gokshura*, or combine the two in equal proportions, using 1 teaspoon of the mixture steeped in a cup of hot water. Drink

Time to See the Doctor

In certain extreme cases, during the last stage of pregnancy the placenta releases toxins and creates a condition characterized by increased blood pressure and swelling of the extremities; proteinurea, convulsions, and coma can develop. This dangerous condition is called eclampsia or pregnancy toxemia. It cannot be treated by home remedies; it requires prompt, expert medical supervision and care.

However, the following herbal formula will help, as an adjunct to treatment, to relieve the convulsions:

brahmi
jatamamsi
shanka pushpi

Mix these herbs in equal amounts. Use $^1/_2$ teaspoon of the mixture to make a tea, and drink it twice a day.

NOTE: If there is ever a generalized swelling of the entire body (including, in men, a swelling of the penis and scrotum), this is a very serious, life-threatening condition that requires immediate treatment.

2 or 3 times a day. This tea will act as a mild diuretic and will remove the swelling.

FOR HIGH BLOOD PRESSURE. Use these herbs:

hawthorn berry
passion flower
arjuna

Mix in equal proportion, and use 1 teaspoon to make a tea. Take twice a day after meals until the situation is normalized. This simple tea will effectively regulate blood pressure. (For more suggestions, see "Hypertension.")

IF THE PROBLEM IS ANEMIA. The swelling may be due to anemia. Folic acid anemia is common during pregnancy, and iron deficiency anemia not uncommon. You can have tests to determine whether you have these deficiencies. If you do, providing the missing ingredients will help reduce or eliminate the swelling. See "Anemia" for suggestions.

PROTEIN DEFICIENCY. Lack of protein may also be the culprit. If you determine that this is the case, eat more protein foods, such as soy products.

ADDITIONAL RECOMMENDATIONS TO RELIEVE EDEMA

EXERCISE. Walking every day for 20 to 30 minutes will improve circulation and help reduce swelling.

AVOID SALT. Salt makes the body retain water and promotes swelling.

RAISE YOUR FEET. When lying down, put a pillow under your feet. This will drain the water and help to gradually decrease the swelling.

Teeth and Gums–Ayurvedic Care

According to Ayurveda, teeth are a by-product of bone. Cavities in the teeth, and receding gums, are signs of aggravation of vata in the skeletal system.

FOR MINERAL DEFICIENCY. Problems with teeth are often related to a deficiency of calcium, magnesium, and zinc. To prevent future problems or to alleviate a deficiency:

- Chew a handful of calcium-rich white sesame seeds every morning. (Then brush your teeth without putting any toothpaste on the brush, so the residue of the sesame seeds can rub against your teeth, polishing and cleaning them.)
- You can also use a mineral supplement containing a daily dose of approximately these amounts: calcium (1,200 mg.), magnesium (600 mg.), and zinc (60 mg.) per tablet.

MASSAGE YOUR GUMS. You can make your teeth healthier and more beautiful by massaging your gums daily with sesame oil. Take a mouthful of warm sesame oil and swish it from side to side for 2 to 3 minutes. Don't swallow it. Spit out the oil, then gently massage your gums with your index finger. This is an excellent preventive measure for receding gums, tooth infection, and cavities.

HERBAL TOOTH CLEANSER. Ayurvedic dentistry recommends the use of bitter and astringent herbs for cleaning the teeth. The main herbs used are *neem,* which is bitter, and *lohdra, kushta,* and *bilva,* which are all astringent. You can make an excellent cleanser for brushing your teeth by mixing the powdered form of *neem* and an equal amount of any of the astringent herbs and use the mixture to brush your teeth as usual. You can also buy commercial toothpastes and powders containing these herbs in natural food stores and from most suppliers of Ayurvedic herbs.

• You may also be able to find powders for the teeth made out of finely ground, roasted almond shells. These are highly beneficial for maintaining the good health of the teeth.

USE TEA TREE OIL FOR RECEDING GUMS AND SENSITIVE TEETH. Receding gums, and sensitivity of teeth to cold and hot temperatures, indicate a bacterial infection in the roots of the teeth.

• To treat the infection, wet a clean toothbrush, and put a few drops of tea tree oil directly onto the brush. Brush your teeth. Then use a cotton swab to apply some tea tree oil to the exposed part of the gums. This treatment will help arrest further infection of the teeth and will take care of pain and sensitivity to hot and cold.

• You can also apply some tea tree oil to your dental floss. This will help you reach some possible deep pockets of infection that the brush doesn't reach. (Commercial floss treated with tea tree oil is also available.)

CHEW WELL. Ayurveda emphasizes the importance of chewing food well. This not only helps the digestive process, but also stimulates the gums.

TRY FIGS. For strengthening teeth and gums, try eating 4 figs and chewing them well, once a day.

TAP YOUR TEETH. *Gently* tap your teeth together 5 or 6 times, almost clenching them—but gently, so that you don't break the crowns! This is said to stimulate the energy meridians related to the teeth.

Tendinitis

In strenuous sports and athletic activities such as running or jumping, a person can pull a muscle and cause inflammation of the tendon, leading to tendinitis or bursitis. This condition can also result from a nonstrenuous activity repeated often enough to become stressful. An example is carpal tunnel syndrome, the result of working for hours a day at a repetitive task such as typing at a computer keyboard.

FOR MILD CONDITIONS

COLD COMPRESS. At the site of tendinitis, apply a cold compress such as an ice pack or a bag of frozen vegetables. That will minimize the inflammation.

APPLY A COOL PASTE. Make a paste of sandalwood and turmeric powder in equal amounts. Mix the powders in enough cold water to form a paste, and apply it on the painful area.

• A paste of salt and turmeric will also be effective.

GENTLE STRETCHING. Careful, gentle stretching of the affected muscles will gradually help to improve circulation and heal the pain and inflammation.

TAKE ANTI-INFLAMMATORY HERBS. Taking some anti-inflammatory herbs will accelerate healing. Make this formula:

kaishore guggulu 2 *parts*
manjistha 2 *parts*
musta 2 *parts*
guduchi 3 *parts*

Take 1/4 teaspoon of this mixture 2 or 3 times a day with warm water after meals.

FOR ACUTE OR CHRONIC CONDITIONS

APPLY HEAT. For both acute tendinitis, where there is much pain, and chronic tendinitis, apply soothing heat, such as a liniment (a penetrating, heating ointment) or a warm water compress. Wet or damp heat is effective to minimize the pain or inflammation.

OIL MASSAGE. Gently massage the affected area with *mahanarayan* oil, and then soak it in warm water.

Tinnitus (Ringing in the Ears)

NOTE: The same line of treatment used to improve hearing is absolutely good to silence tinnitus, or ringing in the ear, so please consult that section ("Hearing Loss") in addition to the following recommendations.

HERBAL REMEDIES. According to Ayurveda, ringing in the ear is a vata disorder. To alleviate this root cause—aggravation of vata in the nervous system—prepare a tea made from equal amounts of comfrey, cinnamon, and chamomile. Steep up to 1 teaspoon of this mixture per cup, and drink 2 or 3 times a day.

• Also, you can take *yogaraj guggulu* (200 mg. 2 or 3 times a day) with warm water, after food.

• Gently rubbing the mastoid bone (behind your ear) with warm sesame oil may be helpful. Try it twice day, morning and evening, for a week, and see if it helps.

• Garlic oil is often effective. Place 3 drops into your ear at night before going to bed. (See appendix 2 for how to prepare oils like garlic oil.)

Toenail Infection

When persons who have thick, tough toenails cut their nails in a convex curve, as the nails grow the edges may start to penetrate the skin and cut the soft tissue. This may lead to inflammation, swelling, pain, and possible infection. Generally, the nails of vata and kapha individuals grow stronger, so they are more prone to toenail infection. Shoes that are too tight can create pressure on the nails, also potentially leading to toenail infection.

The long-term solution is simply to cut the nail straight across, or with a slightly half-moon shape (a concave curve). That allows the nail to grow straight forward instead of into the skin at the sides.

If the nails have already begun to grow under the skin, soak your foot in warm water to soften the nails. When the nails are soft, clean them and apply some tea tree oil mixed half and half with *neem* oil under the nail. Then cut the nail straight across.

To prevent recurrences, wear soft shoes that are not tight, and cut the nails straight across or in a shallow half-moon shape.

Toothache

See also "Teeth and Gums—Ayurvedic Care"; "Gum Disease"

Toothache may be caused by receding gums, cavities, sensitivity due to hyperacidity, and/or infection.

If high acidity is the problem, the person will tend to get heartburn and acid indigestion in addition to toothache. You can control the acidity by following a pitta-soothing diet, particularly avoiding spicy foods, pickles, citrus fruits, and fermented foods (see chapter 8).

When the teeth have cavities or the gums are receding, the roots of the teeth may become exposed. These nerve-filled areas become sensitive to cold or heat. (Sensitivity to cold is a sign of receding gums, while sensitivity to heat indicates infection.)

For any toothache, use a cotton swab to apply a little tea tree oil or clove oil at the site of the pain. Or a small piece of natural, edible camphor (not the synthetic kind, which is poisonous) can be placed next to the painful tooth. The saliva will mix with the camphor and will relieve the toothache. (See appendix 2 for directions on making medicated oils.)

Don't just settle for getting rid of the pain, however. If you have a cavity, be sure to get it taken care of. And to avoid future problems, follow the recommendations for healthy teeth and gums in the section entitled, "Teeth and Gums—Ayurvedic Care."

Ulcers

Ulcers in the gastrointestinal tract are a pitta disorder. Pitta is hot, sharp, and penetrating, and when aggravated, it can erode the surface of internal organs or soft tissues. The mucous membrane lining the esophagus, stomach, duodenum, or colon can develop ulceration because of excess pitta.

Individuals with a pitta constitution or pitta disorder, or whose blood type is O and Rh-positive, are more prone to developing ulcers. A person with ulcers may experience pain, heartburn, nausea, vomiting, midback ache, and shoulder pain.

THE MAIN PRINCIPLE FOR TREATMENT: PACIFY PITTA. Ulcers can be effectively treated by treating the high pitta. If you have ulcers, strictly follow the pitta-pacifying diet: avoid hot spicy food, fermented or sour food, sour fruit, and citrus fruit. (See chapter 8 for complete guidelines.) Stay away from alcohol, tobacco, and coffee. And do not take aspirins or steroids, which can accelerate erosion of the gastric mucosal membrane.

TWO HERBAL FORMULAS. An effective herbal treatment for ulcers is the following formula:

shatavari 5 *parts*
yashti madhu 3 *parts*
shanka bhasma 1/8 *part*
kama dudha 1/8 *part*

Take 1/2 teaspoon of this mixture twice a day, after lunch and dinner, with a little warm water.

• Taking 1 teaspoon of *sat isabgol* (psyllium husks) at bedtime with a cup of warm milk will also be beneficial.

REDUCE STRESS. Stress is often the cause of or a complicating factor in ulcers. To help dissolve stress, make yourself some Tranquillity Tea from these herbs:

jatamamsi
brahmi
shanka pushpi

Combine the herbs in equal proportions, and use about 1/2 teaspoon of the mixture steeped in 1 cup of boiling water to make a tea. Drink it about an hour before going to bed.

YOGA POSTURES. Yoga *asanas* can help you relax and relieve stress, which is beneficial for ulcers. The following positions are particularly recommended for helping with ulcers: Leg Lift, Camel, Cobra, Bow, Bridge, and Spinal Twist. (See illustrations of yoga postures in appendix 4.)

BREATHE AWAY STRESS. *Shitali pranayama,* a breathing exercise that has a cooling, soothing effect, will be helpful. Moon breathing (breathing through the left nostril only) for 5 to 10 minutes has a cooling effect that may also be helpful. Breathing exercises are described in chapter 6.

EAT EARLY IN THE EVENING, AND EAT SMALL MEALS. Persons with ulcers should not eat late at night. They also do best if they eat small, frequent meals. Don't keep the stomach empty for long. At least have breakfast, lunch, and dinner, so the acid secreted in the stomach can be utilized for digestion.

AN EFFECTIVE HERBAL ACID BLOCKER. Today many people use acid-blocking medications for ulcers. The best acid blocker in Ayurveda is a combination of the herbs

brahmi
jatamamsi
yashti madhu

in equal proportions. A tea made from 1/2 teaspoon of these herbs per cup of water, taken after lunch and dinner, can help to inhibit acid secretions and prevent ulceration.

Urinary Incontinence

Urinary incontinence is primarily a vata disorder, caused by weakness of the muscles of the bladder, especially the bladder sphincter. If that becomes weak and uncontrolled, a person may lose voluntary control of urination to a greater or lesser extent.

Another cause of incontinence, especially in the West, seems to be the frequent use of rest rooms. When some people see a rest room, they just use it, whether the need is urgent or not. They apparently think (perhaps subconsciously), "Maybe I won't have another chance for a while." But the bladder muscles become weak and lose the capacity to retain a large amount of urine and pass it out only when really necessary.

Urinary incontinence is more common among women than men, because their urethra is quite short. When women cough, sneeze, or strain, or even when laughing, their bladder may leak a little urine.

This disorder can be controlled by certain herbs, a periodic oil enema, and certain yoga exercises. Let's begin with the latter.

YOGA

ASHWINI MUDRA. This exercise involves using the perineal muscles to suck the anus inward, tightening the gluteal muscles. It will also strengthen the bladder sphincter. Do 10 to 12 repetitions, 2 or 3 times a day (while sitting down).

OTHER POSTURES. Sitting in the Vajrasana pose (see illustration in appendix 4) will help, as will the Forward Bend, Shoulder Stand, and Plow pose.

HERBS

Prepare the following mixture:

ashwagandha 5 *parts*
bala 3 *parts*
vidari 2 *parts*

Take ½ teaspoon with warm water twice a day, after meals.

• Every day eat a handful of white sesame seeds with some jaggery or natural brown sugar. This will strengthen the bladder and help to correct the incontinence.

OTHER REMEDIES AND RECOMMENDATIONS

SESAME OIL ENEMA. Once a week, do a *basti* (enema) using warm sesame oil (see appendix 2). Insert about 1 cup of oil into the rectum, and try to retain it for at least 5 to 10 minutes. If the oil runs out, don't worry. Sesame oil enema is one of the most effective ways to balance vata.

AVOID ALCOHOL AND CAFFEINE. Caffeine is a diuretic and intensifies the need to urinate. Therefore, incontinence and urgency of urination are quite common among coffee drinkers or users of other caffeinated beverages, such as tea or cola. Alcoholic beverages also promote incontinence. So it is better to avoid caffeine and alcohol if you have any problem with urinary control.

VATA-PACIFYING DIET. Since urinary incontinence is largely due to excess vata, following a vata-balancing diet will help. (See the dietary guidelines in chapter 8.)

Yeast Infections

Yeast infections are a result of a mixed pitta and kapha disorder. To heal them, first one has to follow a proper diet, which must not increase either pitta or kapha. Strictly avoid sugar, fermented food, and yeast-containing bread. Ideally, it is best to follow a diet that is pitta-soothing, but not kapha-provoking. The best way to manage this balance is to look in the food charts for each doshic type (see chapter 8) and favor foods in the "yes" column for both kapha and pitta.

EFFECTIVE HERBAL REMEDY. A potent herbal formula that will help to heal a yeast infection is:

turmeric *1/4 teaspoon*
licorice *1/2 teaspoon*
shardunika *1/4 teaspoon*

Take this complete mixture (1 teaspoon of herbs) twice a day with warm water until your symptoms are gone.

DOUCHE FOR VAGINAL YEAST INFECTION. If the yeast infection is vaginal, you will find it helpful to douche with licorice tea. Boil 1 tablespoon of licorice powder in 1 pint of water for 5 minutes. Cool, strain, and use that tea for the douche. You will notice the healing effect quickly.

NOTE: If you have a thick discharge from the genitals, along with an itching and burning sensation, it will be better to do the douche with *triphala* tea instead of licorice. Use the same procedure: take 1 tablespoon of *triphala,* boil it in a pint of water, cool, strain, and use the tea as a douche.

Conclusion

Taking Responsibility for Your Own Health: How to Integrate Ayurveda into Your Life

Ayurveda is a comprehensive approach to health that encompasses all facets of our life and living. Body, mind, and spirit; work and relationships; diet and the external environment; season of the year and daily routine; physical exercise and spiritual practices—all these and many additional factors are treated in the classical Ayurvedic texts.

From our deepest spiritual concerns (Who am I? Where do I come from? What is the purpose of my life?) to the most practical and mundane (How can I heal a sore throat? How much exercise is best for me? What foods should I eat?), the five-thousand-year-old living tradition of Ayurveda has answers that are practical and meaningful.

As a system of natural medicine, Ayurveda is not about curing symptoms, although it certainly accomplishes that. Rather, it is about building a way of life that creates health and healing. To make the best use of Ayurveda—and of this book—you have to put its principles into action. Just to run to the remedies section (Part III) when you have a health problem is truly to miss the richness and beauty of Ayurveda, which is a complete science of life that can enable every individual to be healthy and happy.

I would not be telling the truth if I said that incorporating Ayurveda into your life is totally simple. It is not. You will probably have to learn some new principles, as well as understanding the nature of your constitution, your mind-body type. It is likely that from what you learn, you will want to make changes in your daily routine, such as waking up earlier or changing the amount and type of exercise that you do. You may decide it would be wise to modify your diet, perhaps dropping some favorite foods that may be inappropriate for you. Such changes in our habitual way of living do not happen overnight.

On the other hand, I would also not be

telling the truth if I didn't say that every small step you take toward an Ayurvedic lifestyle will have an immediate and positive effect on your body, mind, and consciousness.

To incorporate Ayurveda into your life, you have to start somewhere. Many people find it easiest to begin by following some of the dietary guidelines for their body type. Then gradually, little by little, you can adopt some of the recommendations for the daily routine, adjusting your daily schedule to be more in tune with nature, or using some of the suggested breathing exercises or meditation practices.

The underlying assumption of Ayurveda is that each individual has the power to heal himself or herself. We each have the ability and the freedom to recover our health if we become ill, or to maintain vitality and joy of living. We can do this by understanding our body and its needs, and by attending to those needs as they change in response to the ever-changing outer environment and our inner world of feelings. For this, consciousness is the key: moment-to-moment awareness of what is happening.

In this book, I discuss more than a hundred health conditions, from acne to yeast infections, from headaches to athlete's foot. Within those major categories of symptoms, I describe literally hundreds of smaller signs and symptoms. These signs and symptoms are nothing but the body's language. By presenting us with a headache, diarrhea, fever, toothache, joint pain, insomnia, emotional anxiety, fear, or insecurity, the body is talking to us, letting us know that something is wrong, something is out of balance and needs our attention. It is the language of *tridosha,* of vata–pitta–kapha.

Ayurveda says that whatever symptom we experience is an expression of doshic imbalance. To restore good health, we have to reestablish balance by juggling the three doshas, favoring this one or pacifying that, in order to attain harmony between *vikruti,* the present doshic state, and *prakruti,* the original state of our constitution.

Ayurveda teaches us how to read this language of signs and symptoms. When, for example, there are signs of excess heat in the body—skin rash, heartburn, a flaring temper—we know that pitta dosha is in excess and needs to be pacified. Similarly, out-of-balance vata may speak to us in terms of insomnia, constipation, or anxiety, while kapha imbalance may communicate its presence as lethargy, overeating, or congestion in the lungs, sinuses, and chest.

We should never disregard this language of *tridosha.* It is the foundation of health and happiness, as well as of ill health.

In this book I have tried to share with you how to take care of those symptoms—not symptomatically but radically, fundamentally, basically. I have tried to show you how to use the symptoms as a catalyst to reestablish balance within the *tridosha,* as well as between body, mind, and consciousness.

By any method, creating balance within body, mind, and consciousness, and within vata–pitta–kapha, is called healing. The purpose of this book is to help you in your healing efforts, so that you can attain total health in your life.

In health and healing, there is an equal sharing of responsibility between the physician and the patient. In this book, really, every reader is taking on both sides of that responsibility. By using your own insight, perception, observation, and judgment, you are becoming your own physician and healer. By following the recommendations given in this book in order to bring healing, you are taking the role of the patient. You are the healer, and you are the person who receives healing.

Use this knowledge well to bring health, harmony, and happiness into your life.

Appendix 1

How to Use the Healing Properties of Metals, Gemstones, Colors, and Aromas

Ayurveda teaches that everything in existence is imbued with the energy and intelligence of Universal Consciousness. That is because all forms of matter, organic and inorganic, are simply the outer manifestations of this most subtle creative energy. Matter is the trapped light of consciousness. The vital force of life flows from the universal source, the essence of all matter, and manifests in the myriad forms and phenomena of nature.

The classic texts of Ayurveda make it clear that all substances in nature contain this cosmic creative intelligence, and thus have a healing value when used in the proper manner. That is why, in its quest to create and maintain perfect health, Ayurvedic medicine makes use of almost everything in nature and in daily life, including food, breathing, exercise, meditation, relationships, yoga, and massage, as well as regulated daily and seasonal routines. It also uses thousands of herbs and herbal formulas.

In addition, Ayurveda utilizes the healing properties of metals, gemstones, colors, and aromas. These contain special, potent forms of energy which may be drawn upon for healing purposes. Most of these methods, clearly described in the ancient textbooks, have been used safely and successfully for healing for thousands of years, though they have been scarcely known and little appreciated in the West until very recently. This appendix will provide a brief introduction to these healing modalities.

Metals

For medicinal purposes, metals are traditionally processed to be taken internally in small doses, after undergoing rigorous and extensive purification to negate any toxic effects upon the body's vital organs. The following recommendations are safe, as they do not involve ingestion of the actual metal.

COPPER

Copper alleviates excess kapha and reduces fat. It is a good tonic for the liver, spleen, and lymphatic system and helps in curing anemia. To treat obesity as well as liver and spleen disorders, thoroughly wash some copper pennies and boil them in a quart of water (or boil a quart of water in a copper vessel) until half the water remains. Take 2 teaspoons of this copper water 3 times a day for a month. It is also helpful to buy a copper drinking glass, fill it every night with pure water, and drink the water in the morning.

GOLD

Gold is strengthening to the nervous system and the heart, improves memory and intelligence, and increases stamina. It is also good for weak lungs. Gold can be helpful for students' pre-exam tension, for arthritis, and for heart arrhythmia.

The energy of gold may be harnessed by preparing gold medicated water. Use pure gold (24 karat is best), such as a gold band. Place the gold into 2 cups of water, and boil until 1 cup evaporates. Take 1 teaspoon of this gold water 2 or 3 times a day to energize the heart, strengthen mental faculties, and awaken pure awareness. (This process won't hurt your gold.)

You can also make golden rice. While cooking rice, place a piece of gold in the rice pot, and cook as usual. When the rice is finished, remove the gold before serving.

NOTE: Gold has heating properties and should be used sparingly by individuals with a pitta constitution.

SILVER

Silver has cooling properties and is beneficial for treating excess pitta. Silver increases strength and stamina and is thus helpful for balancing vata. Emaciation, chronic fever and weakness after fever, heartburn, inflammatory conditions of the intestines, and profuse menstrual bleeding may all be helped by silver. Silver is antiseptic, antibacterial, and disinfectant. Make silver water following the above directions for gold water, and take 1 teaspoon 2 to 3 times a day. Drink warm milk heated in a silver vessel to build up strength and stamina.

IRON

This metal is beneficial for bone marrow, bone tissue, liver, and spleen. It increases the production of red blood cells and helps to cure anemia. Iron also strengthens muscle and nerve tissues and is rejuvenating. For extra iron, try cooking in cast iron pots and pans. However, excess iron in the system is harmful, so be careful about using it. Although women during their menstruating years may be iron-deficient and may benefit from additional iron, very few men in Western society need extra iron. An exception might be longtime strict vegetarians.

Gems and Stones

Gems and precious stones contain healing energies that can be activated by wearing them as ornaments, such as rings or necklaces, or by placing them in water overnight and drinking the water the following day. Gems enliven the vital energy centers in the body (the chakras) and have a direct influence on vata, pitta, and kapha. They may be used to pacify or activate specific organs of the body, or to enhance or neutralize the effects of particular planets in the person's astrological birth chart.

Before we go into the effects of specific gems and stones, here are a few important general points.

• Gems tend to absorb the qualities and energy vibrations of their owners. It is beneficial to purify any stone before using it. Soaking it for two days in saltwater or milk should be sufficient. This will not harm the stone.

• When you wear a gemstone, it should touch the skin through a small window in the setting, so that the subtle energies of the stone can interact directly with the energies of the body.

• Where you wear the stone is important. Here are some recommendations:

diamond—ring finger
pearl—little finger
red coral—ring finger
emerald—little finger
opal—ring finger
yellow sapphire—index finger
blue sapphire—middle finger

Ayurveda generally recommends that rings be worn on the right hand, though in the West, if someone wants to wear their wedding ring on the left hand to conform with tradition, that is all right.

• Processed or chemically treated stones may not have the same healing energy. It is best to get authentic, unprocessed, clean stones without a flaw or crack. When you are considering buying a stone, be sure to use a magnifying glass to examine it for cracks or imperfections.

• Stones should be 3 to 5 karats if possible, but a 1-karat diamond is large enough. A stone that is too small will not produce much of an effect.

• Unless you are knowledgeable both in stones and in Vedic astrology *(jyotish)*, it is wise to consult an expert before investing in a stone. The wrong gem for you, or one worn on the wrong part of the body, can have a negative influence.

Here are some of the characteristics of the main gems and stones.

RUBY

Astrologically, the ruby represents the sun. It is a life-protecting stone that promotes longevity, especially for vata and kapha individuals, and brings prosperity. This gem strengthens concentration and bestows mental power. It also strengthens the heart. Rubies pacify vata and kapha but may elevate pitta. Garnets have the same vibration as rubies; they are the poor man's ruby. Wear both rubies and garnets either in a ring on the ring finger, or in a necklace.

PEARL

As rubies represent the sun, pearls symbolize the moon. They have a cooling effect and a calming, healing vibration. Pearls are balancing to all the doshas, though their cooling action is particularly good for pitta. Pearls confer mental peace and tranquillity. Pearl ash is used internally to effectively treat many ailments. You can gain many of the strengthening effects of pearls by making pearl water. Place 4 or 5 pearls in a glass of water; let it stand overnight, and drink the water in the morning.

YELLOW SAPPHIRE

This precious stone, which represents Jupiter, brings groundedness, stability, and wisdom. It helps to calm both vata and pitta and may slightly increase kapha qualities. It strengthens the heart and also builds lung and kidney energy. Yellow sapphire should always be worn on the index finger, the finger of Jupiter. Yellow topaz, the poor man's sapphire, has many of the same qualities and produces similar benefits.

BLUE SAPPHIRE

This beautiful precious stone represents Saturn and brings the benefits of that very spiritual planet. Saturn, a deity of earth and iron, confers enlightenment. Blue sapphire calms vata and kapha and may stimulate pitta. It builds up muscles and the skeletal system and helps to heal arthritis. Wear blue sapphire on the right middle finger, preferably in a silver setting. Do not wear it with diamonds; this will create disharmony.

LAPIS LAZULI

This stone, which has Saturn-like energy, is heavenly and sacred. It gives strength to the body, mind, and consciousness, and it sensitizes the wearer to higher spiritual vibrations. It strengthens the eyes, calms vata and pitta, and is helpful for anxiety, fear, and weakness of the heart. It is also good for the liver and for skin diseases. Lapis should be set in gold and worn on the little finger, or worn as a necklace.

EMERALD

This powerful precious stone brings prosperity and spiritual awakening. It calms vata and pitta, settles the nervous system, and relieves nervousness. Symbolic of the planet Mercury, emeralds improve writing skills, enhance the power of speech, and promote intelligence. They are best set in gold and worn on the little finger.

DIAMOND

This very powerful gemstone combats premature aging, enhances the span of life, and strengthens immunity. Its energy brings subtle energy vibrations to the heart, brain, and deeper bodily tissues. It is the best stone for rejuvenation. It brings prosperity and is spiritually uplifting.

The doshic effects of diamonds vary according to their color. Red diamonds have a fiery energy that stimulates pitta; blue diamonds are cooling and calm pitta while increasing kapha. Clear, colorless diamonds calm pitta but increase both vata and kapha.

Symbolic of the planet Venus, diamonds actually do help to create a close bond in relationships and are rightfully associated with marriage. These stones stimulate *shukra*, the body's reproductive tissue. Art, music, romance, and sex all go together with this stone. Wear your diamond set in gold, either as a necklace or as a ring on the ring finger. But note: Diamonds of low quality may have negative effects upon the body.

RED CORAL

This gemstone from the sea represents the planet Mars. It calms pitta and helps one to control anger, hatred, and jealousy. Coral gives energy to the liver, spleen, and pericardium. Wear your red coral as a necklace or as a ring set in copper (preferably), silver, or white gold and worn on the ring finger. Red coral is strength-giving and imparts gracefulness.

OPAL

This semiprecious stone represents the planet Neptune. It strengthens *majja dhatu* (bone marrow and nerves) as well as *shukra dhatu* (reproductive tissue). It improves vision, relieves fever, calms pitta, and is good for migraine headaches. Opals enhance spiritual feelings, increase devotion, and help to unfold intuition. This gem is particularly beneficial for individuals with Neptune in their third, fourth, sixth, tenth, or twelfth astrological house. It should be set in gold or silver and worn on the ring finger.

CAT'S-EYE

This stone is good for allergies, repeated colds and congestion, and allergic asthma. It pacifies kapha and vata while slightly increasing pitta. It aids in healing kidney dysfunction. Cat's-eye enhances awareness and helps a person not get caught up in emotions. People working in psychological healing should wear this stone in a gold setting on their ring or little finger; it will help protect them from negative influences.

QUARTZ CRYSTALS

These stones have a Venus-like vibratory energy that is somewhat like that of diamonds. They calm vata, improve the quality of perception, strengthen communication, and enhance intuition. You can wear quartz crystals as a necklace, or set in either silver or gold and worn on the ring finger.

ONYX

This stone is excellent for vata disorders. It is good for old age, debilitating disorders, and neurological dysfunction, and it helps with epilepsy, Parkinson's disease, and even schizophrenia. It induces quiet, deep sleep yet combats lethargy. It is good for memory and promotes positive thinking. Onyx makes life peaceful and happy and enhances love in relationships. It has energy vibrations that are Sun-like and Jupiter-like. This stone should be set in silver and worn on the ring finger. (If your Sun sign is in Sagittarius or Gemini, it is better not to wear this stone.)

JADE

Jade is beneficial for longevity. It strengthens kidney energy and is reputed to bestow success upon its wearer. This stone is also good for the power of speech. It helps to prevent cataracts and is strengthening for the prostate. Wear a jade ring set in silver, on your little finger.

AMETHYST

Amethyst is a stone for the crown chakra and is good for mental clarity. To bring prosperity, it should be set in gold. You can also wear it around the neck on a gold necklace. A person with neuromuscular weakness can be helped by wearing amethysts and by putting them at the four corners of the bed. Some amethysts have a darker color, which gives them a Saturn-like energy similar to blue sapphire. Amethysts bestow dignity, love, compassion, and hope. This gem helps the individual to control emotions and is good for vata and pitta imbalance.

AQUAMARINE

A substitute for emerald, which symbolizes Mercury, aquamarine reduces dullness of mind, promotes happiness and intelligence, enhances the power of speech, and improves memory. This stone also has Venus-like qualities; it is good for married couples to wear aquamarine to enhance love in their relationship. Aquamarine should be set in silver and worn on the little finger.

Remember that in all these cases, simply wearing the correct stone is not enough to take care of a doshic imbalance; you need to watch your diet, meditate, do appropriate exercise and yoga postures, and consciously

Four Inexpensive Stones to Help Balance the Doshas

Though some of the gemstones discussed in this appendix can be obtained for a moderate amount of money, many may be prohibitively priced for you at this time. If so, here are four inexpensive stones you can use to help create balance in your mind and body.

When vata dosha is excessive, you can use *rose quartz* to promote balance. The warming color and energy of rose quartz can bring relief to vata ailments such as nervousness, dry skin, constipation, intestinal gas, and lower back pain.

For aggravated pitta, use *red coral* or *pearls*. Their cooling energy will help with pitta disorders such as angry emotions, various inflammatory conditions and "-itises" such as colitis and conjunctivitis, as well as hyperacidity.

Kapha dosha can be balanced by wearing *garnets*. The deep red color of this stone enlivens the energy in the body and reduces the effects of excess kapha, such as water retention, lethargy, depression, and overweight.

and conscientiously look after your day-to-day and moment-to-moment health.

More information about these and other gemstones, and how to wear them (settings, correct fingers, and so on) is provided in chapter 8 of my book *Secrets of the Pulse* (see the Reading List).

Colors

Ayurvedic treatments also make use of the healing properties inherent in colors. Because the basic colors of the rainbow are correlated with the bodily tissues *(dhatus)* and the doshas, the vibratory energy of the colors may be used to help establish balance in mind and body.

Color is nothing but light, and light is radiant energy imparted from every atom. The source of light and color is the sun. In our solar system, whatever colors we perceive come from sun rays. Every color has a different wavelength, frequency, and vibration. When we put a prism in the sunlight, the seven colors of the rainbow can be separated, but the equal presence of all seven gives white light. The absence of any color is black, darkness. So black is a negative color, and white a positive color.

You can influence your health and happiness by choosing appropriate colors for your clothing and surroundings at home and at work. Also, if you place colored, translucent paper or plastic wrap around a jar or glass of water and place it in sunlight for four hours, the water will become infused with the vibrations of that color. Drinking the water will then bring beneficial results.

RED

Red is warming and stimulating. It relieves aggravated vata and reduces excess kapha. However, because of its heating effect, overexposure to this color may aggravate pitta and result in inflammatory ailments such as conjunctivitis. Red is related to our blood. It stimulates the formation of red blood cells and improves circulation. It also helps to maintain color in the skin and gives energy to nerve tissue and bone marrow. *Pink* has a gentler effect, promoting love and calmness, but it may be conducive to lethargy in kapha individuals.

ORANGE

Like red, orange is warming and has a healing energy. It is a sexually stimulating color that gives energy and strength to the sex organs. Paradoxically, in spiritual seekers who have chosen to be celibate, orange helps with renunciation and transforming sexual energy into Supreme Consciousness. Orange is balancing to both vata and kapha but may be aggravating to pitta. It has antibacterial and bacteriostatic properties; it hinders the growth of bacteria.

YELLOW

Yellow relieves excess vata and kapha. It promotes understanding and intelligence and helps energy rise to the crown chakra for spiritual realization. Yellow is a decongestant that helps to relieve kapha congestion. It also acts as an antibacterial. Overexposure to yellow causes excess bile to accumulate and increases pitta dosha.

GREEN

This color has a calming effect upon mind and body and creates a feeling of freshness. It is soothing to the emotions and brings energy to the heart chakra and feelings of happiness to the heart. Green is calming and pacifying to excess pitta and may aggravate vata and kapha. Green helps to heal ulcers and promotes the growth of granulation tissue.

BLUE

Blue is a cooling color that relieves aggravated pitta. It has a calming effect on the body and mind and helps to correct liver disorders. When a baby has jaundice, placing the baby under a blue light will help it heal faster. Blue is the color of Pure Consciousness. Overexposure to blue may cause aggravation of vata and kapha and may provoke congestion.

PURPLE

This is the color of Cosmic Consciousness and brings an awakening of awareness. It creates lightness in the body and helps to open the doors of perception. Purple relieves excess pitta and kapha but may aggravate vata.

GOLD AND SILVER

Gold, the color of the sun, is a warming color that is beneficial for vata and kapha.

Beneficial Colors for Constitutional Types

For each constitutional type, certain colors are soothing and balancing while others are aggravating. Here is a summary of healthful colors:

- *Vata: Vata* types should minimize the use of dark and cooling colors such as blues, browns, and black. On the other hand, very hot, vivid colors may be overstimulating to vata, which has a tendency toward being hyperactive. So your best bets are warm pastels, sunny yellows, and green, with some warming red and orange.
- *Pitta:* Cool, soft colors are the best for your health and balance of body and mind. Blues and purples/violets are excellent, along with silver (including silver jewelry) and blue-greens. Watch out for reds and oranges, which can inflame pitta dosha, and minimize yellow and gold. Avoid black.
- *Kapha:* Bright, lively, bold colors are good to balance kapha, with its tendency toward lethargy and mental and physical heaviness. Red, yellow, orange, and gold are all good. Even if you feel you look good in green, dark blue, or white, these are not the best for you from a health standpoint.

Silver, associated with the moon, is cooling and soothes pitta.

Aromas

Every human being has five senses, which are associated with the five elements. Sound and hearing are related to the element of space, color and sight to fire, taste to water, smell and aroma to earth, and touch to air. These five senses are the gateways of perception for the human being, and they can be used for healing purposes.

Aromatherapy uses incense and essential oils made from flowers, plants, trees, and grasses to relay fragrances through the olfactory sense to the brain, in order to bring healing energy to mind and body. Ayurveda teaches that smells are directly related to doshic balance and imbalance, and that certain aromas are heating, cooling, or neutral.

Deer musk, for example, and hina, are heating; they calm vata and kapha but may provoke pitta. Camphor is cooling and fragrant, but its aftereffect is heating; it too calms and pacifies vata and kapha but may stimulate pitta. The aroma of sandalwood is anti-inflammatory and cooling; it is calming and soothing for pitta but may increase kapha or vata.

Khus (the essence of khus grass) is grounding, pleasant, and cooling. It has a sweet smell and pacifies pitta, but it may provoke kapha and vata. Jasmine too is cooling and sweet and good for pitta, but it may build up kapha.

The effect of rose depends somewhat on the color of the flower. Dark red roses are warming, while white- and yellow-colored roses are relatively cooling. In general, the aroma of rose flowers is anti-inflammatory and soothing and has an aphrodisiac quality. Rose aroma can be used for cooling pitta but may provoke vata and kapha.

AROMAS AND THE DOSHAS

- Vata can be balanced by using sweet, warming, grounding aromas such as musk, hina, and camphor. Other good fragrances for vata include orange, clove, cardamom, lavender, pine, angelica, and frankincense.
- Pitta is soothed by the use of cooling, calming, sweet aromas such as sandalwood, khus, jasmine, and rose. Rose geranium, lemongrass, fennel, peppermint, gardenia, and mint may also be beneficial.
- Kapha is pacified and balanced by using aromas with a warming, somewhat stimulating effect. Musk, hina, and camphor are helpful. Some more pungent aromas are also helpful for kapha. Some of these are eucalyptus, cinnamon, myrrh, thyme, basil, rosemary, and sage.

Appendix 2

How to Prepare and Use Herbs, Ghees, and Oils

This appendix briefly explains the preparation of herbs and special remedies such as medicated oils and ghees and offers suggestions on their use. For a complete description of herbs and their uses, as well as thorough directions for the preparation of herbal remedies, please refer to *The Yoga of Herbs* by Dr. Vasant Lad and Dr. David Frawley (see Reading List).

Herbal Mixtures

USE WHOLE HERBS AND FOODS

Ayurveda believes strongly in the use of whole herbs, foods, and plants. Isolated active ingredients or chemically produced analogues are not equivalent to natural whole food sources. For sources of herbs, see Resources.

HOW MUCH TO PREPARE

If you are going to be taking an herbal mixture for several days, weeks, or even months, to save time you will probably want to prepare a fairly large quantity. Then each time you use it, take 1/4 to 1/2 teaspoon unless otherwise directed.

In this book formulas for herbal mixtures are given in "parts" rather than in milligrams or teaspoons. For example, a formula may call for

herb 1	2 parts
herb 2	3 parts
herb 3	1/4 part

Choose your own measure, according to how much you want to make. If, for example, you are measuring in teaspoons, you will use

2 teaspoons of herb 1
3 teaspoons of herb 2
$^1/_4$ teaspoon of herb 3

If you are making a large batch for long-term use, you can measure in tablespoons. A 1- to 2-month supply will require 2.5 to 5.0 ounces of herbs, a palm-size quantity. Again, when you take the herb each time, use only $^1/_4$ or $^1/_2$ teaspoon, as recommended.

WHERE TO OBTAIN HERBS

Most of the herbs mentioned in this book can be obtained in bulk or capsules at a good natural foods store. Always try to get organic, nonirradiated herbs. Special Ayurvedic herbs and herbal formulas are available from The Ayurvedic Institute, the suppliers listed in the Resources, and some Indian groceries.

HOW TO TAKE HERBS

Herbs are almost always taken with a vehicle or medium *(anupana)* to facilitate absorption by the body and to carry the quality of the herbs to the specific tissue or site of the disease. The most common vehicles used in Ayurveda are water, milk, honey, aloe vera, and ghee. Raw sugar may also be used at times. The vehicle varies according to the herb, the illness or condition being treated, your constitution, and other factors. Typically, you might take your herbal dose with a spoonful of ghee or honey; mixed in a cup of warm milk; or placed dry on your tongue and then washed down with some warm or room-temperature water.

Most of the recommendations in this book suggest which vehicle to use. If none is suggested, use warm water. I do not recommend using capsules because taste is important (see page 99), but if you must use them, you can buy some empty 00-size vegecapsules (available at most natural food stores) and fill them with the herbal mixture. This is better than not taking the herbs at all, and may be more convenient when you are traveling or at work.

USING TRIPHALA

Triphala ("the three fruits") is a wonderful remedy consisting of three of the most important Ayurvedic herbs: *amalaki, bibhitaki,* and *haritaki. Amalaki* works on pitta dosha, *bibhitaki* on kapha dosha, and *haritaki* on vata dosha. This compound is rejuvenative and strengthening for all three doshas and all seven *dhatus;* it balances *ojas, tejas,* and *prana* and is also an excellent, mild laxative.

Take *triphala* in the evening, at least 1 hour after your evening meal. Add $^1/_2$ to 1 teaspoon *triphala* powder to about 1 cup boiling water. Steep for 10 minutes or until the water is cool enough to drink. You may strain out the herbs before drinking or just leave them at the bottom of your cup.

You may not like the taste of *triphala* at first—it may taste quite bitter. But if you use it regularly, your health is bound to improve, and you will eventually find that the taste becomes less unpleasant.

Triphala can also be taken in these ways:

1. Place $^1/_2$ to 1 teaspoon of dry *triphala* powder on your tongue, and wash it down with warm water.

2. For some people, *triphala* acts as a mild diuretic and may disturb sleep if taken at night. If you are one of these people, drink the tea in the morning and it will act in about one hour.
3. If you really hate the taste, you can mix the *triphala* powder with honey and take it that way.

Ghee

HOW TO MAKE GHEE

Two pounds of butter will make one quart of ghee. Put the butter (sweet and unsalted, organic if available) in a heavy, medium-size pot, turn the heat to medium, and heat until the butter melts, taking care not to burn the butter.

Then turn down the heat, cook until the butter just boils, and continue to cook at this temperature. Do not cover the pot, as it is important to boil the water out and separate the solids. The butter will foam and sputter for a while and then begin to quiet down. Stir it occasionally with a stainless steel spatula, scraping the bottom of the pan.

In 12 to 15 minutes your ghee will begin to smell like popcorn and will turn a lovely golden color. Whitish curds will form and separate from the clear ghee. When these whitish curds turn a light tan color and the boiling quiets down, the ghee is ready. Take it off the heat immediately, for it is most likely to burn at this stage. The cooking time should not be longer than 15 to 20 minutes, depending on the kind of pan and the heat source.

Let the ghee cool until it is just warm. The solid curds will have settled to the bottom of the pot. Decant the clear ghee into a container, and discard the curds left on the bottom.

STORING GHEE

Ghee can be kept on the kitchen shelf. It does not need refrigeration. Its medicinal properties are said to improve with age. Don't ladle out the ghee with a wet spoon or allow any water to get into the container, as this will create the conditions for bacteria to grow and spoil the ghee.

EFFECTS OF GHEE

Ghee increases digestive fire and improves absorption and assimilation. It nourishes *ojas*, the subtle essence of all the body's tissues, strengthens the brain and nervous system, and improves memory. It lubricates the connective tissue and makes the body more flexible. Ghee carries the medicinal properties of herbs to all seven *dhatus*. It pacifies pitta and vata and is okay for kapha in moderation.

> NOTE: People who have high cholesterol or who suffer from obesity should be cautious about using ghee.

HOW TO MAKE MEDICATED GHEES

Ghee is a highly effective *anupana* (vehicle) for carrying herbs to the deeper tissues of the body. Hence many remedies are made by cooking herbs into ghee. Examples include *shatavari* ghee, *brahmi* ghee, *tikta ghrita* (bitter ghee), *triphala* ghee, and many others. The process is quite lengthy, and you will probably prefer to purchase these medicated ghees (and medicated oils as well). But if you wish to make it yourself, proceed as follows:

First, make the ghee, as described above.

Next, make a decoction of the desired herbs by cooking 1 part dry herbs to 16 parts of water, or about $^1/_2$ ounce of herbs per cup (8 ounces) of water. Boil the herbs *slowly* over a low flame until the water is reduced to one-quarter its original amount. For example, 4 cups would be reduced to 1, or 1 cup to $^1/_4$ cup. Then strain out the herbs. This process takes several hours. The liquid can be used as a prepared medicinal decoction, but in this case, you are going to use it for your medicated ghee.

Finally, mix equal parts of ghee and the herbal decoction, and cook it over a low flame until all the water evaporates.

Medicated Oils

Medicated oils (*amla* oil, *brahmi* oil, *bhringaraj* oil, garlic oil, clove oil, and others) are made the same way, except that you use oil instead of *ghee* in the final stage.

NEEM OIL

Neem oil is an herbalized oil made from cooking *neem* leaves in a base of sesame (usually) or some other oil. It is not pure *neem* extract, which would be too strong. *Neem* oil is generally available from suppliers of Ayurvedic products.

How Long to Take a Remedy

The general rule is to use remedies until your symptoms disappear. This may take from a few days to a few months, depending on the severity of the disease or condition, how long you have had it, how motivated you are to get well, and other factors.

In addition to taking your remedies, please also look into the underlying causes of your condition. You may need to rethink your diet, daily routine, exercise program, and so on. Simply taking herbal remedies, without making some changes in your lifestyle, will probably not be sufficient to override the behavior patterns that caused your illness in the first place.

So use your common sense. If the condition is chronic, it is unrealistic to expect that something that has persisted for years is going to disappear in a week or a month. On the other hand, if your condition is serious, and you are diligent with your remedies and make appropriate lifestyle changes, and still the symptoms persist, you need to see your doctor for help.

Appendix 3

Special Ayurvedic Procedures

This brief appendix offers guidelines on some of the Ayurvedic procedures recommended throughout Part III.

Basti (Ayurvedic Enema)

Ayurvedic enema treatment (*basti*) introduces into the rectum medicinals such as sesame oil, or herbal decoctions such as *dashamoola*, in a liquid medium. Medicated enemas pacify vata and alleviate many vata disorders, such as constipation, abdominal distension, insomnia, backache, neck pain, arthritis, sciatica, anxiety, and various nervous disorders. It is said that there are at least eighty vata-related disorders, and that *basti* is a complete treatment for 80 percent of them. *Basti* also is effective for treating chronic fever, sexual disorders, kidney stones, hyperacidity, and numerous other conditions.

NOTE: Medicated enemas are not to be used by anyone suffering from diarrhea, bleeding from the rectum, indigestion, cough, breathlessness, ascites, profuse edema, or active hemorrhoids. Individuals with diabetes or anemia, the aged, and children below the age of seven should also not receive medicated enemas. Oil enemas should not be used if there is acute fever, diarrhea, cold, paralysis, heart pain, severe abdominal pain, or emaciation.

The best times for *basti* are in the morning or evening. The stomach should be empty, so wait at least three hours after eating. Make sure the environment is clean, warm, and comfortable: An area where you can lie down near the toilet is best. You will need an enema bag or syringe, a measuring cup, a hot plate or stove (this doesn't have to be in the bathroom!), the oil and/or herbal substance, and towels.

The usual procedure for *basti* is first to introduce 5 ounces of warm (not hot) sesame oil into the rectum and retain it for 10 minutes. Then, without expelling the oil, introduce a mixture of oil and herbal tea and retain it for at least 30 minutes. The mixture should consist of another 5 ounces of sesame oil, mixed with 16 ounces (1 pint) of tea made from herbs steeped in hot water, then strained and cooled to about body temperature. In this book, the most frequently suggested herbal formula is *dashamoola,* which is particularly effective for balancing vata.

To introduce the fluid into the rectum, first fill the enema bag, which should be suspended about 3 feet above your position. Allow all air to be expelled from the tube, and close the clip on the hose. Then lie on the floor on your left side, your left (bottom) leg extended and your right leg flexed at the knee. (For comfort, prepare a rug or a couple of towels to lie on rather than lying on a bare floor.) Lubricate the tip of the syringe with oil or ghee. Make sure the anal area is clean and lubricated. Carefully and slowly insert the tip of the syringe into the rectum, then release the clip and allow all the fluid to enter. When the enema bag is empty, remove the tip.

Again, try to hold the oil for 10 minutes, and then hold the oil/herbal mixture for another 30 minutes if you can. While holding the fluid inside, assume a hands-and-knees position for a while and elevate the buttocks; this relaxes the colon. Periodically massage the colon area lightly with a counterclockwise motion (as seen when you look down toward your navel). Massage up the left side to the rib cage, across to the right side, and down. (This is opposite to the way food journeys through and serves to propel the enema fluid up into the higher areas of the colon.)

When the fluid has been retained for the suggested time (or if you find you just can't hold it), sit on the toilet and allow the passage of the fluid and fecal matter.

You may wish to wear a sanitary pad of some kind in your underwear for a few hours following *basti,* as there is likely to be some seepage of residual oil.

You may note that for some conditions discussed in this book, only an oil enema, or only a *dashamoola* enema—and occasionally only a warm water enema—is recommended. Follow the recommendations for that condition.

For some individuals, the fluid does not come back out. That simply means that the colon was very dry and that all the liquid has been absorbed. This is entirely natural and is nothing to worry about.

Nasya

Nasya is the nasal administration of herbal oils, ghee, or fine powders. If you were to receive *nasya* in a *panchakarma* treatment at an Ayurvedic clinic, you would lie face up on a table with your head tilted back, nostrils "facing the sky." A small amount of an appropriate powder might be placed into your nostrils, or 3 to 5 drops of a medicated oil or ghee.

When you do *nasya* yourself, simply dip your little finger (clean and with the nail closely trimmed) into ghee or whatever herbalized oil might be recommended, and lightly massage the inside of your nostril with your little finger. Then gently sniff to draw the oil upward.

Nauli

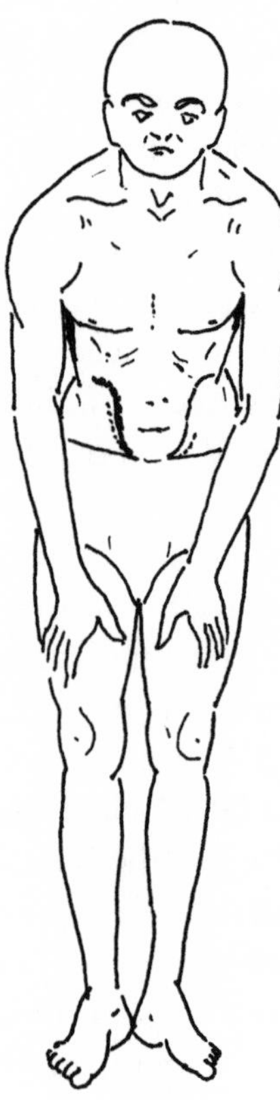

Nauli

Nauli is a simple method of massaging the internal organs, particularly the colon, intestines, liver, and spleen. It also maintains abdominal fire and helps to keep the colon clean.

Stand with your feet about shoulder-width apart, and slightly flex your knees. Bend forward as shown in the diagram, and put each hand on its respective knee. Breathe in, a long deep breath, and gradually exhale it. After a complete exhalation, hold your breath out.

Contract your abdominal muscles so that you form a ropelike structure at the abdominal wall. Then, by alternating the pressure on your right and left hand, you can move the abdominal muscles from right to left and left to right. Do this seven times.

Appendix 4

Yoga Asanas

Throughout this book, I recommend specific yoga *asanas* for vata–pitta–kapha and for various ailments. Although simple illustrations of the recommended postures are provided here, instruction in yoga is not intended and is beyond the scope of this book. You cannot really learn how to do yoga *asanas* properly from written instructions and some illustrations.

If you have already learned how to do yoga *asanas,* these illustrations will serve to refresh your memory. To learn the postures for the first time, please see a qualified yoga instructor.

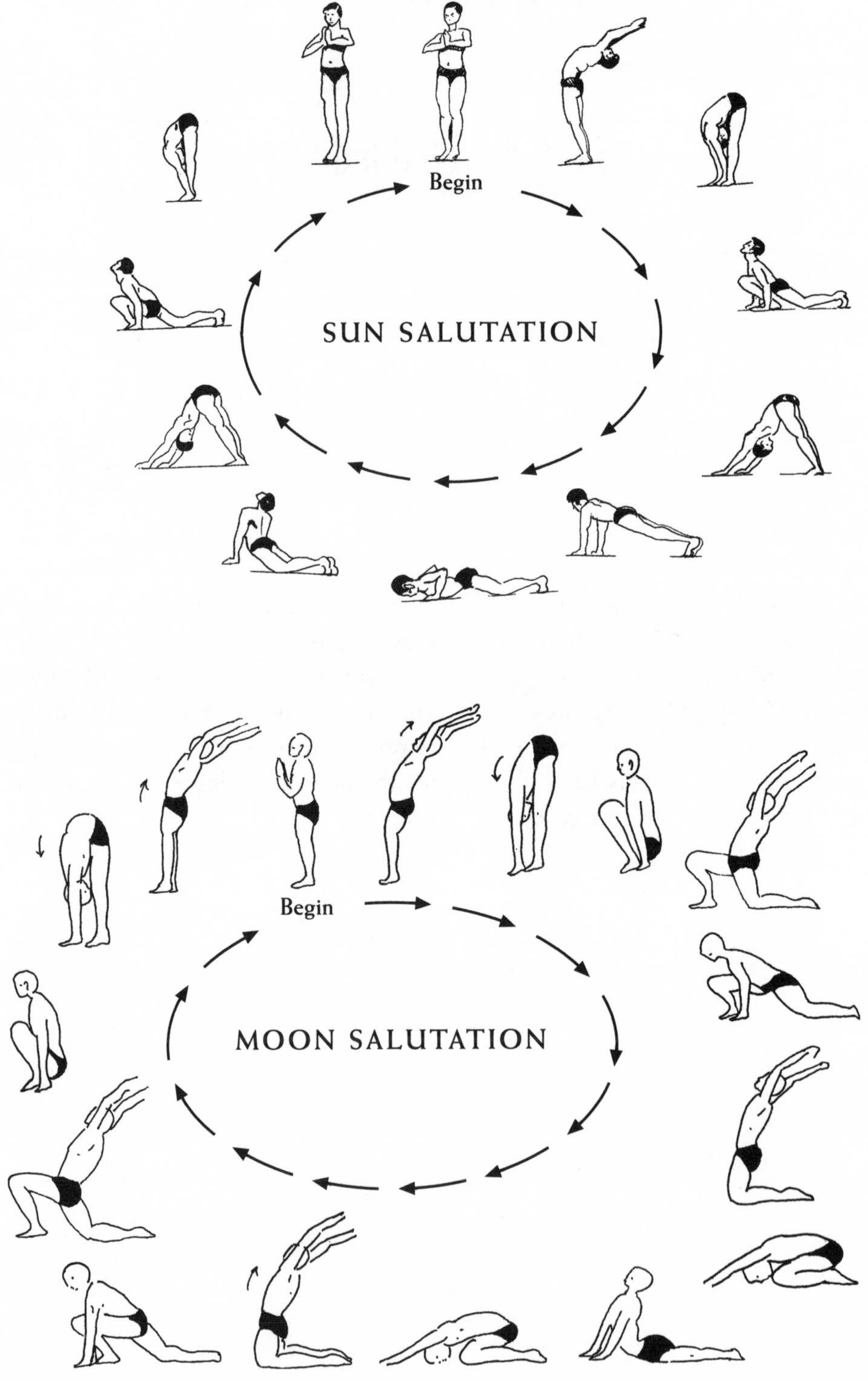
Begin
SUN SALUTATION
Begin
MOON SALUTATION

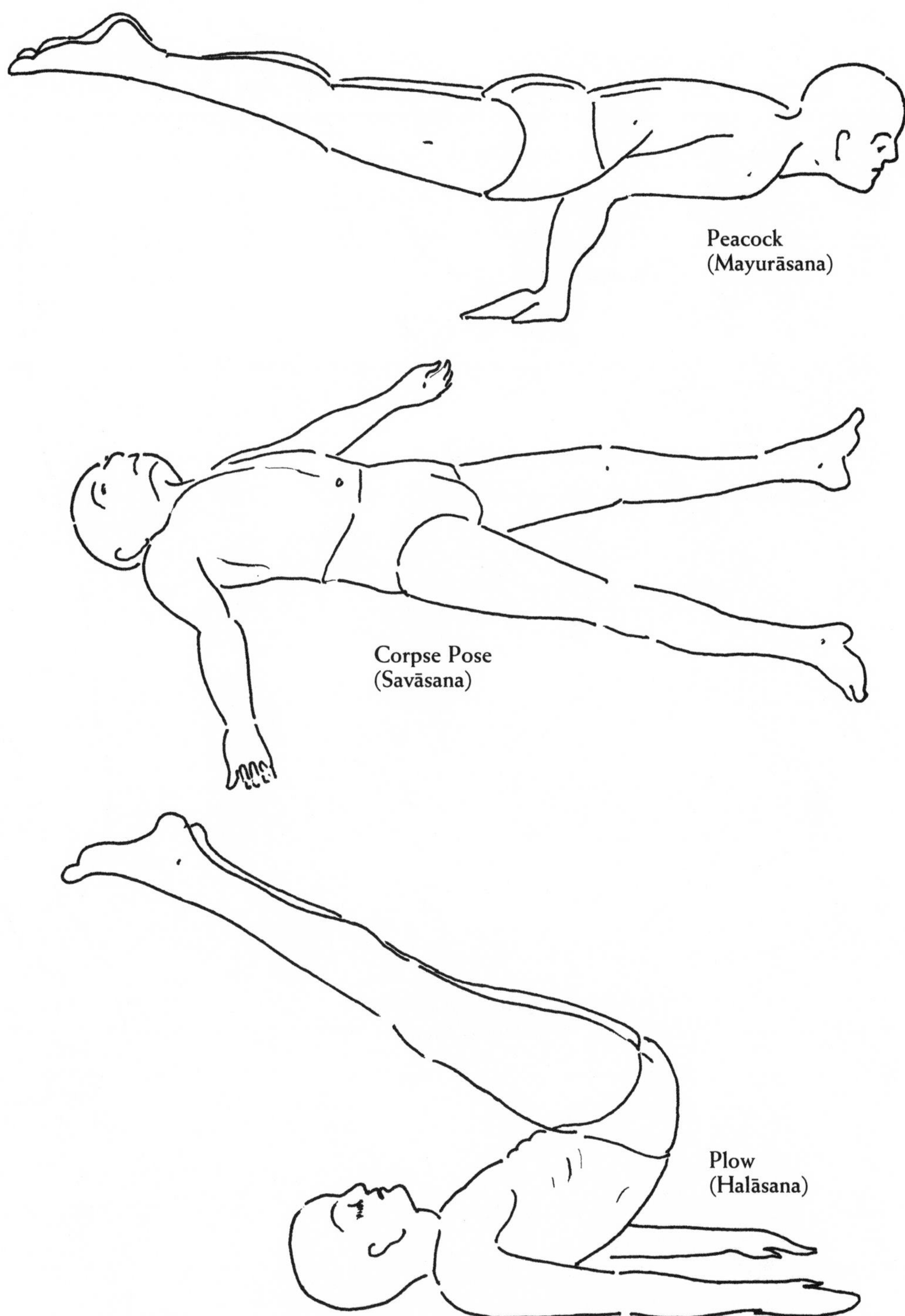

Peacock
(Mayurāsana)

Corpse Pose
(Savāsana)

Plow
(Halāsana)

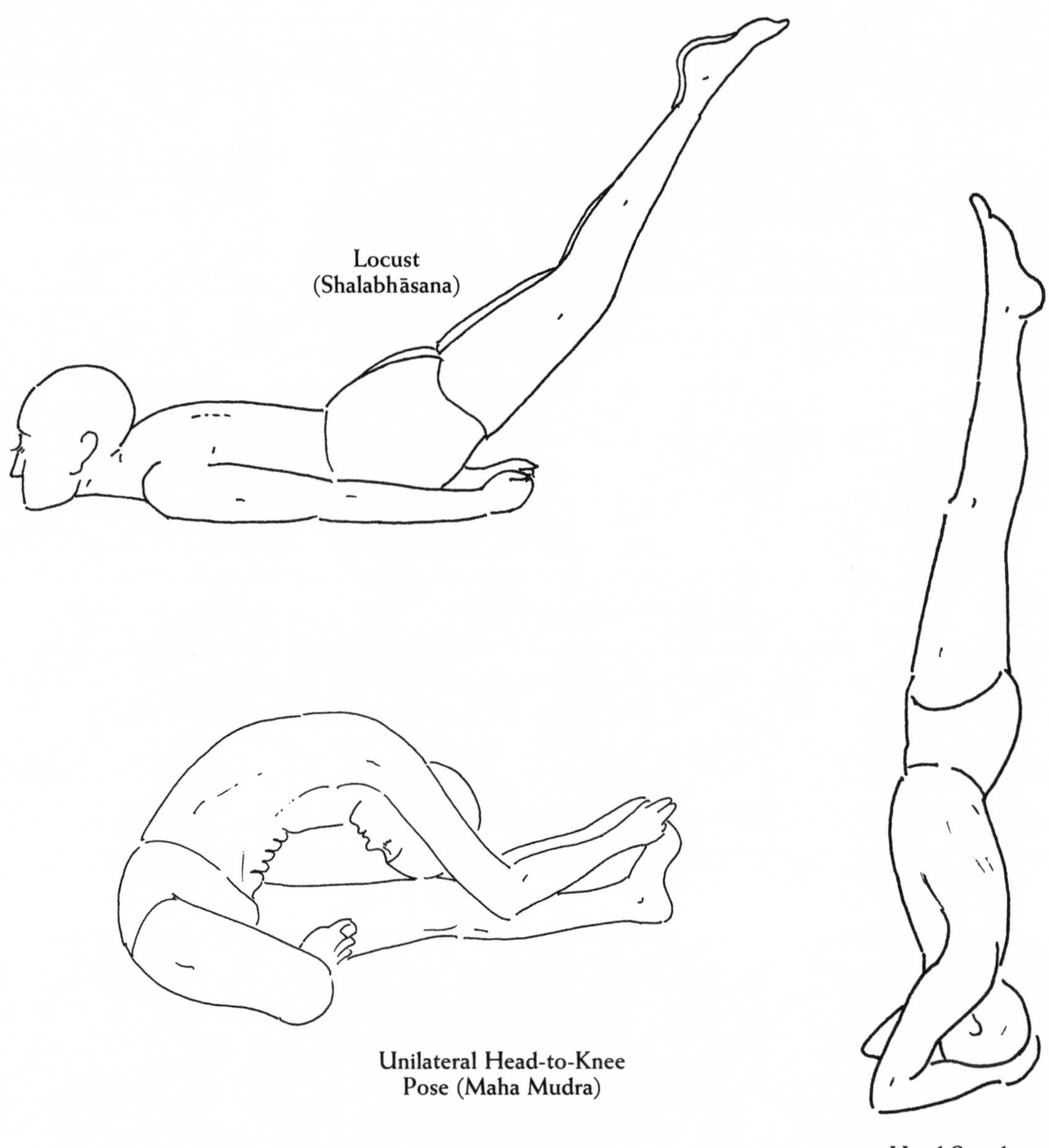

Locust
(Shalabhāsana)

Unilateral Head-to-Knee
Pose (Maha Mudra)

Head Stand
(Shirshāsana)

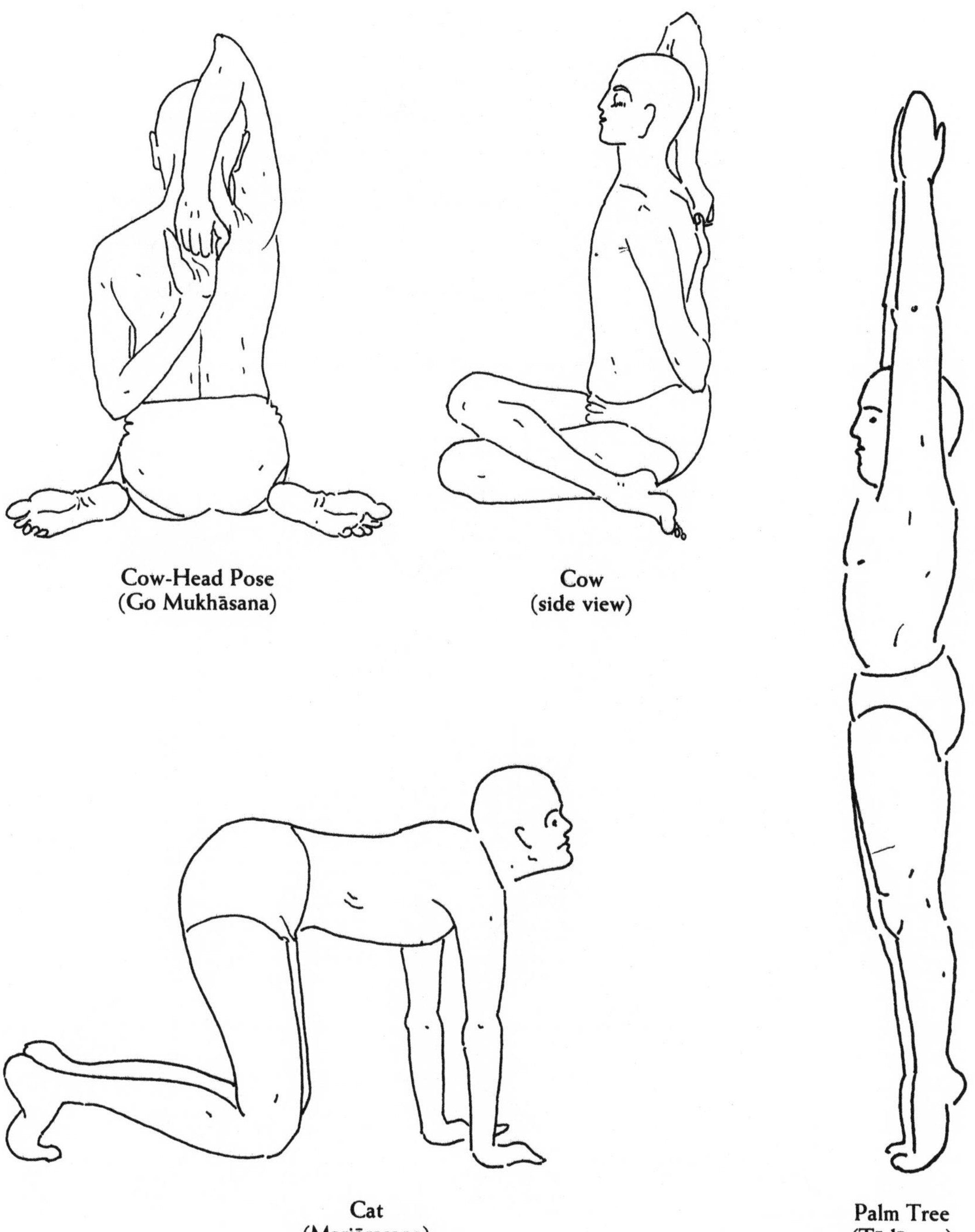

Cow-Head Pose
(Go Mukhāsana)

Cow
(side view)

Cat
(Marjārasana)

Palm Tree
(Tādāsana)

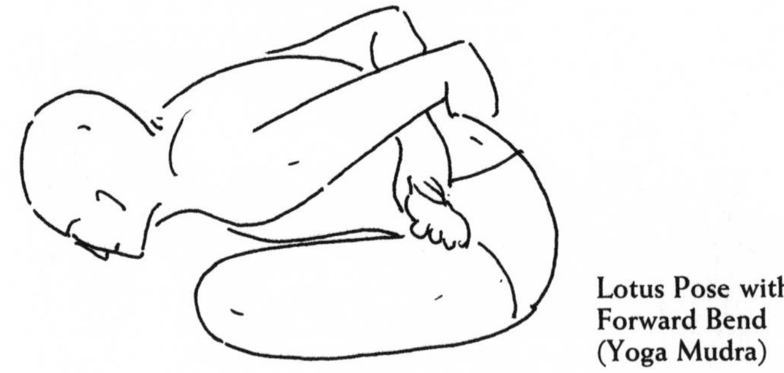

Lotus Pose with Forward Bend (Yoga Mudra)

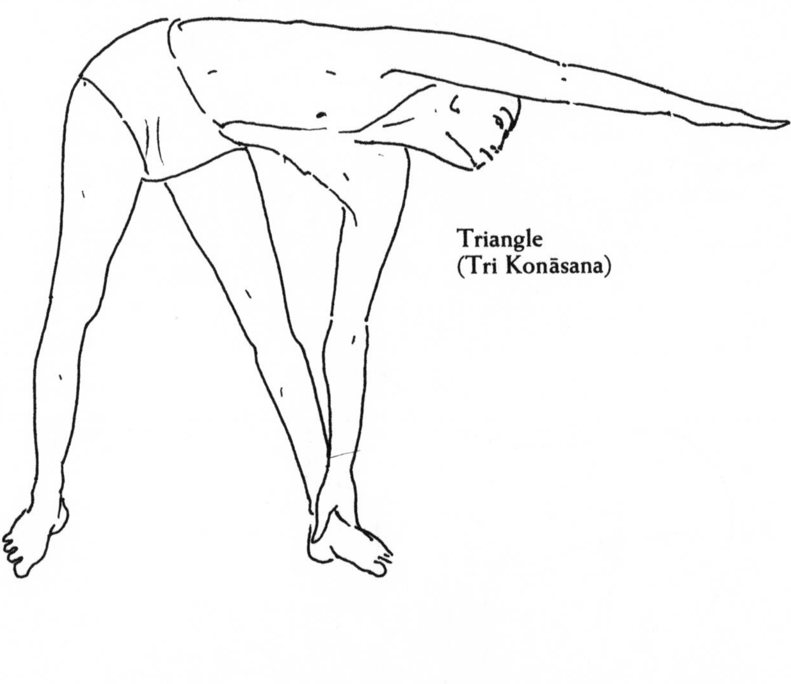

Triangle (Tri Konāsana)

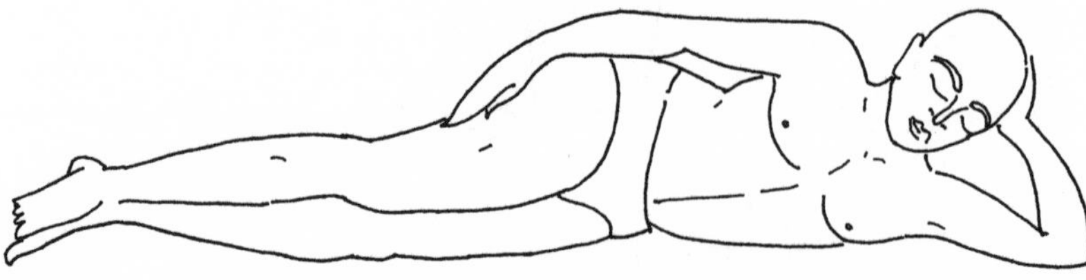

Left Lateral Relaxed Pose with Head Resting on Hand (Narayana)

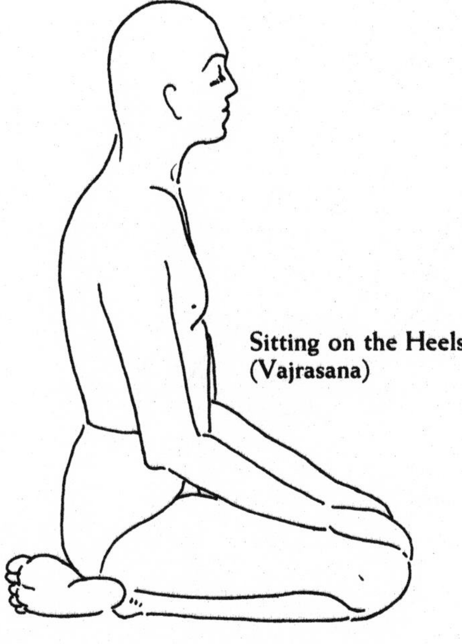

Sitting on the Heels
(Vajrasana)

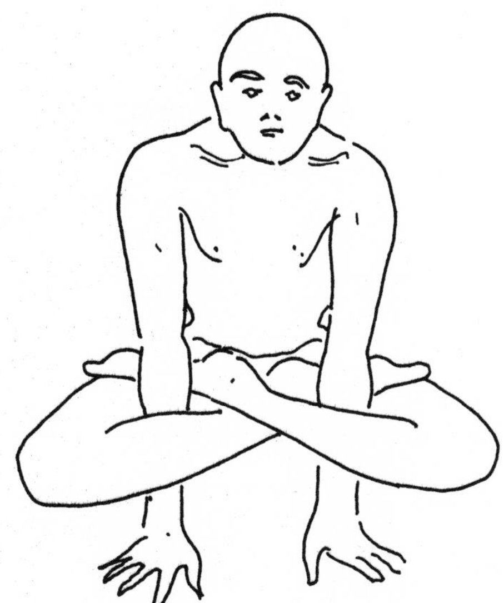

Elevated Lotus
(Kukutasana)

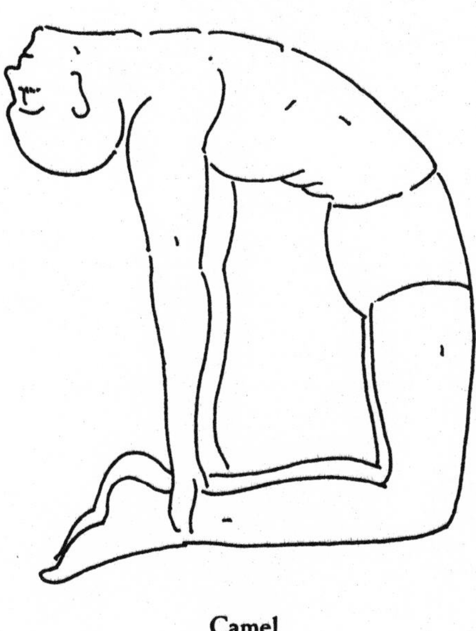

Camel
(Ushtrāsana)

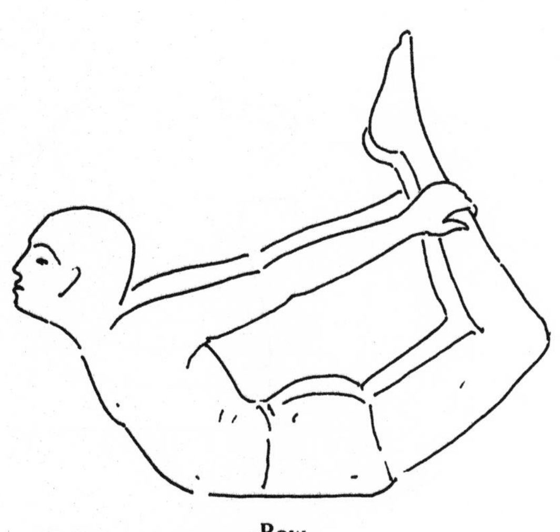

Bow
(Dhanurāsana)

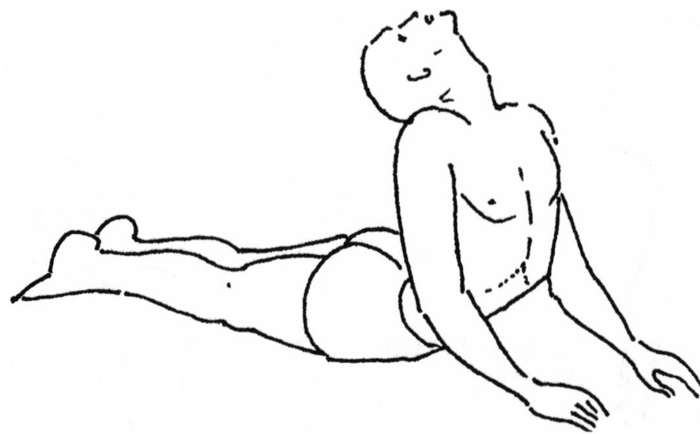

The Cobra Pose
(Bhujangāsana)

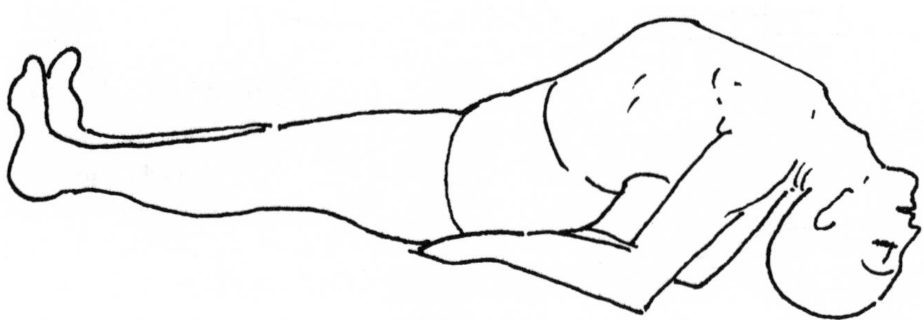

The Fish Pose
(Matsyāsana)

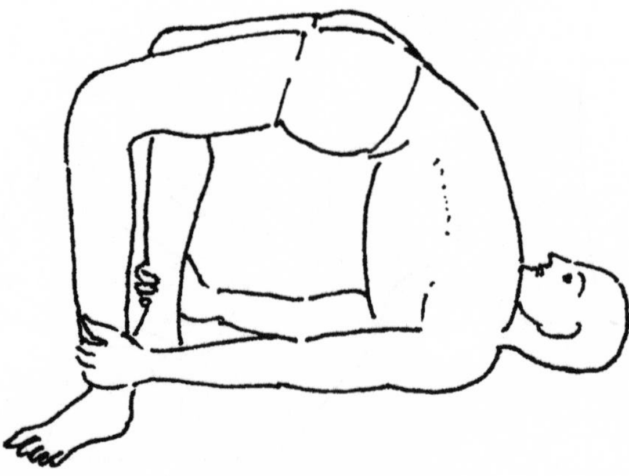

The Bridge Variation
(Setu Bandhāsana)

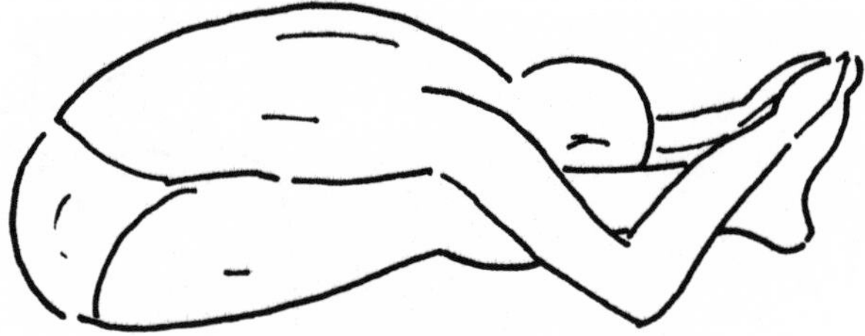

The Forward Bend
(Purvottanāsana)

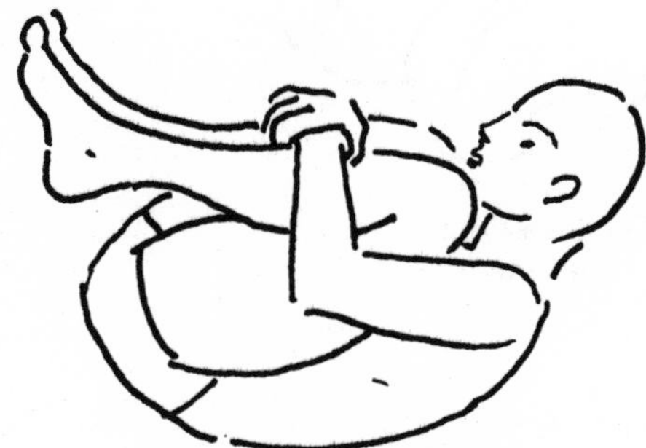

The Knee Chest Pose
(Pavana Muktasana)

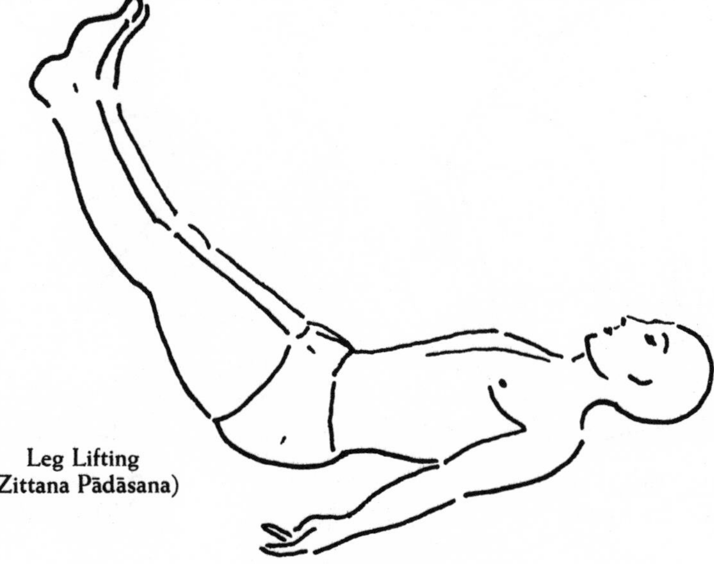

Leg Lifting
(Zittana Pādāsana)

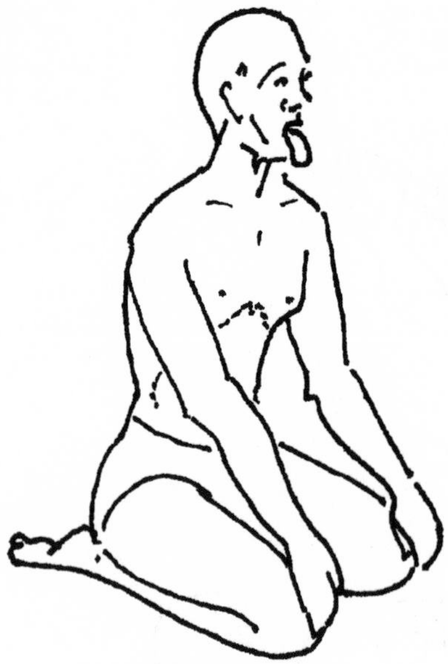

The Lion Pose
(Simhāsana)

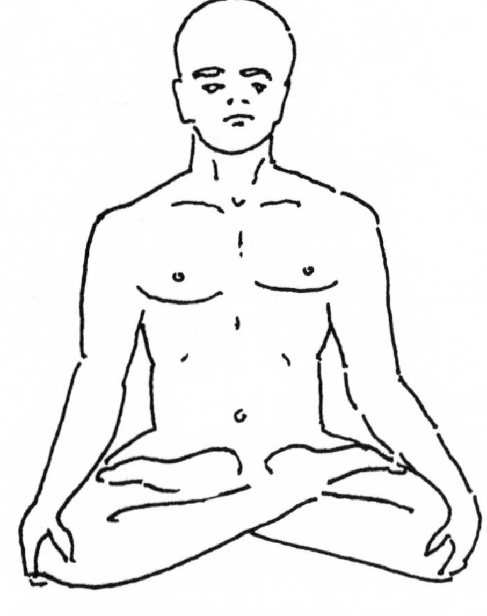

The Lotus Pose
(Padmāsanā)

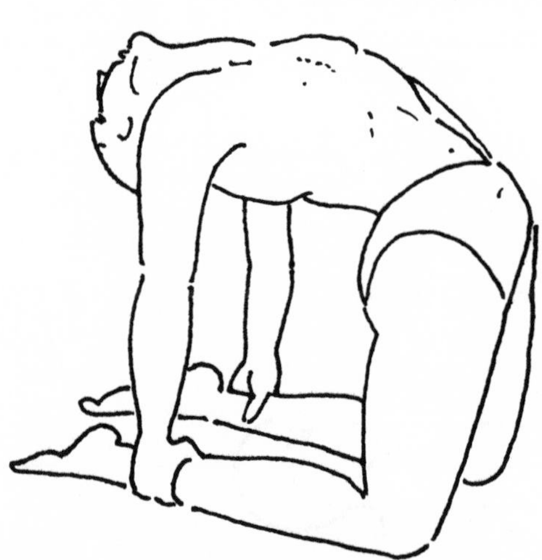

The Kneeling Wheel Pose
(Ardha Chakra Asana)

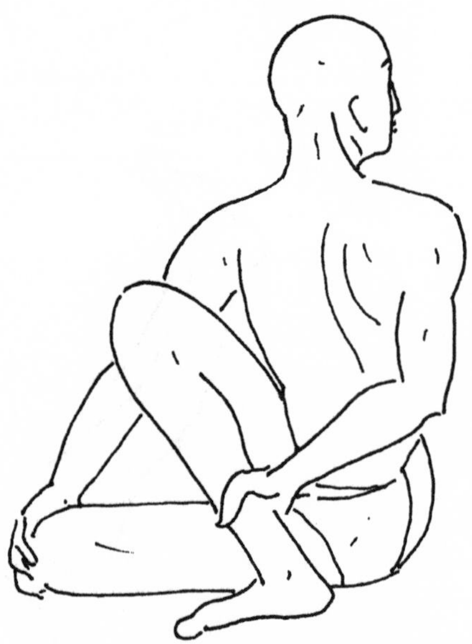

The Spinal Twist
(Matsyendrāsana)

Glossary

AGNI. The biological fire that provides energy for the body to function. Agni regulates body heat and aids digestion, absorption, and assimilation of food. It transforms food into energy or consciousness.

AHAMKARA. Literally, the "I-former"; the ego; sense of separate self; the feeling of "I am."

AMA. A toxic, morbid substance (both systemic and cellular) produced by undigested food which is the root cause of many diseases.

ANUPANA. Substance (such as milk, water, ghee, etc.) that serves as a medium for taking herbs.

ARTAVA DHATU. The female reproductive tissue, one of the seven *dhatus* or bodily tissues.

ASTHI DHATU. One of the seven *dhatus* or bodily tissues; specifically, the bone tissue that supports the body, giving protection, shape, and longevity.

AYURVEDA. The science of life; derived from the Sanskrit words *ayur* meaning life, and *veda,* knowledge or science. The Vedas are the authentic, ancient, spiritual scriptures of India.

BASMATI RICE. A long-grained scented rice originating in the foothills of the Himalayas in India. Easily digestible and nutritious.

BASTI. One of the five important cleansing measures of *panchakarma,* it eliminates excess vata dosha from the system via medicated herbal tea or oil enemas. Helps greatly to heal all vata disorders. The word *basti* literally means bladder. In ancient times, the apparatus used for the procedure was made out of leather.

BHASMA. A specialized Ayurvedic compound prepared and purified by being burned into ash; *bhasmas* have a high potency and release *prana* into the system.

BHASTRIKA. A breathing practice *(pranayama)* in which air is passively drawn in and forcibly pushed out, as in a bellows. Increases heat and improves circulation.

BHRAMARI. A type of breathing practice (*pranayama*) in which a soft humming sound, like a bee, is made during exhalation and/or inhalation. Calms the mind and cools pitta.

CARDAMOM. Pungent spice from a tropical plant.

CHAI. General word for tea; often refers to a spiced black tea made with milk and sugar.

CHAKRAS. The energy centers in the body, related to nerve plexus centers, which govern bodily functions. Each chakra is a reservoir of consciousness.

CHICKPEA FLOUR. A finely ground yellow flour. Also called gram.

CILANTRO. Fresh coriander leaf. This herb is used extensively in Indian cooking and valued for its zesty and cooling taste. Balances spicy dishes.

COCONUT MILK. Made from grating the white flesh of the coconut and mixing with a cup of water.

COCONUT WATER. The natural juice inside the coconut.

DAL. Any type of dried bean, pea, or lentil is called dal. Most dal is husked and split for quick cooking and greater ease of digestion.

DHATU. The structural, building, elemental tissue of the body. There are seven *dhatus* defined in Ayurveda: *rasa* (plasma); *rakta* (blood tissue); *mamsa* (muscle tissue); *meda* (adipose tissue); *asthi* (bone marrow); *majja* (bone and nerves); *shukra* and *artava* (male and female reproductive tissue).

DOSHA. The three main psycho-physiological functional principles of the body (vata, pitta, and kapha). They determine each individual's constitution and maintain the integrity of the human body. The *doshas* govern the individual's response to changes. When disturbed, they can initiate the disease process.

GHEE. Clarified butter; made from unsalted butter that has been gently cooked and the milk solids removed.

GUGGULU. Main ingredient in a number of herbal preparations (*yogaraj guggulu, kaishore guggulu*, etc.). A resin from a small tree, it has many useful medical actions, including benefits for the nervous system, tonification, and anti-inflammatory action on muscle tissues. Helps increase white blood count (good for the immune system) and is a nervine, rejuvenating tonic.

GUNAS. Three qualities influencing all creation: *sattva, rajas,* and *tamas. Sattvic* qualities imply essence, reality, consciousness, purity, and clarity of perception. All movement and activity are due to *rajas. Tamas* brings darkness, inertia, heaviness, and materialistic attitudes. There is a constant interplay among these three *gunas* in all creation. Also refers to the qualities (hard/soft, hot/cold, etc.) of the three doshas, seven *dhatus,* and three *malas.*

JAGGERY. An unrefined sugar made from the juice of crushed sugarcane stalks.

KAPHA. One of the three doshas, combining the water and earth elements. Kapha is the energy that forms the body's structure—bones, muscles, tendons—and provides the "glue" that holds the cells together. It supplies the water for all bodily parts and systems, lubricates joints, moisturizes the skin, and maintains immunity. In balance, kapha is expressed as love, calmness, and forgiveness. Out of balance, it leads to attachment, greed, and envy.

KHAVAIGUNYA. A weak or defective space within an organ or tissue of the body where a pathological condition is likely to begin.

KITCHARI. A cooked mixture of rice and dal and spices that is easy to digest and high in protein. Often used as a nourishing food for a mono-fast.

LASSI. A refreshing drink made from yogurt, water, and spices and often served at the end of a meal as a digestive. Can be sweet or salty.

MAHAT (or ***MAHAD***). The "great principle," intelligence, the cosmic aspect of intellect; also contains the individual intellect, called *Buddhi*.

MAJJA DHATU. One of the seven *dhatus* or bodily tissues; the bone marrow and nerve tissue. It is unctuous and soft. Its main function is to oleate the body, to fill up the bone, and to nourish the *shukra dhatu*. It plays an important role in communication.

MAMSA DHATU. One of the seven *dhatus* or bodily tissues; the muscle tissue. Produced by *rasa* and *rakta*, its main functions are to provide physical strength, coordination, movement, covering, form, and protection.

MANTRA. A sacred word or phrase of spiritual significance and power that transcends the mind and yields bliss.

MARMA. An energy point on the skin that has a door receptor and is connected to the inner pathways of healing.

MUNG DAL. A small bean that has been husked and split. Usually a medium yellow color. Easy to digest.

NASYA. Method of administering medication through the nose; one of the five measures of *panchakarma*.

NIGHTSHADE. Common name for a family of plants including tomatoes, potatoes, eggplant, tobacco, petunias, and belladonna, which have strong medicinal properties. Frequent use may disturb the doshic equilibrium.

OJAS. The pure essence of all the bodily tissues (*dhatus*); the superfine essence of kapha; maintains immunity, strength, and vitality. *Ojas* creates bliss and awareness in the mental faculties and governs the body's immune function. If it is depleted, it can lead to death.

PANCHAKARMA. Five measures for elimination of excess dosha and/or ama from the body. Used for the purpose of internal purification. They are: vomiting (*vamana*); purgation (*virechana*); medicated oil or decoction enema (*basti*); bloodletting (*rakta moksha*); and nasal administration of specific medication (*nasya*).

PIPPALI. *Piper longum*; a close relative of black pepper, which has many medicinal applications, especially for digestion and respiration. A rejuvenative tonic (*rasayana*) for the lungs and liver.

PITTA. One of the three doshas; it corresponds to the elements of fire and water. Sometimes referred to as the fire or bile principle, pitta governs digestion, absorption, assimilation, metabolism, and body temperature. In balance, pitta promotes understanding and intelligence; out of balance pitta arouses anger, hatred, jealousy.

PRAKRUTI. *Prakruti* (spelled with a capital *P*) is the Cosmic Creativity, the primordial matter.

PRAKRUTI. The inherent nature or psychosomatic, biological constitution of the individual, *prakruti* is the fixed constitution of a person, which reflects the proportion of the three doshas (vata, pitta, and kapha) established at conception.

PRANA. The vital life energy. Without it, life cannot exist. The flow of cellular intelligence from one cell to another. Equivalent to the Oriental *Ch'i* or *Ki*.

PRANAYAMA. The control of life energy by various techniques which regulate and restrain breath, through which one can control the mind and improve one's quality of awareness and perception. Helpful with all types of meditation.

PURUSHA. Choiceless, passive awareness; the pure Cosmic Being.

RAJAS. One of the three universal qualities *(gunas)* of *Prakruti*, Cosmic Creativity. *Rajas* is active, mobile, dynamic.

RAKTA DHATU. The second of the seven tissues *(dhatus)*, *rakta* mainly contains red blood cells, which carry life energy *(prana)* to all bodily tissues. This oxygenates, or provides the life function, for all the tissues.

RASA DHATU. The first of the seven *dhatus*, *rasa* (plasma) is nourished from digested food, and after absorption, it circulates in the entire body via specific channels. Its main function is to provide nutrition to each and every cell of the body.

RASAYANA. Rejuvenation therapy which brings about renewal, regeneration, and restoration of bodily cells, tissues, and organs, giving longevity to the cells and enhancing immunity and stamina.

RISHI. A seer, a Vedic sage. The ancient *rishis* perceived and/or recorded the Vedic hymns. These enlightened sages shared their knowledge, medicine, philosophy, and spiritual teachings.

RUDRAKSHA. The "tears of Shiva"; the dried seeds from the fruit of the rudraksha tree. Said to be good for the heart both physically and spiritually, helpful for meditation and for "opening the heart chakra."

SAFFRON. A golden yellow spice that comes from the stigma of a particular crocus. The best quality saffron is grown in Spain and Kashmir.

SAMPRAPTI. The pathogenesis of disease; the entire disease process from its cause through its various stages to the complete manifestation of the disease.

SANKHYA. One of the schools of Indian philosophy, Sankhya denotes both "discriminative knowledge" and "enumeration." It gives a systematic account of cosmic evolution from *Purusha* (Cosmic Spirit) and *Prakruti* (Primordial Matter) through the stages of creation: *Mahad* (Cosmic Intelligence); *Ahamkara* (individuating principle); *Mana* (mind); *Indriyas* (the inner doors of perception); *Tanmatras* (the objects of perception); and *Mahat Bhutas* (five great elements). *Sat* means truth and *khya* means to realize; thus Sankhya means to realize the theory of the creation of the universe in order to realize the ultimate truth of human life. Sankhya reveals the journey of consciousness into matter.

SATTVA. One of the three *gunas* of *Prakruti*, *sattva* denotes light, clarity, purity of perception; it is the essence of pure awareness.

SHITALI. A practice of *pranayama* (breath control) that cools the system. Inhalation is through the curled tongue; exhalation is slow, steady, and complete.

SHUKRA DHATU. The seventh tissue *(dhatu)*; the male reproductive tissue.

SROTAS. Bodily channels.

SUCANAT. A granulated natural sugar made from pure sugarcane juice.

SURYA NAMASKAR. The Sun Salutation, a series of yoga postures done in a flowing sequence with coordinated breathing.

TAMAS. One of the three *gunas* of *Prakruti* or Nature; its characteristics are darkness, inertia, and ignorance; it is responsible for sleep, drowsiness, dullness, unconsciousness.

TEJAS. The pure essence of the fire element; the superfine essence of pitta dosha, which governs the transformation of matter into energy and of food, water, and air into consciousness.

TIKTA GHRITA. "Bitter ghee," a specific Ayurvedic compound made of clarified butter with various bitter herbs; used for medicinal purposes.

TRIDOSHA. The three organizations or codes of intelligence within the body, mind, and consciousness; the three bodily humors: air (vata), fire/bile (pitta), and water (kapha).

TRIKATU. An Ayurvedic compound of ginger, black pepper, and *pippali (piper longum)* that burns ama, detoxifies the body, and improves digestion, absorption, and assimilation.

TRIPHALA. An important Ayurvedic compound consisting of three herbs: *amalaki, bibhitaki,* and *haritaki.* It is the best laxative and bowel tonic and a balanced *rasayana* that is good for vata, pitta, and kapha.

TULSI. Indian holy basil. The sacred plant of Krishna, this herb is said to open the heart and mind, bestowing the energy of love and devotion.

TURBINADO. A granulated sugar made from pure sugarcane.

TURMERIC ROOT. An underground rhizome from a perennial plant native to southern India and Asia. Comes in a red and yellow form, but only the yellow is eaten. One of the most important herbs for both internal and external use, it is also essential in most Indian cooking.

VATA. One of the three doshas, combining the space and air elements; it is the subtle energy associated with bodily movement and governs breathing, blinking, muscle and tissue movement, pulsation of the heart, and all movements in the cytoplasm and cell membranes. In balance, vata promotes creativity and flexibility; out of balance, vata produces fear and anxiety.

VIKRUTI. The current state of the individual, as opposed to the original constitution *(prakruti)* at conception. It may also denote disorder.

YOGA. In its deeper sense, Yoga is union of the lower self with the higher self, of the inner with the outer, mortality with immortality. Yoga postures *(asanas)* promote health, flexibility, and purity toward achieving the state of Yoga.

Resources

This list has been provided courtesy of Lotus Press, P.O. Box 325, Twin Lakes, WI 53181, 1-800-824-6396.

AYURVEDIC HERBS AND SUPPLIES

Auroma International
P.O. Box 1008, Dept. VL
Silver Lake, WI 53170
414-889-8569

The Ayurvedic Institute
P.O. Box 23445
Albuquerque, NM 87192-1445
505-291-9698
Fax: 505-294-7572

Ayush Herbs, Inc.
10025 N.E. 4th Street
Bellevue, WA 98004
800-925-1371

Bazaar of India Imports, Inc.
1810 University Avenue
Berkeley, CA 94703
510-548-4110

Bioveda
P.O. Box 420
Congers, NY 10920

Dr. Singha's Mustard Bath and More
Attn.: Anna Searles
Natural Therapeutic Centre
2500 Side Cove
Austin, TX 78704
800-856-2862

Herbalvedic Products
P.O. Box 6390
Santa Fe, NM 87502

Kanak
P.O. Box 13653
Albuquerque, NM 87192-3653

Internatural (retail)
33719 116th Street, Dept. VL
Twin Lakes, WI 53181
800-643-4221
www.internatural.com

Lotus Herbs
1505 42nd Ave. Suite 19
Capitola, CA 95010
408-479-1667

Lotus Light (wholesale)
P.O. Box 1008, Dept. VL
Silver Lake, WI 53170
414-889-8501

Yoga of Life Center
2726 Tramway N.E.
Albuquerque, NM 87122
505-275-6141

Vinayak Ayurveda Center
2509 Virginia NE, Suite D
Albuquerque, NM 87110
505-296-6522
505-298-2932 (fax)

Maharishi Ayur-Veda Products International Inc.
417 Bolton Road
P.O. Box 54
Lancaster, Mass 01523
800-All-Veda
508-368-7475 (fax)

New Moon Extracts
P.O. Box 1947
Brattleboro, VT 05302-1947

NATURAL INGREDIENTS

Aloe Farms
Box 125
Los Fresnos, TX 78566
800-262-6771
(For aloe vera juice, gel, powder, and capsules)

Arya Laya Skin Care Center
Rolling Hills Estates, CA 90274
(For carrot oil)

Aubrey Organics
4419 North Manhatten Ave.
Tampa, FL 33614
(For rosa mosquita oil and a large variety of natural shampoos and cosmetics)

Body Shop
45 Hosehill Road
Cedar Knolls, NJ 07927-2014
800-541-2535
(Aloe vera, nut and seed oils, cosmetics, makeup, brushes, loofas, and much more)

Culpepper Ltd.
21 Bruton Street
London W1X 7DA
England
(Variety of natural seed, nut, and kernel oils, essential oils, herbs, books, and cosmetics)

Desert Whale Jojoba Co.
P.O. Box 41594
Tucson, AZ 85717
602-882-4195
(For jojoba products and many other natural oils, including rice bran, pecan, macadamia nut, and apricot kernel)

Everybody Ltd.
1738 Pearl Street
Boulder, CO 80302
800-748-5675
(Large variety of oils, oil blends, and cosmetics)

Flora Inc.
P.O. Box 950
805 East Badger Road
Lynden, WA 98264
800-446-2110
(For flaxseed oil, herbal supplements for skin, hair, nails, and cosmetics)

Green Earth Farm
P.O. Box 672
651/2 North 8th Street
Saguache, CO 81449
(For calendula, oil, cream, and herbal bath)

The Heritage Store Inc.
P.O. Box 444
Virginia Beach, Virginia 23458
804-428-0100
(Castor oil, organic ghee, cocoa butter, massage oils, flower waters, essential oils, cosmetics, and natural home remedies)

Janca's Jojoba Oil and Seed company
456 E. Juanita No. 7
Mesa, AZ 85204
602-497-9494
(Jojoba oil, butter, wax, and seeds. Also a large variety of naturally pressed nut and grapeseed. Also have clay, aloe products, essential oils, and their own line of cosmetics.)

Reading List

CLASSICAL AYURVEDIC TEXTS

Caraka Samhita. 4 volumes. Priyavrat V. Sharma, editor-translator. Chowkhamba Sanskrit Series Office: Varanasi, India, 1981–1994.

Caraka Samhita. 3rd edition, 3 volumes. Ram Karan Sharma and Vaidya Bhagwan Dash, editors-translators. Chowkhamba Sanskrit Series Office: Varanasi, India, 1992.

Sushruta Samhita. 4th edition, 2 volumes. Kaviraj Kunjalal Bhishagratna, editor-translator. Chowkhamba Sanskrit Series Office: Varanasi, India, 1991.

Vagbhata, *Ashtanga Hridayam.* 2 volumes. K. R. Srikantha Murthy, translator. Krishnadas Academy: Varanasi, India, 1991–1992.

GENERAL READING

Frawley, David. *Ayurvedic Healing.* Morson Publishing: Salt Lake City, 1989.

Frawley, David, and Vasant Lad. *The Yoga of Herbs.* Lotus Press: Santa Fe, 1986.

Lad, Vasant. *Ayurveda: The Science of Self-Healing.* Lotus Press: Santa Fe, 1984.

Morrison, Judith. *The Book of Ayurveda: A Holistic Approach to Health and Longevity.* New York: Simon and Schuster, 1995.

Svoboda, Robert E. *Ayurveda: Life, Health, and Longevity.* Penguin: London, 1992.

———. *The Hidden Secret of Ayurveda.* Pune, India, 1980. Reprint, The Ayurvedic Press: Albuquerque, 1994.

———. *Prakruti: Your Ayurvedic Constitution.* Geocom Limited: Albuquerque, 1989.

SPECIFIC TOPICS

Lad, Usha, and Dr. Vasant Lad. *Ayurvedic Cooking for Self-Healing.* 2nd edition. The Ayurvedic Press: Albuquerque, 1997.

Lad, Dr. Vasant Dattatray. *Secrets of the Pulse: The Ancient Art of Ayurvedic Pulse Diagnosis.* The Ayurvedic Press: Albuquerque, 1996.

Morningstar, Amadea. *The Ayurvedic Cookbook.* Wilmot: Lotus Press, 1990.

Index

The Ayurvedic Institute with Dr. Vasant Lad, B.A.M.S., M.A.Sc., Ayurvedic Physician, Director

The Ayurvedic Institute was established to promote the traditional knowledge of Ayurveda. In support of this, the Institute also offers programs in the sister disciplines of AyurvedaSanskrit, Yoga, and Jyotisha (Vedic astrology). The Ayurvedic programs reflect the style of sitting with a traditional Indian teacher. The Vedic educational model is quite different from the Western experience with which most of us are familiar. The knowledge is taught with the body, mind, and spiritual components intact, along with practical examples, ceremonies, and stories.

THE EDUCATIONAL DEPARTMENT offers the Ayurvedic Studies Program; the Ayurvedic correspondence course *Lessons & Lectures on Ayurveda* by Dr. Robert E. Svoboda; various introductory, weekend, and intensive seminars; **AyurÉYoga**; and private consultations with Dr. Lad, Dr. Svoboda, Hart deFouw, and others.

AYURVEDIC STUDIES PROGRAM consists of three terms: Introduction to Philosophy and Theory of Ayurveda {Fall}, Introduction to Clinical Assessment {Winter}, and Introduction to Management of Disorders {Spring}. Certificate of completion awarded.

GURUKULA PROGRAM is continuing study with three mornings a week of observation of clinical consultations and one morning of advanced instruction with Dr. Lad. Certificate of completion awarded.

AYURVEDIC CORRESPONDENCE COURSE by Dr. Robert E. Svoboda, B.A.M.S., Ayurvedic Physician, an introduction to the fundamentals of Ayurveda.

WEEKEND AND INTENSIVE SEMINARS on Ayurvedic herbology, pulse assessment, psychology, *panchakarma*, Jyotisha, Vedic palmistry, and other topics.

AYURÉYOGA is an integration of Ayurveda and Yoga, recognizing each person's uniqueness. Classic and restorative Yoga postures, *pranayama* (breathing techniques), and meditation.

THE *PANCHAKARMA* DEPARTMENT offers traditional Ayurvedic procedures for purification and rejuvenation that include oil massage, herbal steam treatment, *shirodhara,* cleansing diet, herbal therapy, lifestyle education, and other treatments.

THE HERB DEPARTMENT carries Ayurvedic and Western herbs, Ayurvedic products, oils, incense, *malas,* books, personal-care products, audio- and videotapes, and a variety of other products. Some of these are formulated by Dr. Lad and produced by the Institute.

THE PUBLISHING DEPARTMENT. The Ayurvedic Press primarily publishes Dr. Lad's new books and articles but also publishes other traditional Ayurvedic and Vedic works.

MEMBERSHIP in the Ayurvedic Institute supports the aims and objectives of the Institute. Members receive the quarterly journal *Ayurveda Today* and a 10 percent discount on seminars and products purchased.

P.O. Box 23445
Albuquerque, NM 87192-1445
505-291-9698; fax 505-294-7572